SANFORD GUIDE®

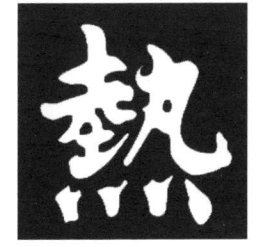
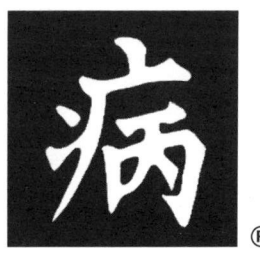

THE SANFORD GUIDE TO HIV/AIDS THERAPY 2009

17th Edition

THE SANFORD GUIDE TO HIV/AIDS THERAPY 2009
17TH EDITION

Jay P. Sanford, M.D.
1928-1996

EDITORS

David N. Gilbert, M.D.
Director of Medical Education & Earl A. Chiles Research
Institute, Providence Portland Medical Center
Professor of Medicine, Oregon Health Sciences University
Portland, Oregon

Robert C. Moellering, Jr., M.D.
Shields Warren-Malinckrodt Professor of Medicine
Harvard Medical School
Boston, Massachusetts

George M. Eliopoulos, M.D.
Chief, James L. Tullis Firm,
Beth Israel Deaconess Hospital
Professor of Medicine
Harvard Medical School
Boston, Massachusetts

Michael S. Saag, M.D.
Professor of Medicine & Director, Division of Infectious DIseases
Director, UAB Center for AIDS Research
University of Alabama
Birmingham, Alabama

Henry F. Chambers, M.D.
Professor of Medicine
Chief of Infectious Diseases
San Francisco General Hospital
University of California at San Francisco
San Francisco, California

CONTRIBUTING EDITOR

Andrew T. Pavia, M.D.
George and Esther Gross Presidential Professor
Chief, Division of Pediatric Infectious Diseases
University of Utah
Salt Lake City, Utah

The Sanford Guides are published annually by

ANTIMICROBIAL THERAPY, INC.
P.O. Box 276, 11771 Lee Highway
Sperryville, VA 22740 USA
Tel 540-987-9480 Fax 540-987-9486
Email: info@sanfordguide.com   www.sanfordguide.com

Copyright © 1992-2008 by Antimicrobial Therapy, Inc.

All rights reserved. No part of this publication may be reproduced, stored in a retrieval system or transmitted in any form or by any means--digital, electronic, mechanical, optical, photocopying, recording or otherwise--without prior written permission from Antimicrobial Therapy, Inc., P.O. Box 276, Sperryville, VA 22740 USA

"SANFORD GUIDE" and "Hot Disease" logo are ® registered trademarks of Antimicrobial Therapy, Inc.

Printed in the United States of America
ISBN 978-10930808-51-5
Library Edition

The SANFORD GUIDE is available from a variety of sources. You may have purchased your copy at a bookstore or directly from us. You may also have received your copy from a pharmaceutical company representative. Regardless of the source, you can be assured that the SANFORD GUIDE has been, and continues to be, independently prepared and published since its inception in 1969. Decisions regarding the content of the SANFORD GUIDE are solely those of the editors and the publisher. We welcome your questions, comments and feedback concerning the SANFORD GUIDE. All of your feedback is reviewed and taken into account in preparing the next edition. Content-related notices are posted on the SANFORD GUIDE website at **www.sanfordguide.com**

Thanks to Lingua Solutions, Inc. for its work on the manuscript design, to Royalty Press for printing and to Fox Bindery for finishing this edition.

IMPORTANT NOTE TO READER

Every effort is made to ensure the accuracy of the content of this guide. However, current full prescribing information available in the package insert for each drug should be consulted before prescribing any product. The editors and publisher are not responsible for errors or omissions or for any consequences from application of the information in this book and make no warranty, express or implied, with respect to the currency, accuracy, or completeness of the contents of the publication. Application of this information in a particular situation remains the professional responsibility of the practitioner.

— TABLE OF CONTENTS —

TABLE 1	Assessment of **HIV Infection Risks** & Recommendations for HIV **Testing**	4
TABLE 2	**Initial Evaluation** of HIV-Infected Adult Patient	7
FIGURE 1	**Life Cycle of HIV** with Sites of Action of Antiretrovirals	8
TABLE 3	**Laboratory Tests** Commonly Used in the Diagnosis & Management of Infection with HIV-1 and HIV-2	9
TABLE 4A	1993 Revised **CDC HIV Classification** System & Expanded AIDS Surveillance Definition for Adolescents & Adults	20
4B	'**Performance Status**' (Karnofsky Scale)/WHO Clinical Staging System	21
TABLE 5	Rapid Oral **TMP/SMX Desensitization**	21
FIGURE 2	**Course** of HIV Infection/Disease in Adults, Clinical Decision Points	22
TABLE 6A	**Antiretroviral Therapy** (ART) in Treatment-Naïve Adults	23
6B	Antiretroviral Drugs & Adverse Effects	38
6C	Drug **Adverse Effects** by Clinical Presentation	41
6D	Overlapping Toxicities Between Antiretrovirals and Other Drugs Commonly Used in HIV Patients	44
6E	Anti-HIV Drugs Available Via Expanded Access Programs	45
6F	Monitoring **Blood Levels** of Antiretroviral Drugs (Therapeutic Drug Monitoring)	46
6G	Antiretrovirals Approved or Tentatively Approved by FDA for International AIDS Relief	47
TABLE 7	Methods for **Penicillin Desensitization**	49
TABLE 8A	HIV/AIDS In **Women/Pregnancy**	50
8B	HIV in the **Fetus & Newborn**	52
8C	HIV Infection in **Children**	53
8D	**Initiation** of Antiretroviral Therapy, P. Carinii Prophylaxis, & Supportive Therapy	54
8E	Clinical Syndromes, Opportunistic Infections, in **Infants & Children**, which Differ from Adults	58
8F	**Selected Drugs** Commonly Used in **Children** with HIV Infection	60
8G	**Prophylaxis** for First Episode of **Opportunistic Disease** in HIV-Infected Infants & Children	68
TABLE 9	**Management of Exposure** to HIV-1 & Hepatitis B/C	69
TABLE 10	Primary **Prophylactic Antimicrobial Agents** Against Opportunistic Pathogens in Adolescents & Adults	72
TABLE 11A	Diagnosis & Differential Diagnosis of **Clinical Syndromes, Opportunistic Infections & Neoplasms**	74
11B	**Immune Reconstitution & Novel Syndromes** Associated with **ARV RX**	119
TABLE 12	Treatment of **Specific Infections**/Microorganisms in HIV+/AIDS Patients	122
FIGURE 3	Activity of Selected **Antifungal Drugs** Against Pathogenic Fungi	135
FIGURE 4	**Activity of Antiviral Agents Against Treatable Pathogenic Viruses**	149
TABLE 13	Drugs Used in Treatment &/or Chronic Suppression of AIDS-Related Infections: **Adverse Effects**, Comments, Cost	159
TABLE 14	Selected **Pharmacologic Features** of Antimicrobial Agents Used in HIV-Associated Infections in Adults	171
TABLE 15A	Dosage of Antimicrobial Drugs in Adult Patients with **Renal Impairment**	174
15B	**No Dosage Adjustment** with Renal Insufficiency, by Category	181
15C	Dosage of Antiretroviral Drugs in Patients with Impaired Hepatic Function	181
TABLE 16A	**Drug/Drug Interactions: Antiretroviral** Drugs & Drugs Used in Treatment of HIV-Associated Infections & Malignancies	182
16B	**Drug-Drug Interactions** Between **Protease Inhibitors**	188
16C	**Drug-Drug Interactions** Between **Non-Nucleoside Reverse Transcriptase Inhibitors (NNRTIs) & Protease Inhibitors**	189
TABLE 17	Antimicrobics in **Pregnancy**	190
TABLE 18	Spectrum & Treatment of HIV/AIDS-Associated **Malignancies**	191
TABLE 19	**Recommendations for Routine Immunization of HIV+ Children**	193
TABLE 20	**Immunization** of HIV+ **Adults** (Asymptomatic & Symptomatic)	194
TABLE 21A	Measures to be Taken by Physicians in Preparing HIV+ Patients & Individuals Likely to Have 'Risky' Behavior for **Overseas Travel**	196
21B	Immunization of HIV+ Adults **Traveling to Developing Countries**	197
TABLE 22	Biologics in Treatment of **Hematocytopenias**	197
TABLE 23	**AIDS Information** & Referral Services	198
TABLE 24	List of **Generic** & Common **Trade Names**	199
INDEX		200

ABBREVIATIONS:

Antibacterial & Antimycobacterial Drugs:
- **AMK** = amikacin
- **Azithro** = azithromycin
- **CIP** = ciprofloxacin
- **Clinda** = clindamycin
- **CLO** = clofazamine
- **Doxy** = doxycycline
- **Erythro** = erythromycin
- **FQ** = fluoroquinolone
- **Gent** = gentamicin
- **INH** = isoniazid
- **IVIG** = intravenous immune globulin
- **Levo** = levofloxacin
- **Metro** = metronidazole
- **Mino** = minocycline
- **Moxi** = moxifloxacin
- **Oflox** = ofloxacin
- **PZA** = pyrazinamide
- **RFB** = rifabutin
- **RFP** = rifapentine
- **RIF** = rifampin
- **SM** = streptomycin
- **TMP-SMX** = trimethoprim sulfamethoxazole
- **Tobra** = tobramycin
- **Vanco** = vancomycin

Antifungal Drugs:
- **Ampho B** = amphotericin B
- **ABCC** = ampho B cholesteryl complex
- **ABCD** = ampho B colloidal dispersion
- **ABLC** = ampho B lipid complex
- **Anidula** = anidulafungin
- **Caspo** = caspofungin
- **Flu** = fluconazole
- **Flucyt** = flucytosine
- **Itra** = itraconazole
- **Keto** = ketoconazole
- **LAB** = liposomal ampho B
- **Mica** = micafungin
- **Posa** = posaconazole
- **Vori** = voriconazole

Antiparasitic Drugs:
- **AP** = atovaquone proguanil
- **CQ** = chloroquine phosphate
- **MQ** = mefloquine
- **PQ** = primaquine
- **Pyri** = pyrimethamine
- **QS** = quinine sulfate

Antiviral Drugs—HIV Drugs By Class:
NRTI = nucleoside reverse transcriptase inhibitor
- **ABC** = abacavir
- **ddI** = didanosine
- **FTC** = emtricitabine
- **Lam** = lamivudine (3TC)
- **d4T** = stavudine
- **TDF** = tenofovir
- **ddC** = zalcitabine, saquinavir
- **ZDV** = zidovudine

NNRTI = non-nucleoside reverse transcriptase inhibitor
- **EFZ** = efavirenz
- **ETR** = etravirine
- **DLV** = delavirdine
- **NVP** = nevirapine

PI = protease inhibitor
- **ATA** = atazanavir
- **DAR** = darunavir
- **FOS-APV** = fosamprenavir
- **IDV** = indinavir
- **LP/R** = lopinavir/ritonavir
- **NFR** = nelfinavir
- **RTV** = ritonavir
- **SQV** = saquinavir
- **TPV** = tipranavir

FI = fusion inhibitor
- **ENF** = enfuviritide

EI = entry inhibitor
- **MVC** = maraviroc

II = integrase inhibitor
- **RAL** = raltegravir

Antiviral Drugs—Non-HIV:
- **ADV** = adefovir
- **ETV** = entecavir
- **LAM** = lamivudine (3TC)
- **Peg-INF** = pegylated interferon

Drug Dosage & Drug Administration:
- **mL** = milliliter
- **mcg** = microgram
- **mg** = milligram
- **gm** = gram
- **DS** = double strength
- **bid** = twice per day
- **tid** = 3 times per day
- **qid** = 4 times per day
- **BW** = body weight
- **DOT** = directly observed therapy
- **AD** = after dialysis
- **div** = divided
- **IP** = intraperitoneal
- **IT** = intrathecal
- **po** = orally (by mouth)
- **dc** = discontinue
- **rx** = treatment

Drug Related:
- **ARV Rx** = antiretroviral therapy
- **G** = generic
- **I** = investigational
- **IA** = injectable agent
- **NB** = name brand
- **NFDA-I** = not U.S. FDA approved indication
- **NUS** = not available in U.S.
- **ASA** = aspirin
- **NSAIDs** = non-steroidal anti-inflammatory drugs
- **TDM** = therapeutic drug monitoring
- **AUC** = area under curve
- **DBPCT** = double blind placebo-controlled trial
- **IVDU** = intravenous drug user
- **Pt** = patient
- **R** = resistant
- **S** = potential synergy in combination with penicillin, ampicillin, vanco & teicoplanin
- **Sens** = sensitive

Disease-Associated:
- **ADC** = AIDS dementia complex
- **AFB** = acid fast bacilli
- **AIDS** = acquired immune deficiency syndrome
- **CAPD** = continuous ambulatory peritoneal dialysis
- **CRRT** = continuous renal replacement therapy
- **CSD** = cat-scratch disease
- **DSP** = distal sensory symmetrical polyneuropathy
- **FUO** = fever of unknown origin
- **HAD** = HIV-associated dementia (HIV-D)
- **Hemo** = hemodialysis
- **HIV** = human immunodeficiency virus
- **IDP** = inflammatory demyelinating polyneuropathy
- **IRIS** = immune response inflammatory syndrome
- **KS** = Kaposi's sarcoma
- **OI** = opportunistic infection
- **PML** = progressive multifocal leuko-encephalopathy
- **STD** = sexually-transmitted disease
- **TBc** = tuberculosis
- **TN** = toxic neuropathy
- **TST** = tuberculin skin test
- **UTI** = urinary tract infection

Organism Associated:
- **CMV** = cytomegalovirus
- **EBV** = Epstein-Barr virus
- **GC** = gonorrhoea
- **HHV** = human herpes viruses
- **HPV** = human papilloma virus
- **HSV** = herpes simplex virus
- **LCM** = lymphocytic choriomeningitis virus
- **MAI** = mycobacterium avium-intracelluare complex
- **M.TBc** = mycobacterium tuberculosis
- **PCP** = pneumocystis carinii pneumonia
- **VZV** = varicella zoster virus

Diagnosis Associated:
- **CD4** = cluster differentiation antigen 4
- **CRF** = circulating recombinant forms
- **CrCl** = creatinine clearance
- **C&S** = culture & sensitivity
- **CSF** = cerebrospinal fluid
- **CXR** = chest x-ray
- **EIA** = enzyme immunoassay
- **ESR** = erythrocyte sedimentation rate
- **LCR** = ligase chain reaction
- **NAAT** = nucleic acid amplification test
- **PCR** = polymerase chain reaction
- **VL** = viral load
- **WB** = western blot
- **PEP** = post-exposure prophylaxis

Organizations:
- **ACIP** = Advisory Committee on Immunization Practices
- **ATS** = American Thoracic Society
- **DHHS** = U.S. Dept of Health and Human Services
- **IDSA** = Infectious Diseases Society of America
- **ICAAC** = Interscience Conference on Antimicrobial Agents & Chemotherapy
- **WHO** = World Health Organization
- **CDC** = U.S. Centers for Disease Control

Journals and Other References:
- **AAC**: Antimicrobial Agents & Chemotherapy
- **AIDS Res Hum Retrovir**: AIDS Research & Human Retroviruses
- **AJG**: American Journal of Gastroenterology
- **AJM**: American Journal of Medicine
- **AJRCCM**: American Journal of Respiratory Critical Care Medicine
- **AJTMH**: American Journal of Tropical Medicine & Hygiene
- **AnIM**: Annals of Internal Medicine
- **AnSurg**: Annals of Surgery
- **ArDerm**: Archives of Dermatology
- **Antivir Ther**: Antiviral Therapy
- **ArIM**: Archives of Internal Medicine
- **ARDD**: American Review of Respiratory Disease
- **BMJ**: British Medical Journal
- **Brit J Derm**: British Journal of Dermatology
- **Can JID**: Canadian Journal of Infectious Diseases
- **CCM**: Critical Care Medicine
- **CID**: Clinical Infectious Diseases
- **CROI**: Conference on Retroviruses & Opportunistic Infections
- **DMID**: Diagnostic Microbiology and Infectious Disease
- **EID**: Emerging Infectious Diseases
- **Gastro**: Gastroenterology
- **Hpt**: Hepatology
- **ICHE**: Infection Control and Hospital Epidemiology
- **IDC No Amer**: Infectious Diseases Clinics of North America
- **JAIDS**: Journal of Acquired Immune Deficiency Syndrome
- **J AIDS & HR**: Journal of AIDS and Human Retrovirology
- **JCI**: Journal of Clinical Investigation
- **J Clin Virol**: Journal of Clinical Virology
- **J Hpt**: Journal of Hepatology
- **J Med Micro**: Journal of Medical Microbiology
- **J Ped**: Journal of Pediatrics
- **JAC**: Journal of Antimicrobial Chemotherapy
- **JAMA**: Journal of the American Medical Association
- **JCM**: Journal of Clinical Microbiology
- **JID**: Journal of Infectious Diseases
- **JTMH**: Journal of Tropical Medicine & Health
- **J Viral Hep**: Journal of Viral Hepatitis
- **Ln**: Lancet
- **Ln ID**: Lancet Infectious Disease
- **Mayo Clin Proc**: Mayo Clinic Proceedings
- **Med Lett**: The Medical Letter
- **Med Myco**: Medical Mycology
- **MMWR**: Morbidity & Mortality Weekly Report
- **NEJM**: New England Journal of Medicine
- **Peds**: Pediatrics
- **PIDJ**: Pediatric Infectious Diseases Journal
- **PLOSMed**: Plos medicine public library of medicine
- **QJM**: Quarterly Journal of Medicine
- **Scand J Inf Dis**: Scandinavian Journal of Infectious Diseases
- **SMJ**: Southern Medical Journal

TABLE 1: ASSESSMENT OF HIV INFECTION RISKS & RECOMMENDATIONS FOR HIV TESTING

I. General

HIV risk assessment is an essential component of primary care for all patients. In talking to patients, avoid medical jargon (e.g., "intercourse"), vague terms ("sexually active"), group designations ("homosexual"), or judgmental terms ("promiscuous"). Learn the language & terminology understood & used by patients. Question responses to the depth necessary to elicit risky behavior & define extent of risk of acquisition & transmission. Eliciting risk is particularly difficult but equally important in resource-limited areas of the world, esp. when working through translators. It is essential that the clinician be knowledgeable about cultural sensitivities, customs & traditions relative to HIV risk behavior.

Risk-reduction counseling works to reduce high-risk behavior in North America, Europe, Africa, & SE Asia. *(Cochrane Database Syst Rev 1: CD001230, 2003; AIDS 16:953 & 2209, 2002; J AIDS 29:284 & 409, 2002; J AIDS 30:S118, 2002; J AIDS 31:2002, 2002; Sex Trans Dis 29:520, 2002; CID 36:1577, 2003; MMWR 152:329, 2003).* Revised CDC Guidelines: *MMWR 50(RR-19):1, 2001.* It is time to include HIV counseling & testing as a critical component of health care maintenance *[MMWR 51(RR-12), 2003].*

II. Specific Behaviors Associated With HIV Transmission

A. **Sexual Behaviors.** The CDC now recommends ART post-exposure prophylaxis within 72 hrs after high risk sexual, injection-drug use, or other non-occupational exposure to HIV *(MMWR Recomm Rep 54:1, 2005)* (See Table 9). Not 100% effective; seroconversion still detected in 1% of 702 exposed individuals *(CID 41:1507, 2005).*

  1. **High-Risk Sexual Partner(s)**
     - HIV-infected partners [especially those with ↑ HIV-RNA *(NEJM 342:921,2000, Sex Trans Dis 29:38, 2002)*]
     - Partners who are at risk but have not been HIV tested [risk of HIV often underappreciated by partners; example, 15.7% crack cocaine smokers HIV+ vs 5.2% in non-smokers in one series, women > men (sex for money or drugs) *(NEJM 331:1422, 1994)* or do not disclose their HIV status to their partners *(MMWR 52:81, 2003)*]
     - Multiple partners: Unsafe sexual activity appears to be ↑ with MSM in American & European cities *(AIDS 16:1537 & 2329, 2002; J AIDS 30:522, 2002; J AIDS 31:63, 2002).*
     - Presence of mucosal ulceration or other STD in either partner *(JID 178:1060, 1998)*

  2. **Sexual Practices**
     a. **High infection risk**
        - Unprotected anal receptive intercourse ("barebacking"): on the rise in young gay males
        - Unprotected vaginal receptive intercourse
     b. **Infection risk documented**
        - Unprotected anal insertive intercourse
        - Unprotected vaginal insertive intercourse (risk may be higher during menses)
        - Unprotected oral receptive intercourse [HIV RNA levels in rectal secretions > serum with & without ART use *(JID 190:156, 2004)*]
        - Unprotected oral insertive intercourse rare *(ArIM 159:303, 1999)*
     c. **Lower infection risk**
        - Any of the above with latex/vinyl condom (vaginal or penile) protection. In 343 HIV-neg. women partners of HIV+ men, seroconversion for those who used condoms with every encounter was 1.1/100 person years while for those who used condoms intermittently or not at all, rate was 7.2/100 person years. In Thailand, aggressive condom campaign reduced seroprevalence from 7.2 to 3.8% in military conscripts. In 1995, rate was 0.55/100 person years *(AIDS 12:F29, 1998).* In U.S., condom use estimated to reduce risk 20-fold *(Sex Trans Dis 29:38, 2002).* However, among female sex workers, 12.5% still became HIV infected during the 100% condom program *(J AIDS 21:313, 1999).* Male condoms are 80–95% effective in ↓ risk of HIV infection *(AmFAR Issue Brief #1, Jan. 2005)*; female condoms 94–97% effective.
        - Cunnilingus, esp. with rubber dam, microwaveable plastic food wrap or other water-impervious barrier
        - Circumcision reduced HIV infection by 60% in a prospective randomized study in 3,274 men in South Africa RR; 0.40 (p<.001) *(PLoS Med e298, 2005)* Two other studies confirmed 50-60% reduction and were stopped early in 2007 *(Ln 369:643, 657, 2007; PLoS Med 4 (7) e223, July 24, 2007).*
        - Microbicides currently in development but data on effectiveness lacking *(JID 193; 36, 2006).* Tenofovir based microbicide safe, acceptable in up to 90% of seronegative women *(Microbicides 2008, Feb. 24-26 New Delhi)*; Nonoxynol-9 actually facilitated transmission *(JAMA 287:1171,2002).*
     d. **Safer**
        - Deep kissing
        - Protected sex with HIV test negative partner
        - Mutual monogamy
        - Mutual masturbation
        - Masturbation or massage
     e. **Safest**
        - Abstinence

  3. **Conditions That Facilitate HIV Sexual Transmission** *(J AIDS 30:73, 2002; JID 191:333, 2005)*

     Male-to-Female Transmission — Relative Risk Reported
     - (a) Oral contraceptives — 2.5–4.5
     - (b) Gonococcal cervicitis — 1.8–4.5
     - (c) Candida vaginitis — 3.3–3.6
     - (d) Genital ulcers — 2.0–4.0
     - (e) Bacterial vaginosis — 2.4 *(J AIDS 29:409, 2002)*
     - (f) HSV-2 — 2.5
     - (g) Vitamin A deficiency — 2.6–12.9
     - (h) CD4 count <200 — 6.1–17.6
     - (i) Depomedroxyprogesterone acetate (DMPA) subdermal implant use as contraceptive — 2.2 *(JID 178:1053, 1998)*
     - (j) Sharing of HLA-B alleles in discordant couples — 2.23 *(Ln 363:2137, 2004)*

     Female-to-Male Transmission
     - (a) Lack of circumcision — 5.4–8.2 risk/coital act ↓ from 1/80 to 1/200 *(Ln 1: 223, 2001; Ln 363:1039, 2004; JID, Feb. 15, 2005)*
     - (b) Genital ulcers — 2.6–4.7
     - (c) Sex during menses — 3.4
     - (d) Herpes simplex type 2 (genital herpes) — 6–16.8 *(JID 187;1513, 2003 & 189;1209, 2004)*

TABLE 1 (2)

↑ **Titers of viral DNA in vaginal secretions** *(JID 175:57, 1997)*
  (a) With low CD4 count — 9.6 (<200 vs >500)
  (b) Vitamin A deficiency — 2.6
  (c) Presence of cervical mucopus — 2.1
  (d) Acute primary HIV infection — ↑
  (e) With ↑ plasma HIV-RNA — ↑ *(JID 177:1100, 1998)*
  (f) Cervicitis — ↑ *(AIDS 15:105, 2001)*
  (g) Peak titer just prior to onset of menses — *(JID 189:2192, 2004)*

↑ **Titers of viral DNA in semen (ejaculate)** *(JID 172:1469, 1995; J AIDS & HR 18:277, 1998)*
  (a) Gonococcal urethritis — 3.2
  (b) Acute primary HIV infection — ↑ *(AIDS 16:1529, 2002)*

Not protective:
  (a) Nonoxynol-9 intravaginally *(Ln 360:971, 2002; AIDS 18:2191, 2004)*
  (b) IUD use

4. **Programs Aimed at Reducing Sexual Transmission**
   The major route of HIV spread worldwide is via heterosexual vaginal intercourse. Efforts to change sexual behavior by reducing number of sexual partners & using safe sex techniques (condoms) have met with varying degrees of success. These are summarized here:
   a. Voluntary counseling & testing (VCT): Prevention based on identifying infected persons & counseling them to prevent transmission to sexual partner(s). Variable success *(AIDS 15:1045, 2001; J AIDS 31:106, 2002; ArIM 162:1818, 2002)*
      (1) In >10,000 pregnant women in Tanzania, ¾ agreed to be tested. 2/3 of those returned for results but only 1/6 of positives disclosed result to sexual partner because of fear of stigma & divorce *(J AIDS 28:458, 2001)*.
      (2) Others reported VCT associated with ↓ risk behaviors & ↓ HIV transmission among discordant couples *(Soc Sc Med 53:1397, 2001)* & both men & women in Thailand *(J AIDS 29:284, 2002; J AIDS 15:493, 2002)*.
      (3) Acceptance ↑ if test results available same day *(Ann NY Acad Sci 918:64, 2000)*.
   b. Counseling & controlling STD in female sex workers: ↓ seroincidence of HIV from 16.3 to 6.5/100 person yrs in 500 subjects in Cote d'Ivoire *(AIDS 15:1421, 2000)* & Benin *(AIDS 16:463, 2002; J AIDS 30:69, 2002)*, & U.S. *(JAMA 292:171, 2004)*
   c. Condom distribution campaigns: Successfully ↓ HIV prevalence in Thailand from 17% in 1992 to 2% in 1999. In South Africa <10% of distributed condoms discarded *(AIDS 15:789, 2001)*.
   d. Prevention campaign focused on education about AIDS & promotion of safer sexual behavior: Appears to have been effective in Uganda, Senegal, Zambia *(J AIDS 25:77, 2000)*, Mexico (among CSWs) *(AIDS 16:1445, 2002)*, & U.S. *(JAMA 292:171, 2004)*.
   e. Delivery of message complex. Examples of communication methods used:
      (1) Radio soap opera (Tanzania, *J Health Comm 5(Suppl):81, 2000*)
      (2) Combination of drama or video reached >85% in Uganda *(Health Educ Res 16:411, 2001)*
      (3) Traditional healers or theater in Sierra Leone *(J Assoc Nurs AIDS Care 12:48, 2001)*
      (4) Folk media in rural Ghana *(Am J Publ Health 91:1559, 2001)*
      (5) Religion has been shown to reduce protective behaviors toward AIDS & suggest a critical need to work with clergy to embrace the prevention message *(AIDS 14:2027, 2000)*
   f. ARV RX ↓ VL in genital secretions & transmission of HIV (by 53%) in Taiwan *(JID 190:879, 2004)*. Studies have not demonstrated ↑ in high-risk heterosexual activity in persons on ARV RX *(JAMA 292:224, 2004)*, but remains a concern.
   g. In 2008, implementation of circumcision programs for young men is being debated by policymakers across Africa and in other countries with high incidence rates for HIV infection.
   h. Concern regarding increased transmission among older heterosexual adults (>55 years old). Many older adults are sexually active *(NEJM 357: 762, 2007)*, and with increased use of erectile dysfunction drugs, higher rates of STDs, including HIV, expected.

B. **Injection (intravenous or "skin popping") Drug Use (IDU) or Smoking Crack Cocaine.** Assess injectable anabolic steroid use! Assess sexual behaviors in all drug users! In one study, infection rates in crack cocaine-smoking women are as high as in men who had sex with men (41% vs 43%). Risk-reduction intervention can ↓ high risk sexual activity in crack cocaine users *(AIDS Edu Prev 15:15, 2003)* & IVDUs *(J AIDS 30:573, 2002)*. IVDU is currently driving explosive spread of syphilis & HIV in Russian cities *(Int J STD AIDS 13:618, 2002; AIDS 16:F25, 2002)*. Interestingly, transmission of drug-resistant HIV ↓ in Amsterdam *(AIDS 18:1571, 2004)*. Buprenorphine, shows promise in reducing opioid-dependence, thus reducing HIV transmission *(CID 41;891, 2005)*.

Drug Use Practices: *(Drug abuse treatment & methadone use programs reduce HIV transmission: AIDS 13:2151 & 1807, 1999)*

1. **Riskiest**
   - **Sharing uncleaned needles,** syringes, other paraphernalia (works), especially in "shooting galleries." HIV DNA found on 85% of needles/syringes & 1/3–2/3 cottons, cookers, wash waters from shooting galleries.
   - Practicing "registering," "booting," or "back loading"

2. **Less risky**
   - Sharing cleaned needles, syringes, works. (Household bleach is effective, especially after washing & when contact time is greater than 5 minutes. It is important to rinse with water after bleach use)
   - Drug paraphernalia used repeatedly but by single user

3. **Least risky**
   - Single use needles, syringes, works (needle exchange programs reduce HIV transmission, [see *MMWR 54;673, 2005* for update of US programs])
   - Sterile needles, syringes, works (needle/syringe exchange appears effective & has not ↑drug use)

C. **Blood Product Infusion Recipient**
   Blood Product Risks:
   1. **Riskiest**
      - Receipt of multiple units of blood products between **1978–1985**
      - Receipt of blood products obtained from donors in countries where screening is unreliable or not done
   2. **Less risky**
      - Receipt of heterologous blood products in U.S. after 1985 (risk per unit 1:450,000 to 1:660,000 units or 1:28,000 after an average of 5.4 units). [This is because of a window (about 20 days) between infection & seroconversion (18–27 donations/yr are in this window).] HIV p24 antigen testing of all blood products (instituted 3/96) reduces the "window" by 6 days & ↓ infectious donations by 25%/yr to 1:600,000-1:880,000 units *[MMWR 45(RR2):1, 1996]*. RhoGAM & hepatitis B vaccine (serum-derived) have never been reported to transmit HIV-1.
      - Receipt of donor-selected blood products in U.S. after 1985 (but no safer than random donors)
   3. **Safest**
      - Receipt of autologous blood products
      - Receipt of genetically engineered blood product substitutes

TABLE 1 (3)

D. **Perinatal Infection:** See Table 8B
E. **Occupational Exposure** *(See Table 9) (CDC Guidelines, MMWR 54 (RR-9):1, 2005; Cochrane Database Syst Rev. 2007 Jan 24;(1) CD002835)*
   Relative Risk Determinants
   1. **Riskiest** [risk may be decreased by glove use, which removes >50% blood from exposure site in some studies but HIV-size microbes can pass through 1/3 of latex gloves tested *(J All Clin Imm 97:575, 1996)*. With double-glove use, blood-hand contacts ↓ from 71 to 32/100 procedures.
      • Deep parenteral inoculation (RR 16.8) via hollow needle of blood from source with high-titer viremia; seroconversion or advanced HIV disease (RR 7.8)
      • Parenteral inoculation of materials containing high titer virus in research laboratory setting
      • Failure to use ARV Rx after inoculation (RR 0.1 when used)
   2. **Less risky**
      • Small volume exposure via non-hollow needle
      • Mucosal exposure/non-intact skin exposure [risk is too low to be quantified in prospective studies; not zero but estimated to be at least a log (90%) lower than needlestick risk. Risk may be increased if large volume or prolonged contact occurs]
   3. **Risk not identified**
      • **Cutaneous contact** (intact skin)
      • Exposure to urine, saliva, sweat, tears
F. **Donor Organ or Tissue Transplantation**
   1. Test potential donors for HIV (note window between infection & seroconversion *(C.2 above)*
   2. Assess donors for risk factors
   3. Evaluate risk/benefits
      • Risk following artificial insemination with semen from HIV+ donor is 3.5% *(Ln 351: 728, 1998)*. HIV testing recommended but **not legally required**

III. Recommendations for HIV Testing
A. In Sept 2006, the CDC issued new guidelines calling for routine universal testing of all Americans between ages 13 & 64 yrs (many experts suggest testing ALL sexually active persons regardless of age). Previously the recommendations had been to test people at risk *(see below)*, however, studies indicated that over 50% of new dx of HIV infection occurred within one yr of a dx of full blown AIDS and the incidence of new cases in the US has recently been estimated upward, now anticipating ~ 60,000 new cases per year (up from 40,000/yr).
The CDC suggested that signed consent for HIV testing be eliminated and included in the general consent for medical care. [Pre-test counseling was not recommended unless pts were from high-risk groups.] Pts should be told verbally that they will be tested as part of their medical care and given the opportunity to opt out of testing. This discussion should include an explanation about HIV infection, how it is transmitted, implications about a positive test. If pt declines, it should be recorded on his chart.
The implications of a positive test [screening & confirmatory *(See Table 2)*] can be profound and have the potential for physical & psychological harm, particularly for women. Counseling & referral services for partner notification should be made available.
While the new recommendations indicate a change in direction, they may conflict with established state laws. Clinicians need to be aware of local regulations regarding consent and counseling. See http://www.hret.org/hret/about/hivmap.html or http: //www.hret.org/hret/about/crossstate.html.*(Ln 369:243, 2007)*.

B. **Post-Test Counseling:**
Rapid HIV antibody tests, which can provide results within 20 minutes has improved the efficiency of point of care testing. However a confirmatory test such as Western Blot is still required. It is critically important to offer counseling to those who test positive. Issues to be discussed should include:
1. Emphasize that HIV infection can now be can be managed successfully as a complicated disease like diabetes
2. Stigma & the fear of disclosure HIV status
3. Need to inform previous/current sexual partner
4. Testing of children & partners at potential risk
5. Strict adherence to safe-sex practices (especially consistent use of condoms)
6. Avoidance of drugs that may cause disinhibition (amphetamines, etc)

TABLE 2: INITIAL EVALUATION OF HIV-INFECTED ADULT PATIENT
(See NEJM 353:16, 2005 for excellent review)

I. **Insist on documentation of a positive HIV antibody test: confirm with a 2nd antibody test, a Western blot, or positive plasma viral quantitation**

II. **History, Review of Systems, & Past Medical History**
   A. **General health status**
      1. General well-being; constitutional symptoms
      2. Infectious diseases (TB, leishmaniasis, cocci, histo, etc.): childhood infections, infections in adult life, previous physician visits, hospitalizations (where, when)
      3. Immunization history, e.g., hepatitis A, B, BCG, pneumococcal
   B. **Drug history**
      1. Medications & dosages
         a. Prescription; non-prescription
         b. Alternative therapies
      2. "Recreational" drug use *(see Table 1, above)*
         a. Intravenous/injection; crack cocaine
         b. Other
         c. Identify partners at risk
      3. Smoking & alcohol history
   C. **Sexual history**
      1. Sexual practices *(see Table 1, page 4)*
      2. Past sexually transmitted diseases
      3. Obstetric/gynecologic history
      4. Contraceptive use
      5. Identify partners at risk
   D. **Past or present HIV-related illness, e.g., candidiasis**
   E. **Risks for opportunistic infections**
      1. Travel history
      2. Geographic location of current/prior residence, e.g., southwest, midwest of USA
      3. Occupational history, e.g., poultry worker
      4. Avocational activities
      5. Tuberculosis status: history of BCG vaccination, family members with &/or treated for tuberculosis, contacts (close) with patients with known tuberculosis, results of previous tuberculin tests &/or chest x-rays if known
      6. Pets, e.g., cats—Bartonella henselae; fish—M. marinum. Cat ownership not associated with toxoplasma antibody seroconversion
   F. **Past history of viral hepatitis, to include type if known, past history of herpes zoster**

III. **Comprehensive Physical Examination**
   A. Document weight & height
   B. Careful funduscopic & oral examination
   C. Dermatologic examination, to include back, buttocks, & extremities, hands, feet
   D. Exam of all lymph node areas: postoccipital, preauricular, cervical, submental, supraclavicular, axillary, epitrochlear, inguinal (measure & record size if palpable, record as negative if not palpable)
   E. Rectal/genital examination, to include pelvic exam with Pap smear in women, inspection for perianal/genital Herpes simplex. Pap smears should be repeated every 12 months.
   F. Assess mental status for evidence of dementia.

IV. **Laboratory Evaluation**
   A. **Baseline**
      1. Complete blood cell count with differential (anemia may complicate zidovudine rx)
      2. Electrolytes, blood sugar (diabetes may complicate use of PIs, which cause insulin resistance), renal function tests: BUN, creatinine (abn renal function may complicate use of tenofovir or adjustment in NRTI/NNRTI dosages)
      3. Liver enzyme tests: serum bilirubin, aspartate aminotransferase (AST, SGOT), alanine aminotransferase (ALT, SGPT), alkaline phosphatase (indinavir & atazanavir can elevate indirect bilirubin levels)
      4. Creatine kinase (inc level may indicate HIV myopathy & baseline to monitor zidovudine which may cause drug-induced myopathy)
      5. Fasting lipid profile (elevated levels may indicate need for dietary/drug therapy or avoidance of certain PIs)
   B. **HIV staging** (Important for all future care decisions including when to initiate ARV RX & prophylaxis)
      1. CD4 & CD8 T-lymphocyte count
      2. Quantitative measurement of plasma HIV RNA *(9)*—"viral load" or plasma "viral burden"
      3. Repeat every 3-4 months.
   C. **Additional studies**
      1. **PPD intermediate** (5TU),or blood assay for M. tbc infection (QuantiFERON-TB GOLD), *MMWR 54 (RR-15), 2005 see Table 12, page 122*
      2. Chest x-ray (baseline important for future care)
      3. VDRL or RPR (tests for syphilis) (evidence of past or recent exposure requires treatment unless there is documentation of adequate course of treatment); repeat annually.
      4. IgG antibody to toxoplasmosis (if + primary prophylaxis indicated when CD4<100
      5. Hepatitis B surface antigen (HBsAg), antibody to Hep B surface Ag (anti-HBsAg), antibody to Hep C (important in consideration of treatment decisions for chronic active infection & ARV RX)
      6. CMV antibody, IgG
      7. G6PD Assay (African-Americans).
      8. Urine nucleic acid amplification test.
      9. Type specific Herpes simplex antibody.

V. **Initial Health Care Maintenance**
   A. HIV risk reduction education *(see Table 1)*
   B. Drug rehabilitation/safer needle use/needle exchange
   C. Smoking cessation (smoking ↑ risk of thrush, hairy leukoplakia, bacterial pneumonia, coronary artery disease)
   D. Partner notification
   E. Reproductive counseling
   F. Psychosocial support
   G. Immunizations *(see Table 20)*. Immunizations transiently ↑ HIV viral load, clinical significance uncertain
      1. Pneumococcal vaccine
      2. Influenza vaccine (annually)
      3. Hepatitis B vaccine, if sexually active or sharing needles; hepatitis A vaccine
   H. Preventive dentistry
   I. If CD4 count <100 cells/mm^3, baseline ophthalmologic evaluation
   J. Cervical Pap smear females; anal Pap smear males

VI. **Primary Care of Patients Infected With HIV**
   Multiple studies demonstrate that physicians & other health care givers who care for large numbers of HIV-infected persons & who make delivery of this care a major focus of their practice, training & continuing education have better outcomes *(see IDSA position statement, CID 26:275, 1998)*. A team approach with coordination of services around patients' needs & integration of acute & long-term care is emerging as the most effective management. 3rd-party payment with private insurance & Medicaid to pay for services remains a challenge

FIGURE 1: Life Cycle of HIV with Sites of Action of Antiretrovirals

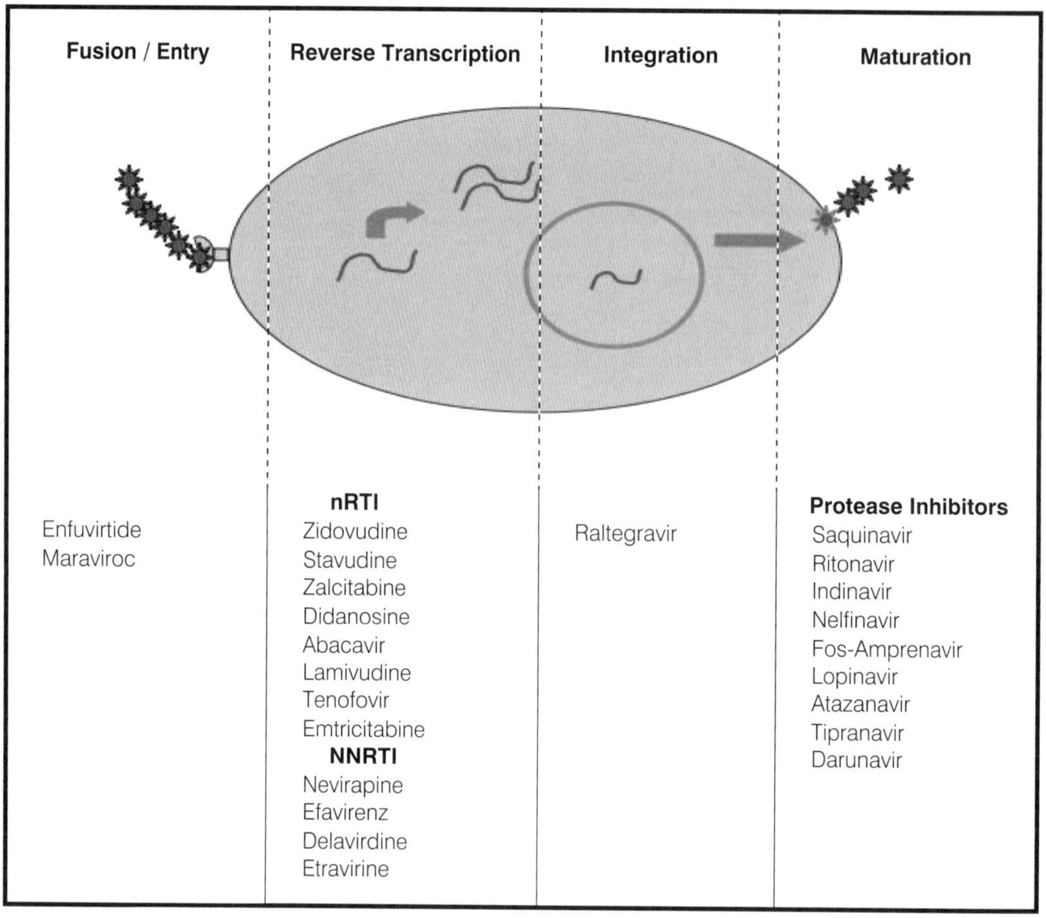

Fusion / Entry	Reverse Transcription	Integration	Maturation
Enfuvirtide Maraviroc	**nRTI** Zidovudine Stavudine Zalcitabine Didanosine Abacavir Lamivudine Tenofovir Emtricitabine **NNRTI** Nevirapine Efavirenz Delavirdine Etravirine	Raltegravir	**Protease Inhibitors** Saquinavir Ritonavir Indinavir Nelfinavir Fos-Amprenavir Lopinavir Atazanavir Tipranavir Darunavir

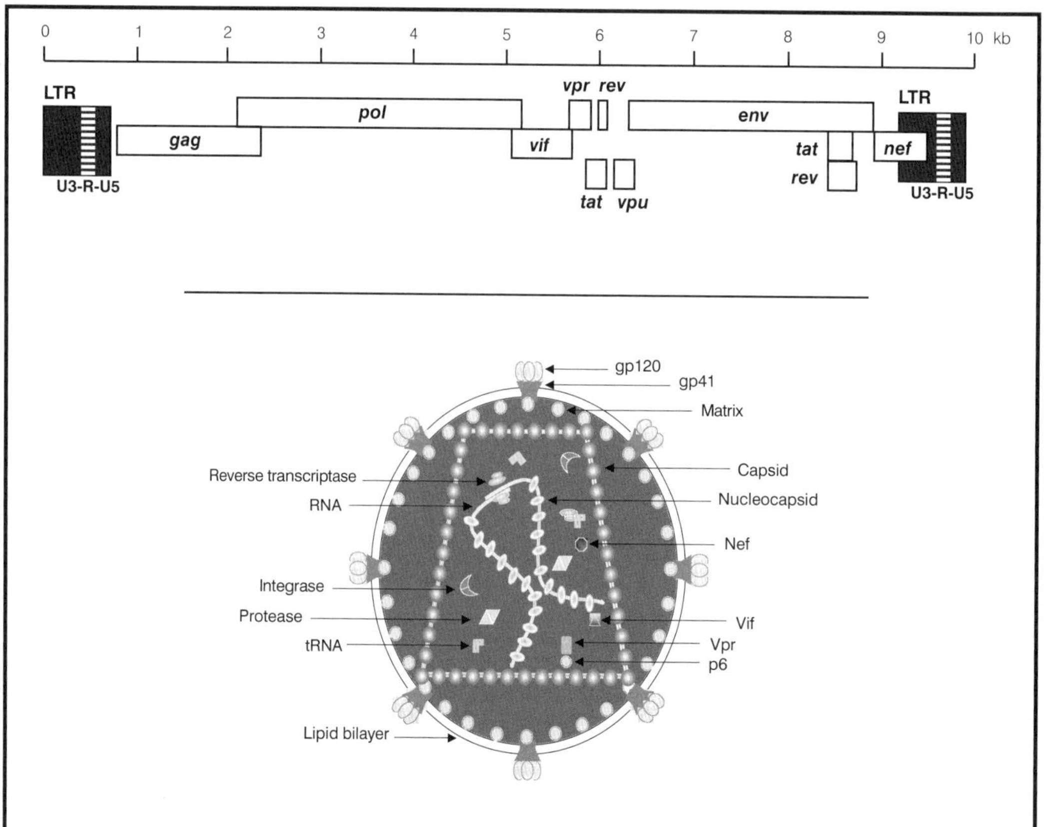

HIV genome (0–10 kb): LTR (U3-R-U5), gag, pol, vif, vpr, tat, rev, vpu, env, tat, rev, nef, LTR (U3-R-U5)

Virion components: gp120, gp41, Matrix, Capsid, Nucleocapsid, Nef, Vif, Vpr, p6, tRNA, Protease, Integrase, RNA, Reverse transcriptase, Lipid bilayer

Contain all necessary elements for reverse transcription

TABLE 3: LABORATORY TESTS COMMONLY USED IN THE DIAGNOSIS & MANAGEMENT OF INFECTION WITH HIV-1 and HIV-2

1. **Classification of HIV-1 genetic forms**
2. **HIV-1 & HIV-2 antibody tests**
   A. Serum antibody detection
      (1) EIA ± Western blot
      (2) Rapid detection methods
      (3) Home test kits
   B. Detection of HIV-1 antibody in other body fluids
      (1) Antibody in saliva
      (2) Antibody in urine
3. **HIV-2 antibody tests**
4. **Indications for Plasma HIV RNA Testing**
5. **Detection/quantitation of HIV**
   A. HIV p24 antigen
   B. Qualitative PCR: Circulating cells or plasma
   C. Quantitative plasma viral "loads"
6. **CD4/CD8 T-lymphocyte counts**
   A. CD4 T-lymphocytes
   B. CD8 T-lymphocytes
7. **Discordant virologic & immunologic responses**
8. **Drug Resistance Testing in the Treatment of HIV Infection**
   A. Mechanism of action & resistance of drugs
   B. When & why to test for resistance?
   C. Who should have HIV resistance testing?
   D. How to test? Genotype or phenotype?
   E. When Not to test?
   F. Does resistance testing predict virologic response?
   G. Genotype resistance testing
   H. Phenotypic drug resistance testing
   I. Interpretation of discordance in drug susceptibility by genotype & phenotype
   J. Summary
9. **Abacavir Hypersensitivity Testing**
10. **Coreceptor Tropism Assays**
    A. When to test for tropism
    B. Interpretation of Results

---

1. Classification of HIV-1—genetic forms. Ref.: Ln ID 2:461, 2002
   A. Three phylogenetic groups:
      M = Main   O = Outlier—Central Africa. Rare   N = Novel: Non-M & Non-O—Central Africa. Rare

      9 subtypes (clades)
      A B C D F G H J K

   B. **Circulating recombinant forms (CRFs)** = Intersubtype recombinant viruses identified in 3 or more epidemiologically unlinked people with full-length genome sequencing. CRFs identified by number (in order of discovery) followed by letters of parental subtypes (CPX = complex: recombinant virus from 3 or more subtypes).
      Examples: CRF01_AE; CRF06_CPX; CRF14_BG.
   C. Geographic distribution of HIV genetic forms

Area	Circulating Genetic Forms	Area	Circulating Genetic Forms
North & Central America	B	Central Africa	A, (CRF02_AG), C, D, F1, F2, G, H, J, (CRF01_AE), O, N
South America	B, F1, (CRF12_BF)	South Africa	C, B
Western Europe	B, G, (CRF14_BG)	South Asia	C, B, A
Eastern Europe	A, B, C, F1, (CRF03_AB)	Southeast Asia	B, (CRF01_AE)
Australia	B	China	B, (CRF07_BC), (CRF08_BC), (CRF01_AE)

2. **HIV-1 antibody tests** (http://hivinsite.ucsf.edu)

A. **Detection of antibody in serum or plasma**

TABLE 3 (2)

Test	Primary Purpose(s)	Sensitivity %	Specificity %	Comment
(1) **Enzyme Immunoassay (EIA) followed by Western blot** for confirmation. All detect antibodies to HIV-1 & HIV-2 (see *Comment* below). For all high-risk groups (*Table 1*); antibody becomes positive approx. 3 wks. post-disease acquisition in majority; 6 mos. after infection, 95% patients antibody-positive. **Western blot** to confirm HIV-1 antibody. Interpretation for HIV-1 result: 1. No antibodies (bands) detected = **negative** 2. Antibody (bands) to Gp41 & Gp120/160 or either of latter plus p24 = **positive.** 3. Any other pattern of positive = **indeterminate**[1]. Proceed to plasma viral load testing. See footnote for HIV-2 Western blot result.	99.9	99.9	EIA detects IgG, IgA, & IgM antibody to HIV-1, Group B subtype. **Most U.S. HIV infections are due to M group, subtype B**. Current EIAs detect nearly all Group M subtypes. Increasing concern, worldwide, regarding circulating recombinant forms (CRFs) of HIV (*Ln ID 2:461, 2002*)—see *Section 1.B, above*. **False-positive** EIA rare; e.g., autoimmune diseases, pregnancy, post-immunization (influenza, HIV vaccine, hepatitis B, rabies) (*ArIM 160:2386, 2000*), *multiple myeloma, chronic renal failure, SLE*. **False-negative EIA** in 1/500,000 units donated blood due to: (1) 1–2wk window between infection & antibody response (*JAMA 284:210, 2000*); (2) agammaglobulinemia; (3) Gp O or N genetic variants. RARE (*AIDS 18:269, 2002*). So far no N group in U.S. EIA negative in 20–30% HIV-2 pts; (4) Post-transplant.
(2) **Rapid HIV Antibody Screening Tests**: See CID 45(Suppl 4):S222, 2007. Results available within 30 minutes. For FDA approved tests—see: www.cdc.gov/hiv/topics/testing/rapid/index.htm. **Need confirmation of pos. results with EIA & Western blot;** for protocol, see *MMWR 53:221, 2004.* **Clinical uses** for all: (a) In labor, no prenatal HIV test (*JAMA 292:219, 2004*); (b) Patient who is source of needlestick injury to health care provider (*JCM 41:3868, 2003*); (c) Evaluation of acutely ill patient with possible PCP; (d) Patients who are unlikely to return for test results.				

Summary of FDA-Approved Rapid HIV Antibody Screening Tests

Test Name	Specimen Type	CLIA* Category	Sensitivity (95% CI)	Specificity (95% CI)	Manufacturer	Approved for HIV-2 Detection
Oraquick Advance Rapid HIV 1/2 Antibody Test	Oral fluid	Waived	99.3% (98-100)	99.8% (99.6-99.9)	Orasure Technologies, Inc. www.orasure.com	Yes
	Whole blood	Waived	99.6% (98.5-99.9)	100% (99.7-100)		
	Plasma	Moderate complexity	99.6% (98.9-99.8)	99.9% (99.6-99.9)		
Uni-Gold Recombigen HIV 1	Whole blood	Waived	100% (99.5-100)	99.7% (99-100)	Trinity Biotech www.unigoldhiv.com	No
	Serum or plasma	Moderate complexity	100% (99.5-100)	99.8% (99.3-100)		

---

[1] Causes of indeterminate Western Blot: Infection (HIV-2, HTLV-1, Schisto), Neoplasms, Dialysis, Ethnicity (Africans), Thyroiditis, Elevated bilirubin, Rheumatologic diseases, Multiple pregnancies, Immunization (tetanus), Nephrotic massive proteinuria, Error in laboratory (IN-DETERMIN).

TABLE 3 (3)

Summary of FDA-Approved Rapid HIV Antibody Screening Tests

Reveal G-3 Rapid HIV-1 Antibody Test	Serum or plasma	Moderate complexity	99.8% (99.7-100)	99.1% (98.8-99.4)	No	Med Mira, Inc. www.medmira.com
	Plasma or serum	Moderate complexity	99.8% (99-100)	99.9% (98.6-100)		
Multispot HIV-1/HIV-2 Rapid Test	Plasma or serum	Moderate complexity	100% (99.9-100)	99.9% (99.8-100)	Yes	Bio-Rad Laboratories
Clearview HIV 1/2 Stat-Pak	Whole blood	Waived	99.7% (98.9-100)	99.9 (98.6-100)	Yes	Chembio Daignostic Systems

* Clinical Laboratory Improvement Initiative

3. **HIV 2 antibody tests**—HIV 1 antibody tests neg. in 20-30% pts with HIV 2 infections. Suspect in patient from West Africa; less than 100 HIV-2 cases reported in U.S.; HIV 2 specific antibody tests available at CDC (used to screen all blood donors)

4. **Indications for Plasma HIV RNA Testing**

Clinical Indication	Information Derived	Use of Result
Illness suggests acute (primary) HIV infection	Establishes diagnosis if HIV antibody test is negative or indeterminate	Establishes diagnosis
Initial evaluation of patient with new HIV infection diagnosis	Establish baseline	Used with CD4 T cell count as basis for starting or deferring therapy
If not on therapy, repeat every 3-4 months	Trend of viral load	Used with CD4 T cell count as basis for starting therapy
Repeat 2-8 weeks after starting antiretroviral therapy	Assessment of drug efficacy	Basis of continuing or changing therapy
Repeat 3-4 months after starting antiretroviral therapy	Assessment of drug efficacy	Basis of continuing or changing therapy
Repeat every 3-6 months while on therapy	Determine durability of efficacy of antiretroviral therapy	Basis of continuing or changing therapy
Significant decrease in CD4 T cells and/or opportunistic infection	Determine change, or absence of change, of viral load	Basis of initiating, continuing or changing antiretroviral therapy

5. **Detection/quantitation of HIV RNA**

Test	Current Use	% Positive	Advantages	Disadvantages	Comment
A. **HIV-1 p24 antigen** (Assumes acid pretreatment to dissociate immune complexes)	Diagnosis of acute HIV syndrome (antibody may not be detectable for 2–6 mos)	% positive depends on method/stage of disease, e.g., in acute retroviral syn.: 100%; if CD4 200–500, 45–70%; if CD4 <200, 75–100%	Detection of infection before antibody appears	Not as good as quant. nucleic acid methods as a measure of effectiveness of therapy	In newborns at risk, HIV DNA PCR (if available) preferable to p24 antigen

TABLE 3 (4)

Test	Current Use	% Positive	Advantages	Disadvantages	Comment
B. **Qualitative HIV nucleic acid by PCR:** circulating cells or plasma	**Use to diagnose primary HIV instead of p24 antigen; also to resolve indeterminate Western blots.** Can use circulating cells or plasma	>99% for HIV variants from U.S. & Europe (subtype B). May fail to detect novel African HIV-1 variants	97% sensitivity & 98% specificity with 1.9% false-pos. & 3.0% false-neg.	Qualitative, not quantitative	Trend is to use quantitative PCR methods.
C. **Quantitative measurement of plasma HIV RNA "viral loads"** Ref.: JID 190:2047, 2004 (1) Can increase ≥10-fold during acute illness; return to baseline within one month	• Clinical uses: (1) Although decision to initiate antiretroviral rx is no longer based primarily on viral load measurements, high levels (>50,000/ml) may signal more rapid decline in CD4 counts & poor prognosis. (2) Monitor response to antiretroviral rx. (3) Predict likelihood of transmission of HIV from mother to fetus. (4) Diagnose infection in newborn.		At least 3 competing methods. Test availability varies with locale. Ability to accurately quantitate low levels of viremia (<40–50 viral RNA equivalents/ml). Changes in viral burden of ≤0.3 log (2-fold) may be just technical variation; changes ≥0.5 log (3-fold) reflect real changes in viral burden (see Section 7, next page). Recommend repeat use of same test method for individual patients because of discrepancies between the different techniques. In developing countries, can collect dried whole blood on filter paper, rather than plasma, for HIV viral loads (Ln 362:2067, 2003).		
(2) Due to assay differences, use same assay repeatedly for a given patient. Results with RT-PCR & NASBA consistently greater than bDNA (MMWR 50:RR-20, 2001).	• Current methods:		**Reportable ranges (copies/ml)**	**Preferred anticoagulant[1]:**	
(3) For given assay, significant difference is a change of ≥0.5 log$_{10}$ (3-fold)	(1) Couples RNA reverse transcription (RT) to a **DNA PCR amplification (RT-PCR)** (Roche Ampicor HIV-1 Monitor, Version 1.5). NOTE: Ideally collect with EDTA & separate plasma within 6hrs. Freeze plasma until assayed.	>98	Standard 400–750,000; Ultrasensitive assay 50–100,000	ACD/EDTA	Quantifies group M subtypes A-H. **Values roughly 2x higher than bDNA.** RT-PCR is less efficient than bDNA at quantitation of subtypes (JAIDS 29:330, 2002).
(4) NOTE: Use standard EDTA tubes; use of "plasma separation tubes" can result in fictitious low-level viremia (CID 41:1671, 2005)	(2) Amplification of RNA of HIV; **a nucleic acid sequence-based amplification** (NASBA) (bioMerieux NucliSens., HIV-1 QT). Freeze plasma until assayed.	>98	NucliSens: 176–3,400,000. Can quantify HIV in CSF, seminal fluid, breast milk, saliva, vaginal fluid.	ACD/EDTA/HEP	For information, call bioMerieux (800-682-2666). May under-estimate viral burden if subtype C
	(3) Identification of HIV RNA, **then signal amplification by DNA branched-chain technique** (referred to as bDNA) (Bayer Versant HIV-1 RNA Quantiplex 3.0 Assay). Freeze plasma until assayed.	>98	Version 3.0:75–500,000	EDTA	For information, call Bayer (800-434-2447). Detects subtypes A to G.
	(4) Real-time RT-PCR (COBAS Ampliprep/COBAS Tag Man HIV-1, Roche Diagnostics	>98	48-10,000,000 copies/mL	EDTA	Quantifies group M subtypes A-H
	(5) Real-time RT-PCR (RealTime HIV-1, Abbott Molecular)	>98	48-10,000,000 copies/mL	EDTA	Quantifies all group M subtypes, group O and recombinants

[1] **ACD** = acid citrate dextran; **EDTA** = ethylenediaminetetraacetic acid; **HEP** = heparin

D. **Interpretation:** Changes of ≥50% (3-fold or 0.5 $\log_{10}$ copies/mL) are considered significant.
   (1) **A guide to logarithmic changes;** for a person **starting with 100,000 copies/mL** of HIV-RNA:

$\log_{10}$ copies/mL	n-Fold Change	Copies of HIV RNA Remaining
-0.3	2-fold	50,000
-0.5	3-fold	33,000
-1.0	10-fold	10,000
-1.5	30-fold	3,300
-2.0	100-fold	1,000

   (2) **Factors that increase viral load:**
       a. Progressive uncontrolled HIV infection due to non-adherence or ineffective regimen
       b. Active non-HIV infection, e.g., tuberculosis (5–160 fold ↑), pneumococcal pneumonia (3–5 fold ↑) and other acute illnesses
       c. Immunization, e.g., influenza, pneumococcal
   (3) **Falsely low viral loads:**
       a. Non-B subtype not detected with Amplicor assay
       b. HIV-2 infection

TABLE 3 (5)

6. **CD4/CD8 antigen T-lymphocyte counts (CD=cluster differentiation)**—CDC Guidelines for absolute CD4 T cell counts: *MMWR 52(RR-2):1–13, 2003*

Test	Current Use	Results	Advantages	Disadvantages	Comment
A. **CD4 T-lymphocyte count (T-helper lymphocyte)** Principles of flow cytometry: *Crit. Care Med.* 33 (Suppl):S426, 2005. Cost: $60-$150 Discussion of CD4 lymphocyte % vs. absolute CD4 lymphocyte count: see *JID* 192:945 & 950, 2005.	(1) Decision to initiate antiretroviral rx (200–350/mm³ (Table 6B); (2) Assess magnitude of injury to host immune system; (3) Changes used to monitor effectiveness of antiretroviral rx. **Normals: CD4 500–1400/mm³. CD8 180–865/mm³; CD4/CD8 ratio 1.1–3.5;** (4) Initiation of prophylaxis vs opportunistic infections (Table 10).	Results expressed as both absolute CD4 T-lymphocyte count & % CD4 cells. **In HIV negative patients with hepatic cirrhosis low absolute CD4 count but normal % CD4 cells:** (CID 44:431 & 438, 2007).	Generally available. Rate of ↓ in absolute CD4 count or % CD4 lymphocytes correlates with HIV disease progression (*JID* 195:425, 2007). New method (reference above): flow cytometry with 3 different monoclonal antibodies measures absolute CD4 count in single step.	Test must be done ≤18 hrs after blood collection. **Absolute CD4 counts may ↓ due to:** time of day, time of year, lab doing test, intercurrent infection, & corticosteroids. **Absolute CD4 levels may ↑ due to:** HTLV-1 co-infection, splenectomy.	Fluoresceinated monoclonal antibodies are added to pt blood & the % fluorescent cells counted in cell sorter. CD4 count calculated as: WBC × % lymphocytes × % CD4 cells. **To avoid influence of change in WBC, can use % CD4s** (≥29% = CD4 count of >500; 14–28% = CD4 200–499; <14% = CD4 <200/mm³).
B. **Total lymphocyte count (TLC)** CD4 surrogate in resource-poor areas	TLC <750/mm³ correlates with CD4 count of <200 cells/mm³ *For review & meta-analysis: Ln 366:1868, 2005.*	No applicable			
C. **CD8 T-lymphocyte count (T-suppressor/cytotoxic lymphocyte)**	Often measured in parallel with CD4, even though role in disease process less well defined—see Comment		3–4 wks following infection, both CD4 & CD8 counts ↑ but CD8 ↑ is greater with inversion of normal CD4/CD8 ratio. CD8 cells believed to play a role in control of viral replication in many cells including CD4 cells.		

7. **Discordant virologic (HIV viral load, RNA copies per ml) & immunologic responses (CD4 T-lymphocyte count) to antiretroviral therapy** *(J Clin Virol 33:110, 2005; JAC 58:506, 2006).*

	CD4 Count	Viral Loads	Possible Explanations
A.	Increases	Decreases	Expected response to antiretroviral therapy
B.	Fails to ↑ or decreases	Decreases	Drug Toxicity: e.g., combination of tenofovir & didanosine (*AIDS* 19:1107, 2005); Deficiency in CD4 cell redistribution from lymphoid tissue, regeneration, and/or increased apoptosis (*JID* 191:1670, 2005)
C.	Increases	Remains high	Drug resistant virus; drug-induced defective virus with reduced replicative capacity (*JID* 191:1670, 2005; *Pediatrics* 114:604, 2004)
D.	Fails to increase	Increases	Non-adherence to therapy; drug-resistant HIV

TABLE 3 (6)

8. **Drug Resistance Testing in the Treatment of HIV Infection** (*Topics in HIV Med 16:62, 2008; www.iasusa.org; http://hivdb.stanford.edu*)
   A. **Mechanism of action & resistance of drugs used to treat HIV infection**

Drugs	Mechanism of Action	Mechanism of Resistance
Nucleoside analogues (NRTIs): Abacavir Didanosine Emtricitabine/lamivudine Stavudine Zalcitabine Zidovudine	Analogues of nucleosides; Active when triphosphorylated; Incorporated into new viral DNA; & Prematurely terminate synthesis of HIV DNA	a. Thymidine analogue (stavudine & zidovudine) mutations promote ATP- & pyrophosphate- mediated **excision** of incorporated chain terminator b. Other mutations **impair incorporation** of nucleoside analogues into new HIV DNA
Nucleotide analogue (Nucleotide RTI): Tenofovir	Same as nucleosides	Specific mutation impairs incorporation into HIV DNA
Non-nucleoside reverse-transcriptase inhibitors (NNRTIs): Delavirdine Efavirenz Etravirine Nevirapine	Binds to hydrophobic pocket of HIV, type 1 reverse transcriptase; HIV, type 2 resistant (ETV active vs HIV-2) Blocks polymerization of viral DNA	Mutations decrease affinity for the enzyme; & Single mutation can lead to high level of resistance, except ETV, usually, >1 mutation
Protease inhibitors (PIs): Atazanavir Darunavir Fosamprenavir Indinavir Lopinavir Nelfinavir Ritonavir Saquinavir Tipranavir	Binds to, & interferes with, the active site of the protease	Mutations reduce affinity of inhibitors for the protease; & High level resistance usually requires multiple mutations
Fusion inhibitor: Enfuvirtide	Interferes with glycoprotein 41-dependent membrane fusion	Mutations in a portion of glycoprotein 41
CCR5 Inhibitor: Maraviroc	Binds to and interferes with the attachment of HIV to CCR5 co-receptor on CD4+ T-lymphocyte	Unmasking of low-level pre-existent population of dual-mixed tophic virus; mutations in V3 loop of gp120 not fully characterized yet
Integrase Inhibitor: Raltegravir	Interferes with integration of HIV into host genome, likely at strand transfer step	Unknown. Likely a change in ability of enzyme to function

B. **When & why to test for resistance?**
   (1) **Always test while on therapy except acute HIV.** Off therapy ≥2 wks, wild type virus "emerges." Once resistant, always resistant.
   (2) Results identify drugs to avoid.
   (3) Past history of clinical resistance better predictor than laboratory evidence of resistance.

C. **Who should have HIV resistance testing?**
   (1) All pts with **primary (acute) HIV infection.** *(JAMA 288:181, 2002; NEJM 347:385 & 438, 2002): Determine if drug-resistant virus transmitted.*
   (2) **Chronic HIV infection** & no prior therapy: Pretreatment resistance to one drug class is 6-16% *(JID 189:2174, 2004).*
   (3) **Treatment failure:** Recommend testing. See *definition of treatment failure below.*[1]
   (4) **Pregnancy:** Recommend testing.

---

[1] **Definition of rx failure:** (1) Failure to ↓ viral load (VL) >0.5–0.7 $\log_{10}$ copies/ml (≥3-fold) by 4 wks of rx ; (2) failure to ↓ VL >1 $\log_{10}$ copies/ml (10-fold) by 8 wks of rx; OR (3) failure to achieve <400 copies/ml by week 24 or <50 copies/ml by week 48.

TABLE 3 (7)

D. **How to test? Genotype or phenotype?**
   (1) Genotype identifies specific mutations. Can use genotype to predict a "virtual" phenotype. Results available within 1-2 weeks.
   (2) Phenotype exposes virus to drugs in tissue culture system. Results in 2-3 weeks or longer. More expensive than genotype.
   (3) Prefer genotyping during failure of 1st or 2nd regimen; many prefer phenotyping of highly-treated pts with many PI mutations; some data support genotyping in these pts also (CID 188:194, 2003).

E. **Tropism Testing.** Necessary for all patients prior to initiating maraviroc therapy.

F. **When Not to test?** Do not test if viral load is <1000 copies per ml because amplification of virus is unreliable.

G. **Does resistance testing predict virologic response?** *(Antivir Ther 8:427, 2003; CID 38:723, 2004).*
   (1) Using **genotypic & phenotypic** testing to guide treatment results in:
   - **EXTRA 0.5–0.6 log10 copies/ml (approx. 30,000 copies/ml or 3-fold) ↓ in viral load**
   - **EXTRA 10–20% of patients with viral loads below 200–500 copies/ml**
   (2) Improved longterm virologic outcome in treatment-experienced pts (CID 38:723, 2004)
   Fair ability to predict phenotype from genotype (CID 41:92, 2005).

H. **Genotype resistance testing** *(Ref: CID 42:1608, 2006).*
   (1) **DETECTS MUTATIONS IN TARGET PROTEINS THAT ARE ASSOCIATED WITH DRUG RESISTANCE. EXPERT ADVICE ON INTERPRETATION IMPROVES VIROLOGIC RESPONSE**
   a. Use PCR to amplify HIV protease & reverse transcriptase genes; some labs do not detect mutations in the envelope gene or integrase gene.
   b. Sequence genes. Report mutations found. Pattern of mutations used to predict response to antiretrovirals.
   c. **Mutation pattern updates on the internet: www.iasusa.org or http://hivdb.stanford.edu**
   d. Selected mutations, or combinations of mutations, may ↓ the **replication capacity** of HIV clinical isolates. **Definitions: Replication capacity** = number of progeny produced per round of infection per unit time. **Fitness** = relative reproductive success of various subtypes of HIV. **Virulence** = ability to destroy CD4 lymphocytes or impair immune system function.
   (2) **Commercial assays** (www.hivresistanceweb.com) for genotype resistance testing:
   a. Approx. cost $300–500; results in approx. 2wks
   b. Companies:

Test Name	Manufacturer	Website	Phone	Minimum Viral Load for Testing
Trugene	Visible Genetics	www.visgen.com	877-786-8446	1000
ViroSeq	Applied Biosystems	www.appliedbiosystems.com	800-327-3002	1000–2000
GeneSeq HIV	Monogram Biosciences	www.monogramhiv.com	800-777-0177	500
Gen Chec	Virco	www.vircolab.com	800-325-7504	200–400; combines genotype & phenotype

(3) **Nucleoside analog derivation of drugs:** Important as predictor of cross-resistance: e.g., resistance to one cytidine analog forecasts resistance to all cytidine analogs

Drug	Analog of:	Drug	Analog of:	Drug	Analog of:	Drug	Analog of:
Abacavir	Guanosine	Lamivudine	Cytidine	Zalcitabine	Cytidine	Tenofovir	Adenosine
Didanosine	Deoxyadenosine	Stavudine	Thymidine	Zidovudine	Thymidine	Emtricitabine	Cytidine

(4) **Description of resistant mutations:** Gene (codon) numbers plus amino acid change
   a. In addition to above gene numbers, the resulting change in amino acid may be indicated by:
   i.   A prefix letter code indicating amino acid encoded in wild-type virus
   ii. A letter code after the codon (gene) number indicating amino acid encoded in the mutant virus, e.g., M46I = at codon (gene) 46, isoleucine has replaced methionine

TABLE 3 (8)

b. Amino acid codes

Code Letter	Amino Acid	Code Letter	Amino Acid	Code Letter	Amino Acid	Code Letter	Amino Acid
A (Ala)	Alanine	G (Gly)	Glycine	M (Met)	Methionine	S (Ser)	Serine
C (Cys)	Cytosine	H (His)	Histidine	N (Asn)	Asparagine	T (Thr)	Threonine
D (Asp)	Aspartic acid	I (Ile)	Isoleucine	P (Pro)	Proline	V (Val)	Valine
E (Glu)	Glutamic acid	K (Lys)	Lysine	Q (Gln)	Glutamine	W (Trp)	Tryptophan
F (Phe)	Phenylalanine	L (Leu)	Leucine	R (Arg)	Arginine	Y (Tyr)	Tyrosine

c. To save space, specifics of amino acid substitutions deleted in some of the tables below. For full & updated data, see www.iasusa.org.

(5) **Selected Genotype Mutations that Result in Resistance to NRTIs** (www.iasusa.org/resistancemutations; *Topics in HIV Med* 15:119, 2007)

Mutation	Selected By	Mechanism	Effects On Other NRTIs	Comment
M184V	Lamivudine, Emtracitabine	Impairs drug incorporation	Decreased susceptibility to lamivudine & emtracitabine; Increased susceptibility to zidovudine, stavudine & tenofovir	Presence delays appearance of thymidine analogue mutations (TAMs). TAMs + M184V decreases response to abacavir
Thymidine analogue mutations (TAMS) E40F, M41L, D67N, K70R, L210W, T215Y/F, K219 Q/E/N/R	Zidovudine, stavudine	Mutation leads to excision of drug from DNA chain terminus	Decreased suscept to all NRTIs; the more TAMs, the more resistance.	TAM acquisition slowed by presence of M184V. May increase susceptibility to NNRTIs.
Q151M complex, T69 insertion	(Zidovudine/didanosine) or (Stavudine/didanosine)	Impairs drug incorporation	Q151M complex: resistance to all NRTIs except tenofovir; T69 insertion: resistance to all NRTIs	
K65R	Tenofovir, abacavir, didanosine	Impairs drug incorporation	Variable decreased suscept. To abacavir, didanosine, lamivudine/ emtracitabine & especially tenofovir	Increases suscept to zidovudine & stavudine
L74V	Abacavir, didanosine, tenofovir		Decreased suscept to abacavir, didanosine & tenofovir	Prevented by presence of zidovudine in treatment regimen
E44D, V118I	Zidovudine, stavudine		Decreased suscept to all NRTIs	

(6) **Mutations in Non-Nucleoside Reverse Transcriptase Inhibitors (NNRTIs). Cross-resistance is the rule.** Amino acid substitutions shown only once per codon (gene) number.

Multi-NNRTI resistance[1]:								
Multi-NNRTI resistance mutations[2]:	L100I	K103N	V106M V106A	Y181C/I	Y188L	G190S/A	P225H	M320L	P236L
Delavirdine		103	106	181	188				
Efavirenz[3]	100	103	106 108	181	188	190			
Nevirapine	100	103	106 108	181	188	190			
Etravirine	100 101 90 98		106	179 181		190	225	320	236

[1] K103N most common & usually occurs first
[2] Expect cross-resistance among all NNRTIs
[3] New NNRTIs in development

TABLE 3 (9)

(7) Mutations in the Protease Gene Associated with Resistance to Protease Inhibitors (PIs)—major mutations in bold print; others "minor"

   a. In general, multiple mutations needed for high-level resistance
   b. Cross-resistance common: e.g. mutations at codons 82, 84, 90; EXCEPTIONS–no cross-resistance: D30N nelfinavir & I50L atazanavir mutations
   c. Specific amino acid substitutions shown only once to avoid clutter

Multi-PI resistance mutations:																									
	10																								
Atazanavir/Riton*	10	16	20	24	32	33	34	36		46	48	**I50L**	53	54	60	62	64	71	73			82	**I84**	**88**	90	93
Darunavir/Riton*		11			32	33				47		**I50V**		**54**					73	**76**			**84**		89	
Fosampren/Riton*	10				32				46	47		**I50V**		54					73	76		82	**84**		90	
Indinavir/Riton*	10		20	24	32			36		**M46I/L**	**I47V/A**		50	53	54				71	73	76	77	**82**	84		90	
Lopinavir/Riton*	10		20	24	**V32I**	33				46	**I47V/A**	50	53	54		63			71	73	76		**V82A**	84		90	
Nelfinavir	10						**D30N**	36		46												77	82	84	88	**L90M**	
Saquinavir/Riton*	10			24							**G48V**			54		62			71	73		77	82	–	84	**90**	
Tipranavir/Riton*	10	13				**L33F**	35	36	43	46		47		54	58			69			74		82	83	84	90	

*Protease inhibitors customarily boosted by ritonavir (riton)

(8) Mutations in Gp41 Envelope Gene Associated with Resistance to Enfuvirtide *(JID 195:318, 2007):*

   Enfuvirtide   G36D/S   I37V   V38A/M/E   Q39R   40   42   43   In HR1 Region

(9) Maraviroc: Requires presence of virus that utilizes host CCR5 co-receptor (see Section 10 below). Virus with mutations in the V3 loop of gp120 remain CCR5 tropic but have decreased susceptibility to maraviroc *(J Virol 81:2359, 2007)*.

(10) Mutations in integrase gene associated with resistance to Raltegravir: Q148H/K/R & N155H

(11) Virtual Phenotype: Genotype used to project a phenotype based on a large library of compared genotypic & phenotypic test results.
See next section for phenotypic drug resistance testing.

I. **Phenotypic drug resistance testing: Measures susceptibility of recombinant viruses to an individual drug in cell culture**

   (1) **Indications for phenotypic testing**
      a. After multiple treatment failures
      b. Genotype shows many & complex mutation patterns
      c. Evaluate suscept to a new drug
      d. Patient infected with nonsubtype-B HIV

   (2) **General Comments**
      a. Methods & interpretation evolving
      b. Results reflect combination of:
         i.   Accumulated genetic mutations
        ii.   Variables in assay system
        iii.   End-point (cutoff) used—*see below*
      c. Compared to genotyping, phenotypic resistance assays:
         i.   Take longer (2–8wks); easier to interpret; quantitative degree of resistance
        ii.   Cost more ($800–1000)
        iii.   **Need minimal viral burden of 500–1000 RNA HIV equivalents/ml of plasma to perform test**
        iv.   If circulating drug-resistant virus represents less than 10% of plasma virus load, resistant virus probably not detected.
        v.   Only detect resistance to single drug, not combinations

TABLE 3 (10)

(3) **Method Comments**
  a. Overview of laboratory procedure:
   Genes for reverse transcriptase & protease from patients circulating HIV are inserted into laboratory clone of HIV → HIV inserted into CD4 cells → HIV replication in various drug concentrations measured by expression of a reporter gene → results compared to replication of laboratory strain of HIV.
  b. **Results expressed as fold increase (or fold resistance)**
   IC_{50} = drug concentration that inhibits viral replication by 50%
   IC_{50} patient virus/IC_{50} reference virus = fold increase (or fold resistance)
  c. **Definition of phenotypic resistance; consultation with a specialist recommended**
   i. Phenotypic resistance definition varies with cutoff value used; "cutoff" is separation of sensitive from resistant virus—3 levels of cutoffs in use:
   ii. **3 resistance cutoffs.** Ref.: *J AIDS 31:128, 2002*
    (a) **Technical or reproducibility cutoffs:** Based on variability of repeated testing of patient samples
     (1) Definition: lowest fold difference for which susceptible isolates reliably separated from reference laboratory HIV strains
     (2) Sensitive <4-fold increase IC_{50} patient/IC_{50} lab HIV in presence of test drug
      Intermediate 4-10-fold increase
      Resistant >10-fold increase
     (3) Technical cutoffs now rarely used
    (b) **Biologic cutoffs:** Based on variability of wild-type virus from patients
     (1) Determined by study of IC_{50} concentration of test drug vs HIV from wild type (treatment-naive) patients. Cutoff defined as IC_{50} above mean +250 (99% percentile).
     (2) More relevant but still arbitrary—see *Clinical cutoffs*
     (3) Cutoffs vary from one commercial assay to another
    (c) **Clinical cutoffs: Correlation with outcome data from clinical trials**
     (1) Determined by correlation of in vitro IC_{50} with virologic response in clinical trial
     (2) **Best definition of phenotypic resistance but most difficult to obtain.** Examples of validated clinical cutoffs:
      Abacavir: 4.5 "fold increase" = resistance (0.5–6.5, some pts may have at least 0.5 log ↓ in viral load)
      Didanosine & stavudine: 1.7 fold increase = reduced susceptibility
      Lopinavir: >10 fold increase = reduced susceptibility; >40-fold increase = resistance
      Tenofovir: 1.4 fold increase = reduced susceptibility (*JID 189:837, 2004*)
      Indinavir & ritonavir: >10 fold increase = reduced susceptibility
     (3) Difficult to determine—need large-scale trials
     (4) With multi-drug regimen, individual drug response influenced by other drugs used

(4) **Commercial labs**

Test Name	Manufacturer	Website	Phone	Minimum Viral Load
Virco Type HIV-1	Virco (Belgium)	www.vircolab.com	800-325-7504	1000 copies/ml; combines genotype & phenotype
PhenoSense HIV	Monogram Biosciences (USA)	www.monogrambio.com	800-777-0177	500 copies/ml; also offers combined genotypic/phenotypic testing and replication capacity
Phenoscript	Specialty Labs & Viralliance (France)	www.specialtylabs.com	800-421-7110	500 copies/ml

J. **Interpretation of discordance in drug susceptibility by genotype & phenotype**

TABLE 3 (11)

Genotype	Phenotype	Cause	Interpretation
Resistant	Susceptible	Mixture HIV subtypes	Resistant
Resistant	Susceptible	Hypersusceptibility	Resistance mutation, e.g., 184, that predicts "R" some drugs with increased susceptibility to others—see Section 8.F.5. above.
Not available	Susceptible or resistant	New drug	Phenotype result valid
Susceptible	Resistant	Novel drug	Resistant due to new mechanism of resistance

K. In summary, failure to respond to treatment depends on:
   (1) % of viral population that is drug-resistant
   (2) Plasma viral load
   (3) Compliance with prescribed treatment regimen
   (4) Low drug potency
   (5) Poor pharmacokinetics
   (6) High plasma protein binding

9. **Abacavir Hypersensitivity Testing** (NEJM 358:568, 2008; JAIDS 45:1, 2007; JAC 59:591, 2007)
   A. Immunologic hypersensitivity reaction in 5-8% of patients in first 6 weeks of therapy.
      1. Fever, rash, N/V, diarrhea, respiratory symptoms.
      2. Reversible with discontinuation.
      3. **Rechallenge reactions severe and can be life-threatening.**
   B. Presence of major histocompatibility complex class I allele **HLA-B*5701** correlates with **abacavir hypersensitivity.**
      1. If possible/available should screen for **HLA-B*5701** before starting abacavir.
      2. Screening reduced reactions from 7.8% to 3.4% (NEJM 358:568, 2008).
   C. Methodology: Use PCR and sequence-specific oligonucleotide probes.
      1. Available from Lab Corp: 800-533-1037 (approximately $165).
      2. Whole blood or 4 buccal swabs.

10. **Coreceptor Tropism Assays**
    A. HIV enters cells by attachment to CD4 receptor and then binding to either CCR5 or CXCR4 molecules.
    B. CCR5 inhibitor drugs (maraviroc, vicriviroc) bind to CCR5 & prevent viral entry.
    C. **Perform coreceptor tropism assay before prescribing a CCR5 inhibitor drug.**
    D. Co-receptor assays are phenotypic: Tropism assays use lab generated pseudovirus that expresses gp120 & gp41.
       1. Trofile assay, Monogram Biosciences, San Francisco, 800-777-0177 **(Expensive).**
       2. Trofile takes 2 weeks, need >1000 HIV RNA copies/mL.
       3. Trofile detects X4 and D/M minor variants with 100% sensitivity down to a frequency of 0.3%.
       4. Results reported as: R5 (CCR5 tropic), X4 (CXCR4 tropic) or D/M (dual mixed) or non-phenotypable/non-reportable (NP/NR).
       5. % positive for CCR5 receptor only: 50-85% in various studies, higher proportion in naive and earlier stage disease.

TABLE 4A: 1993 REVISED CDC HIV CLASSIFICATION SYSTEM & EXPANDED AIDS SURVEILLANCE DEFINITION FOR ADOLESCENTS & ADULTS
(MMWR 41:RR-17, Dec. 18, 1992)

The revised system emphasizes the importance of CD4 lymphocyte testing in clinical management of HIV infected persons. The system is based on 3 ranges of CD4 counts & 3 clinical categories giving a matrix of 9 exclusive categories. This system is less valuable in clinical decision making today because of availability of measures of viral RNA.

CRITERIA FOR HIV INFECTION: Persons 13 years or older with repeatedly (2 or more) reactive screening tests (ELISA) + specific antibodies identified by a supplemental test, e.g., Western blot ["reactive" pattern = + vs any two of p24, gp41, or gp120/160 (*MMWR 40:681, 1991*)]. Other specific methods of diagnosis of HIV-1 include virus isolation, antigen detection, & detection of HIV genetic material by PCR or branched DNA assay (bDNA).

CLASSIFICATION SYSTEM

CD4 Cell[§] Category	Clinical Category A	Clinical Category B	Clinical Category C
(1) ≥500/mm^3	A1	B1	C1
(2) 200-499/mm^3	A2	B2	C2
(3) <200/mm^3	A3	B3	C3

* See table for clinical definitions. Shaded area indicates expansion of AIDS surveillance definition. Cats. A3, B3 & C require reporting as AIDS.

§ There is a diurnal variation in CD4 counts averaging 60/mm^3 higher in the afternoon in HIV+ individuals. Blood for sequential CD4 counts should be drawn at about the same time of day each time (*J AIDS 3:144, 1990*). The equivalence between CD4 counts & CD4 % of total lymphocytes is ≥500 = ≥29%, 200-499 = 14-28%, <200 = <14%.

Clinical Categories

Clinical Category A	Clinical Category B	Clinical Category C
Asymptomatic HIV infection Persistent generalized lymphadenopathy (PGL)[1] Acute (primary) HIV illness	Symptomatic, not A or C conditions. Examples include but not limited to: Bacillary angiomatosis Candidiasis, vulvovaginal: persistent >1 month, poorly responsive to rx Candidiasis, oropharyngeal Cervical dysplasia, severe or carcinoma in situ Constitutional sx, e.g., fever **(38.5°) or diarrhea >1 month** The above must be attributed to HIV infection or have a clinical course or management complicated by HIV.	Candidiasis: esophageal, trachea, bronchi Coccidioidomycosis, extrapulmonary Cryptococcosis, extrapulmonary [†]Cervical cancer, invasive Cryptosporidiosis, chronic intestinal (>1 month) CMV retinitis, or CMV in other than liver, spleen, nodes HIV encephalopathy Herpes simplex with mucocutaneous ulcer >1 month, bronchitis, pneumonia Histoplasmosis: disseminated, extrapulmonary Isosporiasis, chronic, >1 month Kaposi's sarcoma Lymphoma: Burkitt's, immunoblastic, primary in brain M. avium or M. kansasii, extrapulmonary M. tuberculosis,[†] pulmonary or extrapulmonary Pneumocystis carinii pneumonia [†]Pneumonia, recurrent (≥2 episodes in 1 year) Progressive multifocal leukoencephalopathy Salmonella bacteremia, recurrent Toxoplasmosis, cerebral Wasting syndrome due to HIV

* These are the 1987 CDC case definitions contained in the 1987 definition (*MMWR 36:15, 1987*). The 1993 *CDC Expanded Surveillance Case Definition* includes all conditions contained in the 1987 definition (*above*) plus persons with documented HIV infection & any of the following: (1) CD4 T-lymphocyte count <200/mm^3 (or CD4 <14%), (2) pulmonary tuberculosis,[†] (3) recurrent pneumonia[†] (≥2 episodes within 1 year) or (4) invasive cervical carcinoma.[†] There are no CDC definitions utilizing viral load available to date.

---

[1] Nodes in 2 or more extrainguinal sites, at least 1cm in diameter for ≥3mos

TABLE 4B: "PERFORMANCE STATUS" (KARNOFSKY SCALE)/WHO CLINICAL STAGING SYSTEM

PERFORMANCE STATUS (Karnofsky Scale)			WHO CLINICAL STAGING SYSTEM	
Able to carry on normal activity; no special care is needed	100	Normal; no complaints; no evidence of disease	WHO Clinical Stage 1	No clinical symptoms May have persistent generalized lymphadenopathy (PGL) Performance scale 1 * Normal activity
	90	Able to carry on normal activity; minor signs or symptoms of disease		
Unable to work; able to live at home & care for most personal needs; a varying amount of assistance is needed	80	Normal activity with effort; some signs or symptoms of disease	WHO Clinical Stage 2	Weight loss <10% Minor skin rash Herpes zoster Recurrent upper respiratory infection Performance scale 2 * Symptomatic but normal activity
	70	Cares for self; unable to carry on normal activity or to do active work		
	60	Requires occasional assistance but is able to care for most needs		
	50	Requires considerable assistance & frequent medical care	WHO Clinical Stage 3	Weight loss >10% Chronic diarrhea >1 month Recurrent fevers >1 month Oral thrush Pulmonary tuberculosis Performance scale 3 * Bedridden <50% of the day during the last month
Unable to care for self; requires equivalent of institutional or hospital care; disease may be progressing rapidly	40	Disabled; requires special care & assistance		
	30	Severely disabled; hospitalization is indicated although death not imminent		
	20	Very sick; hospitalization necessary; active supportive treatment necessary	WHO Clinical Stage 4	Cryptococcal meningitis Toxoplasmosis of the brain Kaposi sarcoma Dementia Performance scale 4 * Bedridden >50% of the day during the last month
	10	Moribund; fatal processes progressing rapidly		
	0	Dead		

NOTE that patients may move from a later stage to an earlier stage if the presenting opportunistic infection is treated.

See *HIV Infection*, Ed. E. Katabira, M.R. Kamya, F.X. Mubiru, N.N. Bakyaita. Makevere Univ. Printery, 2000. 2nd Edition.

TABLE 5: RAPID ORAL TMP/SMX DESENSITIZATION

HOUR	DOSE TMP/SMX (mg)	HOUR	DOSE TMP/SMX (mg)	COMMENT
0	0.004/0.02	3	4/20	Perform in hospital or clinic. Use oral suspension [40 mg TMP/200 mg SMX/5 ml (tsp.)].
1	0.04/0.2	4	40/200	Take 6 oz. water after each dose. Corticosteroids, antihistamines NOT used.
2	0.4/2	5	160/830	Refs.: *CID* 20:849, 1995; *AIDS* 5:311, 1991

FIGURE 2: COURSE OF HIV INFECTION/DISEASE IN ADULTS, CLINICAL DECISION POINTS

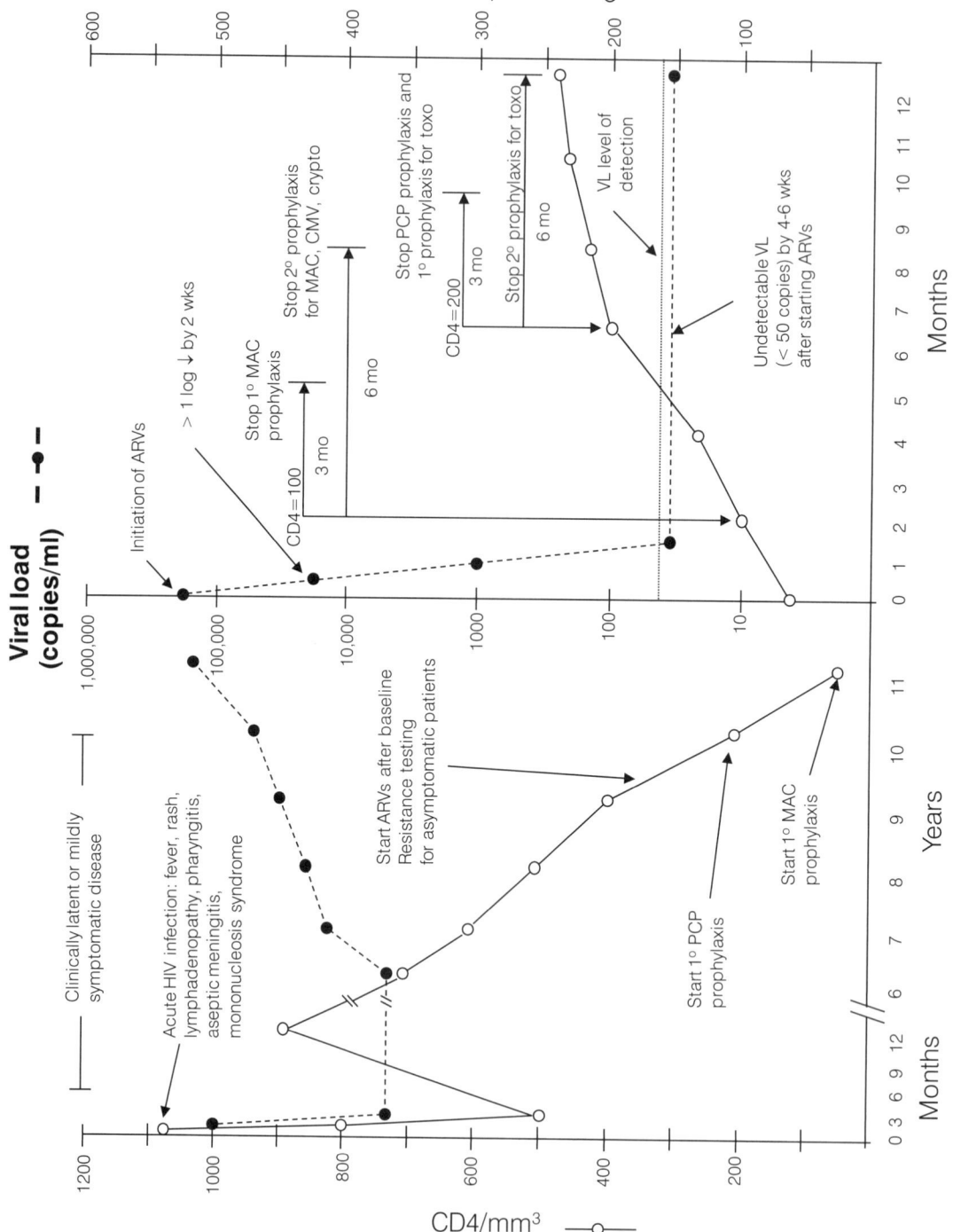

TABLE 6A: ANTIRETROVIRAL THERAPY (ART) IN TREATMENT-NAÏVE ADULTS

The U.S. Dept of Health & Human Svcs (DHHS) updated guidelines for treatment of adults and adolescents infected with HIV-1 in late 2007 and again in early 2008. These, as well as recommendations for anti-retroviral (ARV) therapy in pregnant women and in children, are available at www.adsinfo.nih.gov. These documents provide detailed recommendations and explanations, drug characteristics, and additional alternatives concerning the use of ARV therapy. The 2008 DHHS guidelines include significant changes from prior recommendations. These include: (1) recommendations to start therapy at CD4 <350 cells/mm³ for asymptomatic patients; (2) resistance testing for all treatment-naïve patients at initial care, even if ARV rx is to be deferred; (3) listing of abacavir + lamivudine as a preferred NRTI option for pts who test negative for HLA-B*5701. In addition, several previous alternative ARV choices are no longer recommended. Since the prior version of this guide additional ARVs have been approved: the first of 2 novel classes, a CCR5 co-receptor antagonist, and an integrase inhibitor, as well as a new NNRTI. Note **that immune reconstitution syndromes** (IRS or IRIS) may result from initiation of any ARV therapy, and may require medical intervention.

The following principles and concepts guide therapy:
- **The goal of rx is to inhibit maximally viral replication, allowing re-establishment & persistence of an effective immune response that will prevent or delay HIV-related morbidity.**
- **Fully undetectable levels of virus (<50 copies/ml) is the target of therapy for ALL patients, regardless of stage of disease or number / type of prior regimens.**
- **The lower the viral RNA can be driven, the lower the rate of accumulation of drug resistance mutations & the longer the therapeutic effect will last.**
- **To achieve maximal & durable suppression of viral RNA, combinations of potent antiretroviral agents are required, as is a high degree of adherence to the chosen regimens.**
- **Treatment regimens must be tailored to the individual as well as to the virus. Antiretroviral drug toxicities can compromise adherence in the short term & can cause significant negative health effects over time. Carefully check for specific risks to the individual, for interactions between the antiretrovirals selected & between those & concurrent drugs, & adjust doses as necessary for body weight, for renal or hepatic dysfunction, & for possible pharmacokinetic interactions.**

A. **When to start therapy?** (www.aidsinfo.nih.gov)

HIV Symptoms	CD4 cells/μl	Start Treatment	Comment
Yes	Any	Yes	New recommendation
No	<350	Yes	
No	>350	Not generally*	*Some pts may benefit from rx at CD4 ≥350 (see *discussion in www.aidsinfo.nih.gov*). Treatment is indicated for any patient with Hepatitis B Co-infection, HIV associated renal disease, and pregnant women. Whether there is long-term immunological benefit of starting ART at CD4>350 is a topic of investigation (*CID 44:441, 2007*). DHHS also recommends ARV rx irrespective of CD4 count for (1) pregnant women, (2) pts with HIV-associated nephropathy, and (3) pts requiring rx of HepB (ie, if any agent used for HBV can select for HIV resistance, then a full HIV rx regimen should be employed).

B. **Acute HIV Infection.** The benefits of ARV treatment in acute HIV infection are uncertain, but may include improved immunological response to the virus and decreased potential for transmission. However, treatment also exposes the patient to risks of drug adverse events, and the optimal duration of rx is unknown. Therefore, treatment is considered optional and is best undertaken in a research setting. Optimal regimens in this setting have not yet been defined. An observational study of acute or early HIV-1 infection showed comparable results from either PI-based or NNRTI-based regimens (*CID 42:1024, 2006*), although some feel that the higher barrier to resistance of PIs might be advantageous (*JAMA 296:827, 2006*). **Perform resistance testing** to guide design of ARV regimen because of appreciable risks of acquisition of virus with resistance to one or more ARV. DHHS guidelines recommend that a PI-based regimen be used if rx is started before resistance test results are known. Perform genotypic resistance testing for later reference even if rx is deferred.

23

TABLE 6A (2)

C. **Approach to constructing ARV regimens for treatment naïve adults.** (From Guidelines for the Use of Antiretroviral Agents in HIV-1-Infected Adults and Adolescents at www.aidsinfo.nih.gov. See that document for explanations, qualifications and further alternatives.)

Design a regimen consisting of
[either an NNRTI *OR* a Protease Inhibitor] *PLUS* [a dual-NRTI component]

- See Section D of Table 6A for specific regimens and tables which follow for drug characteristics, usual doses, adverse effects and additional details
- Selection of components will be influenced by many factors, such as
  - Co-morbidities (e.g., lipid effects of PIs, liver or renal disease, etc)
  - Pregnancy (e.g., avoid efavirenz, particularly in the first trimester when the neural tube is forming —pregnancy class D)
  - HIV status (e.g., avoid nevirapine in women with CD4 >250)
  - Results of viral resistance testing (recommended for all patients prior to initiation of ARV therapy)
  - Potential drug interactions or adverse drug effects; special focus on tolerability (even low grade side effects can profoundly effect adherence)
  - Convenience of dosing

Co-formulations increase convenience, but sometimes prescribing the two constituents individually is preferred, as when dose-adjustments are needed for renal disease.

Preferred components by class

NNRTI	Protease Inhibitor (alphabetical order)	Dual-NRTI (alphabetical order)
Efavirenz	Atazanavir + ritonavir or Fosamprenavir + ritonavir (twice-daily regimen) or Lopinavir/ritonavir (co-formulated, twice-daily regimen)	Abacavir/Lamivudine (for patients who test negative for HLA-B5701 or Tenofovir/ Emtricitabine (co-formulated)

Alternative components by class

NNRTI	Protease Inhibitor (alphabetical order)	Dual-NRTI (order of preference)
Nevirapine	Atazanavir or Fosamprenavir or Fosamprenavir + ritonavir (once-daily regimen) or Lopinavir/ritonavir (co-formulated, once-daily regimen) or Saquinavir/ritonavir	Zidovudine/ Lamivudine (co-formulated) or (less preferred alternative) Didanosine + (emtricitabine or lamivudine)

TABLE 6A (3)

D. **Examples of Initial Treatment Regimens that might be used for Untreated Chronic HIV-1 Infection based on DHHS agent grouping.** Doses & use assume normal renal & hepatic function unless otherwise stated. See *additional comments, Section G. (For pregnancy, Section D.4 below & Table 8B; for additional explanation & alternatives, see www.aidsinfo.nih.gov)*

1. **Regimens Employing "Preferred" Components** *(note: additional options exist; see www.aidsinfo.nih.gov)*

	Regimen	Pill strength (mg)	Usual Daily Regimen (oral)	No. pills/day	Comment (See also *individual agents & Table 6B*)
a.	(Tenofovir + Emtricitabine) + Efavirenz	(300 + 200) + 600	(Combination—Truvada 1 tab q24h) + 1 tab q24h at bedtime, empty stomach	2	At 48-wks of ongoing trial, superior virus suppression, higher CD4 & fewer AEs of tenofovir/ emtricitabine/ efavirenz as compared to ZDV/3TC/efavirenz (*NEJM 354:251, 2006*). Tenofovir: reports of renal toxicity (*CID 42:283, 2006*). **Renal function MUST be evaluated prior to dosing with tenofovir; if est. CrCl < 50 ml/min, tenofovir should be dosed every other day;** cannot use Atripla in that setting. Avoid efavirenz in pregnancy or in women who might become pregnant **(Pregnancy Category D).** Food may ↑ serum efavirenz concentration, which can lead to ↑ adverse events. See Section F.2 re how to stop efavirenz. Dosing efavirenz at night minimizes side effects (dysphoria; may have 'weird dreams' or nightmares)
	OR as a single tablet (Tenofovir + Emtricitabine + Efavirenz)		Combination—Atripla 1 tab q24h at bedtime, empty stomach	1	
b.	(Abacavir + Lamivudine) + Efavirenz	(600 + 300) + 600	(Combination-Epzicom 1 tab q24h) without regard to food + 1 tab q24h at bedtime, empty stomach	2	Low pill burden. **Risk of abacavir hypersensitivity reaction;** obtain HLA-B*5701 testing before use *(see Comment Table 6B).* Comparison of abacavir/lamivudine with tenofovir/emtricitabine as backbone in rx-naive pts under study; *see Table 6A, Section F* regarding possible limitations of ABC/3TC. Avoid efavirenz in pregnancy or in women who might become pregnant **(Pregnancy Category D).** Food may ↑ serum efavirenz concentration, which can lead to ↑ adverse events.
c.	(Tenofovir + Emtricitabine) + Lopinavir/ Ritonavir	(300 + 200) + 200/50	(Combination—Truvada 1 tab q24h) + (Combination—Kaletra 2 tabs bid) without regard to food	5	Tenofovir: reports of renal toxicity (*CID 42:283, 2006*). One study found ↓ renal function decline at 48-wk in pts receiving TDF with a PI (mostly lopinavir/ritonavir) than an NNRTI (*JID 197:102, 2008*). Preferred regimens use lopinavir/ritonavir twice daily. As an alternative regimen, lopinavir/ritonavir can be given as 4 tabs once daily in rx-naïve pts. Lop/Rit inferior to EFV based regimen ACTG5142 (*NEJM 358:2095, 2008*).
d.	(Tenofovir + Emtricitabine) + Atazanavir + Ritonavir	(300 + 200) + 300 + 100	(Combination—Truvada 1 tab q24h) + 1 cap q24h + 1 cap q24h both with food	3	Tenofovir: reports of renal toxicity (*CID 42:283, 2006*). *See comment re TDF+PI in section above.* Atazanavir ↑ tenofovir exposure; watch for adverse effects. Do not use unboosted atazanavir with TDF. Atazanavir may ↑ EKG PR interval & bilirubin. Acid-lowering agents can markedly ↓ absorption; avoid unboosted atazanavir with PPIs or H₂ blockers OK; boosted atazanavir may be used under some circumstances (*see Section F.3 of this table*).
e.	(Abacavir + Lamivudine) + Lopinavir/ Ritonavir	(600 + 300) + 200/50	(Combination-Epzicom 1 tab q24h) without regard to food + (Combination—Kaletra 2 tabs bid) without regard to food	5	**Risk of abacavir hypersensitivity reaction;** obtain HLA-B*5701 testing before use *(see Comment Table 6B).* See *Table 6A, Section F,* regarding possible limitations of ABC/3TC. Preferred regimens use lopinavir/ritonavir twice daily. As an alternative regimen, lopinavir/ritonavir can be given as 4 tabs once daily in rx-naïve pts.
f.	(Abacavir + Lamivudine) + Fosamprenavir + Ritonavir	(600 + 300) + 700 + 100	(Combination-Epzicom 1 tab q24h) without regard to food + 1 tab bid fed or fasting + 1 cap bid fed or fasting	5	**Risk of abacavir hypersensitivity reaction;** obtain HLA-B*5701 testing before use *(see Comment Table 6B). See Table 6A, Section F,* regarding possible limitations of ABC. Fosamprenavir contains sulfa moiety. Alternative fosamprenavir regimens available for rx-naïve pts, including fosamprenavir without ritonavir & once-daily fosamprenavir/ritonavir *(see label for use & doses)*.

TABLE 6A (4)

2. **Regimens Employing "Alternative" Components** (For additional alternatives, see Comments sections below, Table 6C., and www.aidsinfo.nih.gov)

	Regimen	Pill strength (mg)	Usual Daily Regimen (oral)	No. pills/day	Comment (See also individual agents & Table 6B)
a.	(Zidovudine + Lamivudine) + Efavirenz	(300 + 150) + 600	(Combination—Combivir 1 tab bid) + 1 tab q24h at bedtime, empty stomach	3	Good efficacy; low pill burden. Avoid efavirenz in pregnancy or in women who might become pregnant **(Pregnancy Category D)**. Food may ↑ serum efavirenz concentration, which can lead to ↑ adverse events. See Section F.2 re how to stop efavirenz.
b.	(Zidovudine + Lamivudine) + Lopinavir/ Ritonavir	(300 + 150) + 200/50	(Combination—Combivir 1 tab bid) + (Combination—Kaletra 2 tabs bid) without regard to food	6	Good virologic efficacy & durable effect. Tolerable AEs. *Preferred regimen* is to use lopinavir/ritonavir twice daily. As an alternative regimen, lopinavir/ritonavir can be given as 4 tabs once daily in rx-naïve pts.
c.	(Zidovudine + Lamivudine) + Atazanavir + Ritonavir	(300 + 150) + 300 + 100	(Combination—Combivir 1 tab bid) + 1 cap q24h + 1 cap q24h both with food	4	As an alternative regimen, atazanavir can be used without ritonavir, at a dose of 400 mg q24h with food, in combination therapy for Rx-naïve patients. Lower potential for lipid derangement by (unboosted) atazanavir than w/other PIs. May ↑ EKG PR interval & bilirubin. Acid-lowering agents can markedly ↓ absorption; avoid unboosted atazanavir with PPIs or H_2 blockers; boosted atazanavir OK in some circumstances (see Section F of this table).
d.	(Zidovudine + Lamivudine) + Fosamprenavir + Ritonavir	(300 + 150) + 700 + 100	(Combination—Combivir 1 tab bid) + 1 tab bid fed or fasting + 1 cap bid fed or fasting	6	Can take without regard to meals. Skin rash, GI symptoms. Fosamprenavir contains sulfa moiety. Alternative fosamprenavir regimens available for rx-naïve pts, including fosamprenavir without ritonavir & once-daily fosamprenavir/ritonavir regimens (see label for use & doses).
e.	Didanosine EC + Lamivudine + Efavirenz	400 + 300 + 600	1 cap q24h at bedtime, fasting + 1 tab q24h + 1 tab q24h at bedtime, empty stomach **Didanosine dosage shown for ≥60 kg**	3	Low pill burden. Potential didanosine AEs (pancreatitis, peripheral neuropathy). Avoid efavirenz in pregnancy or in women who might become pregnant **(Pregnancy Category D)**. Food may ↑ serum efavirenz concentration, which can lead to ↑ adverse events. Can substitute emtricitabine 200 mg po q24h for lamivudine 300 mg po q24h.
f.	[(Zidovudine + Lamivudine) or (Tenofovir + Emtracitabine)] + Saquinavir + Ritonavir	(300 + 150) or (300 + 200) + 500 + 100	(Combination—Combivir 1 tab bid) (Combination—Truvada 1 tab qd) + 2 tabs bid + 1 capsule bid	8 or 7	Use saquinavir only with ritonavir. Watch for drug interactions with CYP3A4 metabolized drugs

TABLE 6A (5)

3. **Triple nucleoside regimen:** Due to inferior virologic activity, use only when preferred or alternative regimen not possible. Seek expert advice about alternatives.

	Regimen	Pill strength (mg)	Usual Daily Regimen (oral)	No. pills/day	Comment (See also *individual agents & Table 6B*)
a.	(Zidovudine + Lamivudine + Abacavir)	(300 + 150 + 300)	(**Combination-Trizivir** 1 tab bid)	2	Reduced activity as compared with preferred or alternative regimens. Potentially serious abacavir AEs (*see comments for individual agents*).

4. **During pregnancy. Expert consultation mandatory.** Timing of rx initiation & drug choice must be individualized. Viral resistance testing should be strongly considered. Long-term effects of agents unknown. Certain drugs hazardous or contraindicated. (*See Table 17*). For additional information & alternative options, see www.aidsinfo.nih.gov. For regimens to prevent perinatal transmission, see *Table 8A*. See *JID 193:1191, 2006* re pre-term delivery with PIs.

	Regimen	Pill strength (mg)	Usual Daily Regimen (oral)	No. pills/day	Comment
a.	(Zidovudine + Lamivudine) + Nevirapine	(300 + 150) + 200	(Combination-Combivir 1 tab bid) + 1 tab bid fed or fasting [after 14-day lead-in period of 1 tab q24h]	4	See especially nevirapine **Black Box warnings**—among others ↑ risk of **potentially fatal hepatotoxicity** in women with CD4 >250 and men with CD4 count >400. Avoid in this group unless benefits clearly > risks; monitor intensively if drug must be used.
b.	(Zidovudine + Lamivudine) + Lopinavir/ritonavir	(300 + 150) + 200/50	(Comination—Combivir 1 tab bid) + 2 tabs bid without regard to food	6	*Optimal dose in 3rd trimester unknown. May need to monitor levels as ↑ dose may be required. Once-daily dosing of lopinavir/ritonavir not recommended.*
c.	(Zidovudine + Lamivudine) + Nelfinavir	(300 + 150) + 625	(Combination-Combivir 1 tab bid) + 2 tabs bid with food	6	Nelfinavir-associated diarrhea in 20%. Contraindicated with drugs highly dependent on CYP3A4 elimination where ↑ levels may cause life-threatening toxicity. Time to loss of virological response shorter than for lopinavir/ritonavir (studied in non-pregnant pts)(*NEJM 346:2039, 2002*).

E. Antiretroviral Therapies That Should NOT Be Offered *(Modified from www.aidsinfo.nih.gov)*

TABLE 6A (6)

1. Regimens not recommended

	Regimen	Logic	Exception
a.	Monotherapy with NRTI	Rapid development of resistance & inferior antiviral activity	Perhaps ZDV to reduce peripartum mother-to-child transmission. See *Perinatal Guidelines* at www.aidsinfo.nih.gov and Table 8B
b.	Dual NRTI combinations	Resistance and Inferior antiretroviral activity compared with standard drug combinations	Perhaps ZDV to reduce peripartum mother-to-child transmission. See *Perinatal Guidelines* at www.aidsinfo.nih.gov and Table 8B
c.	Triple NRTI combinations	Triple-NRTI regimens have shown inferior virologic efficacy in clinical trials: (tenofovir + lamivudine + abacavir) & (didanosine + lamivudine + tenofovir) & others	(Zidovudine + lamivudine + abacavir) or (zidovudine + lamivudine + tenofovir) might be used if no alternative exists.

2. Drug, or drugs, not recommended as part of antiretroviral regimen

	Regimen	Logic	Exception
a.	Saquinavir hard gel cap or tab (Invirase) as single (unboosted) PI	Bioavailability only 4%; inferior antiretroviral activity	No exceptions
b.	Stavudine + didanosine	High frequency of toxicity: peripheral neuropathy, pancreatitis & mitochondrial toxicity (lactic acidosis). In pregnancy: lactic acid acidosis, hepatic steatosis, ± pancreatitis	Toxicity partially offset by potent antiretroviral activity of the combination. Use only when potential benefits outweigh the sizeable risks.
c.	Efavirenz in pregnancy or in women who might become pregnant	Teratogenic in non-human primates. **Pregnancy Category D—may cause fetal harm**	Only if no other option available; major risk would be 1st trimester. Note that oral contraceptives alone may not be reliable for prevention of pregnancy in women on ART or other medications (see *Safety & Toxicity of Individual Agents in Pregnancy* at www.aidsinfo.nih.gov).
d.	Stavudine + zidovudine	Antagonistic	No exceptions
e.	Atazanavir + indinavir	Additive risk of hyperbilirubinemia	No exceptions
f.	Emtricitabine + lamivudine	Same target and resistance profile	No exceptions
g.	Abacavir + tenofovir	Rapid development of K65R mutation; loss of effect	Can avoid if zidovudine also used in the regimen; might be an option for salvage therapy but not earlier lines of therapy.
h.	Tenofovir + didanosine	Reduced CD4 cell count increase; concern of K 65R development	Use with caution

F. **Selected Characteristics of Antiretroviral Drugs**

1. **Selected Characteristics of Nucleoside or Nucleotide Reverse Transcriptase Inhibitors (NRTIs)**
   All agents have Black Box warning: Risk of lactic acidosis/hepatic steatosis. Also, labels note risk of fat redistribution/accumulation with ARV therapy. For combinations, see warnings for component agents.

TABLE 6A (7)

Generic/Trade Name	Pharmaceutical Prep.	Usual Adult Dosage & Food Effect	% Absorbed, po	Serum T½, hrs	Intracellular T½, hrs	Elimination	Major Adverse Events/Comments (See Table 6B)
Abacavir (ABC; Ziagen)	300 mg tabs or 20 mg/ml oral solution	300 mg po bid or 600 mg po q24h. Food OK	83	1.5	20	Liver metab., renal excretion of metabolites, 82%	**Hypersensitivity reaction:** fever, rash, N/V, malaise, diarrhea, abdominal pain, respiratory symptoms. (Severe reactions may be ↑ with 600 mg dose.) **Do not rechallenge!** Report to 800-270-0425. **Test HLA-B*5701 before use. See Comment Table 6B.** Study raises concerns re ABC/3TC regimens in pts with VL ≥ 100,000 (www3.niaid.nih.gov/news/newsreleases/2008/actg5202bulletin.htm). Recent report suggests possible ↑ risk of cardiac event in pts with other cardiac risk factors (*2008 CROI, abstr. 957c*).
Abacavir/lamivudine/ zidovudine (Trizivir)	Film-coated tabs: ABC 300 mg + 3TC 150 mg + ZDV 300 mg	1 tab po bid (not recommended for wt <40 kg or CrCl <50 mL/min or impaired hepatic function)	(See individual components)				(See *Comments for individual components*) Note: **Black Box warnings** for ABC hypersensitivity reaction & others. Should only be used for regimens intended to include these 3 agents. Black Box warning— limited data for VL >100,000 copies/mL. Not recommended as initial therapy because of inferior virologic efficacy.
Didanosine (ddI; Videx or Videx EC)	125, 200, 250, 400 enteric-coated caps; 100, 167, 250mg powder for oral solution;	≥60kg: Usually 400mg enteric-coated po q24h 0.5 hr before or 2hrs after meal. Do not crush. <60 kg: 250 mg EC po q24h. Food ↓ levels. See *Comment*	30–40	1.6	25–40	Renal excretion, 50%	**Pancreatitis,** peripheral neuropathy, lactic acidosis & hepatic steatosis (rare but life-threatening, esp. combined with stavudine in pregnancy). Retinal, optic nerve changes. **The combination ddI + TDF is generally avoided, but if used,** reduce dose of ddI-EC from 400mg to 250mg EC q24h (or from 250mg EC to 200mg EC for adults <60kg). **Monitor for ↑ toxicity & possible ↓ in efficacy of this combination; may result in ↓ CD4.**

29

TABLE 6A (8)

Generic/Trade Name	Pharmaceutical Prep.	Usual Adult Dosage & Food Effect	% Absorbed, po	Serum T½, hrs	Intracellular T½, hrs	Elimination	Major Adverse Events/Comments (See Table 6B)
Emtricitabine (FTC, Emtriva)	200 mg caps; 10 mg per mL oral solution.	200 mg po q24h. Food OK	93 (caps), 75 (oral sol'n)	Approx. 10	39	Renal excretion 86%, minor biotransformation, 14% excretion in feces	Well tolerated; headache, nausea, vomiting & diarrhea occasionally, skin rash rarely. Skin hyperpigmentation. Differs only slightly in structure from lamivudine (5-fluoro substitution). **Exacerbation of Hep B reported in pts after stopping FTC.** Monitor at least several months after stopping FTC in Hep B pts; some may need anti-HBV therapy.
Emtricitabine/tenofovir disoproxil fumarate (Truvada)	Film-coated tabs: FTC 200 mg + TDF 300 mg	1 tab po q24h for CrCl ≥50 ml/min. Food OK	92/25	10/17	—	Primarily renal/renal	See *Comments for individual agents* **Black Box warning—Exacerbation of HepB after stopping FTC;** but preferred therapy for those with Hep B.
Emtricitabine/tenofovir/efavirenz (Atripla)	Film-coated tabs: FTC 200 mg + TDF 300 mg + efavirenz 600 mg	1 tab po q24h on an empty stomach, preferably at bedtime. Do not use if CrCl <50 ml/min	(See individual components)					Not recommended for pts <18yrs. (See warnings for individual components). **Exacerbation of Hep B** reported in pts discontinuing component drugs; some may need anti-HBV therapy (preferred anti-Hep B therapy). **Pregnancy category D**- may cause fetal harm. Avoid in pregnancy or in women who may become pregnant.
Lamivudine (3TC; Epivir)	150, 300 mg tabs; 10 mg/ml oral solution	150 mg po bid or 300 mg po q24h. Food OK	86	5–7	18	Renal excretion, minimal metabolism	**Use HIV dose, not Hep B dose.** Usually well-tolerated. **Risk of exacerbation of Hep B after stopping 3TC.** Monitor at least several months after stopping 3TC in Hep B pts; some may need anti-HBV therapy.
Lamivudine/abacavir (Epzicom)	Film-coated tabs: 3TC 300 mg + abacavir 600 mg	1 tab po q24h. Food OK Not recommended for CrCl <50 ml/min or impaired hepatic function	86/86	5–7/1.5	16/20	Primarily renal/metabolism	See *Comments for individual agents.* **Note abacavir hypersensitivity Black Box warnings** (severe reactions may be somewhat more frequent with 600 mg dose) and 3TC Hep B warnings. Test HLA-B*5701 before use.
Lamivudine/zidovudine (Combivir)	Film-coated tabs: 3TC 150 mg + ZDV 300 mg	1 tab po bid. Not recommended for CrCl <50 ml/min or impaired hepatic function Food OK	86/64	5–7/0.5–3	—	Primarily renal/metabolism with renal excretion of glucuronide	See *Comments for individual agents.* See **Black Box warning**—exacerbation of Hep B in pts stopping 3TC

TABLE 6A (9)

Generic/Trade Name	Pharmaceutical Prep.	Usual Adult Dosage & Food Effect	% Absorbed, po	Serum T½, hrs	Intracellular T½, hrs	Elimination	Major Adverse Events/Comments (See Table 6B)
Stavudine (d4T; Zerit)	15, 20, 30, 40 mg capsules; 1 mg per mL oral solution	≥60 kg: 40 mg po bid <60 kg: 30 mg po bid Food OK	86	1.2–1.6	3.5	Renal excretion, 40%	Not recommended by DHHS as initial therapy because of adverse reactions. **Highest incidence of lipoatrophy, hyperlipidemia, & lactic acidosis of all NRTIs.** Pancreatitis. Peripheral neuropathy. (See *didanosine comments*.)
Tenofovir disoproxil fumarate (TDF; Viread)—a nucleotide	300 mg tabs	CrCl ≥50 ml/min: 300 mg po q24h. Food OK; high-fat meal ↑ absorption	39 (with food) 25 (fasted)	17	>60	Renal excretion	Headache, N/V. **Cases of renal dysfunction reported:** avoid concomitant nephrotoxic agents. One study found ↑ renal function at 48-wk in pts receiving TDF with a PI (mostly lopinavir/ritonavir) than with a NNRTI (*JID* 197:102, 2008). Must adjust dose of ddI (↓) if used concomitantly but best to avoid this combination (see *ddI Comments*). Atazanavir & lopinavir/ritonavir ↑ tenofovir concentrations: monitor for adverse effects. **Black Box warning—exacerbations of Hep B reported after stopping tenofovir.** Monitor several months after stopping TDF in Hep B pts; some may need anti-HBV Rx.
Zidovudine (ZDV, AZT; Retrovir)	100 mg caps, 300 mg tabs; 10 mg per mL IV solution; 10 mg/mL oral syrup	300 mg po q12h. Food OK	64	1.1	11	Metabolized to glucuronide & excreted in urine	Bone marrow suppression, GI intolerance, headache, insomnia, malaise, myopathy.

2. **Selected Characteristics of Non-Nucleoside Reverse Transcriptase Inhibitors (NNRTIs)**

Generic/Trade Name	Pharmaceutical Prep.	Usual Adult Dosage & Food Effect	% Absorbed, po	Serum T½, hrs	Elimination	Major Adverse Events/Comments
Delavirdine (Rescriptor)	100, 200 mg tabs	400 mg po three times daily. Food OK	85	5.8	Cytochrome P450 (3A inhibitor). 51% excreted in urine (<5% unchanged), 44% in feces	Rash severe enough to stop drug in 4.3%. ↑ AST/ALT, headaches. **Use of this agent is not recommended.**

TABLE 6A (10)

Generic/Trade Name	Pharmaceutical Prep.	Usual Adult Dosage & Food Effect	% Absorbed, po	Serum T½, hrs	Elimination	Major Adverse Events/Comments
Efavirenz (Sustiva) **(Pregnancy Category D)**	50, 100, 200 mg capsules; 600 mg tablet	600 mg po q24h at bedtime, without food. Food may ↑ serum conc., which can lead to ↑ in risk of adverse events.	42	40–55 See *Comment*	Cytochrome P450 2B6 (3A mixed inducer/ inhibitor). 14–34% of dose excreted in urine as glucuronidated metabolites, 16–61% in feces	Rash severe enough to dc use of drug in 1.7%. High frequency of diverse CNS AEs: somnolence, dreams, confusion, agitation. Serious psychiatric symptoms. Certain CYP2B6 polymorphisms may predict exceptionally high plasma levels with standard doses (*CID 45:1230, 2007*). False-pos. cannabinoid screen. **Pregnancy Category D—may cause fetal harm—avoid in pregnant women or those who might become pregnant.** (Note: No single method of contraception is 100% reliable). Very long tissue T½. **If rx to be discontinued, stop efavirenz 1–2 wks before stopping companion drugs.** Otherwise, risk of developing efavirenz resistance, as after 1–2 days only efavirenz in blood &/or tissue. Some authorities bridge this gap by adding a PI to the NRTI backbone if feasible after efavirenz is discontinued. (*CID 42:401, 2006*)
Etravirine (Intelence)	100 mg tabs	200 mg twice daily after a meal	Unknown (↓ systemic exposure if taken fasting)	41	Metabolized by CYP 3A4 (inducer) & 2C9, 2C19 (inhibitor). Excreted into feces (> 90%), mostly unchanged drug.	For pts with HIV-1 resistant to NNRTIs & others. Active in vitro against most such isolates. Rash common, but rarely can be severe. Potential for multiple drug interactions. Generally, multiple mutations are required for high-level resistance (*JAC 2008: advanced access, June 19*). Because of interactions, do not use with boosted atazanavir, boosted tipranavir, unboosted PIs, or other NNRTIs.
Nevirapine (Viramune)	200 mg tabs; 50 mg per 5 mL oral suspension	200 mg po q24h x14 days & then 200 mg po bid (see *Comments* & ***Black Box warning***) Food OK	>90	25–30	Cytochrome P450 (3A4, 2B6) inducer; 80% of dose excreted in urine as glucuronidated metabolites, 10% in feces	**Black Box warning—fatal hepatotoxicity.** Women with CD4 >250 esp. vulnerable, inc. pregnant women. Avoid in this group unless benefits clearly > risks (www.fda.gov/ cder drug/advisory/nevirapine.htm). If used, intensive monitoring required. Men with CD4 >400 also at ↑ risk. Rash severe enough to stop drug in 7%, **severe or life-threatening skin reactions** in 2%. Do not restart if any suspicion of such reactions. 2wk dose escalation period may ↓ skin reactions. As with efavirenz, because of long T½, consider continuing companion agents for several days if nevirapine is discontinued.

TABLE 6A (11)

3. **Selected Characteristics of Protease Inhibitors (PIs).**

All PIs: Glucose metabolism: new diabetes mellitus or deterioration of glucose control; fat redistribution; possible hemophilia bleeding; hypertriglyceridemia or hypercholesterolemia. Exercise caution re: potential drug interactions & contraindications. QTc prolongation has been reported in a few pts taking PIs; some PIs can block HERG channels in vitro (*Lancet* 365:682, 2005)

Generic/Trade Name	Pharmaceutical Prep.	Usual Adult Dosage & Food Effect	% Absorbed, po	Serum T½, hrs	Elimination	Major Adverse Events/Comments (See *Table 6B*)
Atazanavir (Reyataz)	100, 150, 200, 300 mg capsules	400 mg po q24h with food. Ritonavir-boosted dose (atazanavir 300 mg po q24h + ritonavir 100 mg po q24h), with food, is recommended for ARV rx-experienced pts. The boosted dose is also used when combined with either efavirenz 600 mg po q24h or TDF 300 mg po q24h. If used with buffered ddI, take with food 2 hrs pre or 1 hr post ddI.	Good oral bioavailability; food enhances bioavailability & ↓ pharmacokinetic variability. Absorption ↓ by antacids, H₂-blockers, proton pump inhibitors. Avoid unboosted drug with PPIs/H2-blockers. Boosted drug can be used with or > 10hr after H2-blockers or > 12hr after a PPI, as long as limited doses of the acid agents are used (see 2008 drug label changes).	Approx. 7	Cytochrome P450 (3A4, 1A2 & 2C9 inhibitor) & UGT1A1 inhibitor; 13% excreted in urine (7% unchanged), 79% excreted in feces (20% unchanged)	Lower potential for ↑ lipids. . Asymptomatic unconjugated hyperbilirubinemia common;jaundice especially likely in Gilbert's syndrome (*JID* 192:1381, 2005). Pro- Headache, rash, GI symptoms. Prolongation of PR interval (1st degree AV block) reported. Caution in pre-existing conduction system disease. Efavirenz ↓ tenofovir ↓ atazanavir exposure: use atazanavir/ritonavir regimen; also, atazanavir ↑ tenofovir concentrations—watch for adverse events. In rx-experienced pts taking TDF and needing H2 blockers, atazanavir 400 mg with ritonavir 100 mg can be given; do not use PPIs. Rare reports of renal stones
Darunavir (Prezista)	300 mg, 600 mg tablets	[600 mg darunavir + 100 mg ritonavir] po bid, with food	82% absorbed (taken with ritonavir). Food ↑ absorption.	Approx 15 hr (with ritonavir)	Metabolized by CYP3A and is a CYP3A inhibitor	Contains sulfa moiety. Rash, nausea, headaches seen. Coadmin of certain drugs cleared by CYP3A is contraindicated (*see label*). Use with caution in pts with hepatic dysfunction. (Recent FDA warning about occasional hepatic dysfunction early in the course of treatment). Monitor carefully, esp. first several months and with pre-existing liver disease. May cause hormonal contraception failure.

TABLE 6A (12)

Generic/Trade Name	Pharmaceutical Prep.	Usual Adult Dosage & Food Effect	% Absorbed, po	Serum T½, hrs	Elimination	Major Adverse Events/Comments (See Table 6B)
Fosamprenavir (Lexiva)	700 mg tablet, 50 mg/ml oral suspension	1400 mg (two 700 mg tabs) po bid **OR** with ritonavir: [1400 mg fosamprenavir (2 tabs) + ritonavir 200 mg] po q24h **OR** [1400 mg fosamprenavir (2 tabs) + ritonavir 100 mg] po q24h **OR** [700 mg fosamprenavir (1 tab) + ritonavir 100 mg] po bid	Bioavailability not established. Food OK	7.7 Amprenavir	Hydrolyzed to amprenavir, then acts as cytochrome P450 (3A4 substrate, inhibitor, inducer)	Amprenavir prodrug. Contains sulfa moiety. Potential for serious drug interactions (see label). Rash, including Stevens-Johnson syndrome. Once daily regimens: (1) not recommended for PI-experienced pts, (2) additional ritonavir needed if given with efavirenz (see label). Boosted twice daily regimen is recommended for PI-experienced pts.
Indinavir (Crixivan)	100, 200, 400 mg capsules Store in original container with desiccant	Two 400 mg caps (800 mg) po q8h, without food or with light meal. Can take with enteric-coated Videx. [If taken with ritonavir (e.g., 800 mg indinavir + 100 mg ritonavir po q12h), no food restrictions]	65	1.2–2	Cytochrome P450 (3A4 inhibitor)	**Maintain hydration. Nephrolithiasis,** nausea, inconsequential ↑ of indirect bilirubin (jaundice in Gilbert syndrome), ↑ AST/ALT, headache, asthenia, blurred vision, metallic taste, hemolysis. ↑ urine WBC (>100/hpf) has been assoc. with nephritis/medullary calcification, cortical atrophy.
Lopinavir + ritonavir (Kaletra)	(200 mg lopinavir + 50 mg ritonavir), and (100 mg lopinavir + 25 mg ritonavir) tablets. Tabs do not need refrigeration. Oral solution: (80 mg lopinavir + 20 mg ritonavir) per mL. Refrigerate, but can be kept at room temperature (≤77°F) x2 mos.	(400 mg lopinavir + 100 mg ritonavir)—2 tabs po bid. Higher dose may be needed in non-rx-naive pts when used with efavirenz, nevirapine, or unboosted fosamprenavir. [Dose adjustment in concomitant drugs may be necessary; see Table 16B & Table 16C]	No food effect with tablets.	5–6	Cytochrome P450 (3A4 inhibitor)	Nausea/vomiting/diarrhea (worse when administered with zidovudine), ↑ AST/ALT, pancreatitis. Oral solution 42% alcohol. Lopinavir + ritonavir can be taken as a single daily dose of 4 tabs (total 800 mg lopinavir + 200 mg ritonavir), except in treatment-experienced pts or those taking concomitant efavirenz, nevirapine, amprenavir, or nelfinavir.
Nelfinavir (Viracept)	625, 250 mg tabs; 50 mg/gm oral powder	Two 625 mg tabs (1250 mg) po bid, with food	20–80 Food ↑ exposure & ↓ variability	3.5–5	Cytochrome P450 (3A4 inhibitor)	Diarrhea. Not recommended in initial regimens because of inferior efficacy. Should not be used in patients with moderate or severe liver impairment. Coadministration of drugs which are highly dependent on CYP34A for clearance for which elevated plasma concentrations are associated with serious and/or life-threatening events is contraindicated.

TABLE 6A (13)

Generic/Trade Name	Pharmaceutical Prep.	Usual Adult Dosage & Food Effect	% Absorbed, po	Serum T½, hrs	Elimination	Major Adverse Events/Comments (See Table 6B)
Ritonavir (Norvir)	100 mg capsules; 600 mg per 7.5 mL solution. Refrigerate caps but not solution. Room temperature for 1 mo. is OK.	Full dose not recommended (see comments). **With rare exceptions, used exclusively to enhance pharmacokinetics of other PIs, using lower ritonavir doses.**	Food ↑ absorption	3–5	Cytochrome P450. Potent 3A4 & 2D6 inhibitor	Nausea/vomiting/diarrhea, extremity & circumoral paresthesias, hepatitis, pancreatitis, taste perversion, ↑ CPK & uric acid. **Black Box warning**— potentially fatal drug interactions. Many drug interactions—see Table 16A–Table 16C
Saquinavir (Invirase—hard gel caps or tabs) + **ritonavir**	Saquinavir 200 mg caps, 500 mg film-coated tabs; ritonavir 100 mg caps	[2 tabs saquinavir (1000 mg) + 1 cap ritonavir (100 mg)] po bid with food	Erratic, 4 (saquinavir alone)	1–2	Cytochrome P450 (3A4 inhibitor)	Nausea, diarrhea, headache, ↑ AST/ALT. Avoid rifampin with saquinavir + ritonavir: ↑ hepatitis risk. **Black Box warning**—Invirase to be used only with ritonavir.
Tipranavir (Aptivus)	250 mg caps. Refrigerate unopened bottles. Use opened bottles within 2 mo. 100 mg/mL solution	[500 mg (two 250 mg caps) + ritonavir 200 mg] po bid with food.	Absorption low, ↑ with high fat meal, ↓ with Al⁺⁺⁺ & Mg⁺⁺ antacids.	5.5–6	Cytochrome 3A4 but with ritonavir, most of drug is eliminated in feces.	Contains sulfa moiety. **Black Box warning—reports of fatal/nonfatal intracranial hemorrhage,hepatitis, fatal hepatic failure.** Use cautiously in liver disease, esp. hepB, hepC; contraindicated in Child-Pugh class B-C. Monitor LFTs. Coadministration of certain drugs contraindicated (see label). **For highly ART-experienced pts or for multiple-PI resistant virus.**

TABLE 6A (14)

4. Selected Characteristics of Fusion Inhibitors

Generic/Trade Name	Pharmaceutical Prep.	Usual Adult Dosage	% Absorbed	Serum T½, hrs	Elimination	Major Adverse Events/Comments (See Table 6B)
Enfuvirtide (T20, Fuzeon)	Single-use vials of 90 mg/mL when reconstituted. Vials should be stored at room temperature. Reconstituted vials can be refrigerated for 24 hrs only.	90 mg (1 ml) subcut. bid. Rotate injection sites, avoiding those currently inflamed.	84	3.8	Catabolism to its constituent amino acids with subsequent recycling of the amino acids in the body pool. Elimination pathway(s) have not been performed in humans. Does not alter the metabolism of CYP3A4, CYP2D6, CYP1A2, CYP2C19 or CYP2E1 substrates.	Local reaction site reactions 98%, 4% discontinue; erythema/induration ~80–90%, nodules/cysts ~80%. **Hypersensitivity reactions reported** (fever, rash, chills, N/V, ↓ BP, &/or ↑ AST/ALT)—do not restart if occur. Including background regimens, peripheral neuropathy 8.9%, insomnia 11.3%, ↓ appetite 6.3%, myalgia 5%, lymphadenopathy 2.3%, eosinophilia ~10%. ↑ incidence of bacterial pneumonias: Alone offers little benefit to a failing regimen (NEJM 348:2249, 2003).

5. Selected Characteristics of CCR-5 Co-receptor Antagonists

Generic/Trade Name	Pharmaceutical Prep.	Usual Adult Dosage	% Absorbed	Serum T½, hrs	Elimination	Major Adverse Events/Comments (See Table 6B)
Maraviroc (Selzentry)	150 mg, 300 mg film-coated tabs	Without regard to food: 150 mg bid if concomitant meds include CYP3A inhibitors including PIs (except tipranavir/ritonavir) and delavirdine (with/without CYP3A inducers) 300 mg bid without significantly interacting meds including NRTIs, tipranavir/ritonavir, nevirapine 600 mg bid if concomitant meds include CYP3A inducers, including efavirenz, (without strong CYP3A inhibitors)	Est. 33% with 300 mg dosage	14–18	CYP3A and P-glycoprotein substrate. Metabolites (via CYP3A) excreted feces > urine.	**Black Box Warning-Hepatotoxicity**, may be preceded by rash, ↑ eos or IgE. NB: no hepatotoxicity was noted in MVC trials. Black box inserted owing to concern about potential CCR5 class effect. Data lacking in hepatic/renal insufficiency; ↑concern with either could ↑ risk of ↓BP. Currently for treatment-experienced patients with multi-resistant strains. Document CCR-5-tropic virus before use, as treatment failures assoc. with appearance of CXCR-4 or mixed-tropic virus.

6. Selected Characteristics of Integrase Inhibitors

Generic/Trade Name	Pharmaceutical Prep.	Usual Adult Dosage	% Absorbed	Serum T½, hrs	Elimination	Major Adverse Events/Comments (See Table 6B)
Raltegravir (Isentress)	400 mg film-coated tabs	400 mg po bid, without regard to food	Unknown	~9	Glucuronidation via UGT1A1, with excretion into feces and urine. (Therefore does NOT require ritonavir boosting)	For treatment experienced pts with multiply-resistant virus. Generally well-tolerated. Nausea, diarrhea, headache, fever similar to placebo. CK↑ & rhabdomyolysis reported, with unclear relationship to drug.

TABLE 6A (15)

G. Other Considerations in Selection of Therapy
Caution: Initiation of ARV therapy may result in immune reconstitution syndrome with significant clinical consequences. *(AIDS Reader 16:199, 2006).*

1. Resistance testing: Given current rates of resistance, resistance testing is recommended in all patients prior to initiation of therapy, including those with acute infection syndrome (may initiate therapy while waiting for test results and adjusting Rx once results return), at time of change of therapy owing to antiretroviral failure, when suboptimal virologic response is observed, and in pregnant women. **Resistance testing NOT recommended if pt is off ARV therapy for > 4 weeks or if HIV RNA is < 1000 c/ml.**
2. Drug-induced disturbances of glucose & lipid metabolism *(see Table 6C)*
3. Drug-induced lactic acidosis & other FDA "box warnings" *(see Table 6C)*
4. Drug-drug interactions *(see Table 16A)*
5. Risk in pregnancy *(see Table 17)*
6. Use in women & children *(see Table 8A)*
7. Dosing in patients with renal or hepatic dysfunction *(see Table 15B)*
8. Other special populations *(see www.aidsinfo.nih.gov)*

   a. **Injection drug users.** Active drug use may compromise adherence. Potentially co-existing neuropsychiatric symptoms & ↑ prevalence of Hep B & C add to risk of drug toxicities. Drug interactions may potentially cause ↑ or ↓ blood levels of ART drugs, & of methadone or drugs of abuse *(Mt Sinai J Med 67:429, 2000; see Table 16A)*.

   b. **Co-infection with Hep B &/or C.** Co-infection with Hepatitis B is an indication for treatment of HIV. Lamivudine, emtricitabine & tenofovir are active against HBV *(CID 39:1062, 2004)*. Two active agents are recommended for the treatment of HIV in HBV co-infected patients. **Therefore the use of TDF/FTC or TDF/3TC are the nucleoside backbones of choice in HIV/HBV co-infected pts** because of concerns about emergence of HBV resistance should TDF be used without support of FTC or 3TC and vice versa. If uncertain how to treat, seek expert consultation.
   Severe hepatitis flare *(see Black Box warnings)* may occur in pts with chronic Hep B after stopping any of these 3 drugs used for HIV therapy. In HCV/HIV co-infected pts, ↑ rate of progression to cirrhosis. Proper sequencing of rx for HIV/HCV important to avoid ↑ toxicities *(see Table 12, pg 152–156)*.
   Some experts find that an NRTI backbone of [tenofovir + (emtricitabine or lamivudine)] is better tolerated in this population than one of [zidovudine + lamivudine], whether used with a PI- or NNRTI-based regimen. It is suggested that PI-based rx may slow fibrosis progression, while nevirapine may ↑ fibrosis *(JAC 55:417, 2005)*. Changes in ART drug elimination with hepatic dysfunction may necessitate dosing changes *(CID 40:174, 2005; see Table 15B)*. Therapeutic drug monitoring should be considered when there is significant liver dysfunction.

   c. **Adolescents:** Adult guidelines for ARV use are generally appropriate for post-pubertal adolescents. Dosage should be prescribed according to Tanner staging of puberty and not on the basis of age. If Tanner Stage I and II, dose according to Pediatric dosing recommendations; if late puberty Tanner V, dose according to Adult dosing recommendations. Youth in a growth spurt should continue with pediatric dosing initially. Adherence to medication is particularly challenging in adolescent populations and need to be managed carefully. Efavirenz should be used with caution among female adolescents owing to potential teratogenicity concerns.

H. Response to Antiviral Therapy

1. **Adequate response to antiviral therapy: Continue current regimen**
   a. 0.5–0.75 log$_{10}$ ↓ in plasma HIV RNA by 4 weeks but generally effective rx ↓ VL by >1 log (90% or 10-fold ↓) within 2 weeks
   b. Undetectable levels by 4–6 months
   c. A sustained ↑ in CD4 counts: counts typically ↑ ≥50 cells/ml at 4 to 8 weeks after rx initiated or changed followed by 50–100 cells/ml per year thereafter

2. **Virologic/clinical failure to antiretroviral therapy: Confirm adherence. If OK, suspect resistance. Check susceptibility & change current regimen.**
   a. <0.5–0.75 log$_{10}$ ↓ in plasma HIV RNA by 4 weeks
   b. <1 log$_{10}$ ↓ in plasma HIV RNA by 8 weeks
   c. Failure to suppress plasma HIV RNA to below 400 copies/ml by 24 weeks or 50 copies/ml by 48 weeks
   d. Repeated detection of significant level of virus in plasma after initial suppression to undetectable levels, suggesting the development of resistance
   e. Persistent decline in CD4 counts, as measured on at least 2 separate occasions
   f. Clinical deterioration or progression

I. Changing Treatment Regimens Due to Intolerance or Failure *(www.aidsinfo.nih.gov)*

1. For drug intolerance to a specific antiretroviral agent, it is acceptable to substitute a single alternative agent.
2. For failure to achieve complete viral suppression or with sustained reappearance of virus after initial suppression, goal is to re-establish suppression to preserve immunologic function & minimize accumulation of drug resistance. This is easiest in less antiretroviral-experienced patients & with early intervention.
3. Review history for potential impediments to maximal adherence. If adherence seems good & no other explanations, could consider therapeutic drug monitoring (PI or NNRTI trough concentrations) if any concerns about absorption (e.g., GI disease) or too-rapid elimination (e.g., from drug interactions)
4. Review history of antiretroviral use (for clue to archived mutant virus) & perform resistance testing (genotype &/or phenotype) while on failing regimen.
5. Possible approaches to treatment for pts who are not extensively treatment-experienced:
   a. Most aggressive approach for relatively treatment-inexperienced patients is switch from NNRTI-based regimen to PI-based regimen, or vice versa. Select new NRTIs from resistance testing results & history. Pts on PI-based regimen could also be switched to an alternative PI (with appropriate NRTIs) based on resistance testing.
   b. For patients with partial suppression (low-detectable viral loads), consider intensification of regimen with additional agents (e.g., tenofovir if not on a TDF-based regimen) or boosting a PI-based regimen with ritonavir
   c. If possible, avoid adding only one active drug to a failing regimen.
   d. In failing, adherent patient with no or minimal demonstrable genotypic or phenotypic resistance, consider measuring plasma drug levels (therapeutic drug monitoring)
   e. If resistant to multiple licensed drugs, investigate available clinical trials or agents available through expanded access program

TABLE 6B: ANTIRETROVIRAL DRUGS & ADVERSE EFFECTS (See also www.aidsinfo.nih.gov; for combinations, see individual components)

DRUG NAME(S): GENERIC (TRADE)	MOST COMMON ADVERSE EFFECTS	MOST SIGNIFICANT ADVERSE EFFECTS
Nucleoside Reverse Transcriptase Inhibitors (NRTI) (Black Box warning for all nucleoside/nucleotide RTIs: **lactic acidosis/hepatic steatosis, potentially fatal**. Also carry Warnings that fat redistribution has been observed)		
Abacavir (Ziagen)	Headache 7-13%, nausea 7-19%, diarrhea 7%, malaise 7-12%	**Black Box warning-Hypersensitivity reaction (HR)** in 8% with malaise, fever, GI upset, rash, lethargy & respiratory symptoms most commonly reported; myalgia, arthralgia, edema, parethesia less common. **Rechallenge contraindicated; may be life-threatening.** Severe HR may be more common with once-daily dosing. **HLA-B*5701 allele** predicts ↑ risk of HR in Caucasian pop.; excluding pts with B*5701 markedly ↓'d HR incidence (NEJM 358:568, 2008; CID 46:1111-1118, 2008). DHHS guidelines recommend testing for B*5701 and use of abacavir-containing regimens only if HLA-B*5701 negative; Vigilance essential in all groups. Possible increased risk of MI under study (www.fda.gov/CDER).
Didanosine (ddI) (Videx)	Diarrhea 28%, nausea 6%, rash 9%, headache 7%, fever 12%, hyperuricemia 2%	**Pancreatitis 1–9%. Black Box warning—Cases of fatal & nonfatal pancreatitis** have occurred in pts receiving ddI, especially when used in combination with d4T or d4T + hydroxyurea. Fatal lactic acidosis in pregnancy with ddI + d4T. Peripheral neuropathy in 20%, 12% required dose reduction. Rarely, retinal changes. Possible increased risk of MI under study (www.fda.gov/CDER).
Emtricitabine (FTC) (Emtriva)	Well tolerated. Headache, diarrhea, nausea, rash, skin hyperpigmentation	Potential for lactic acidosis (as with other NRTIs). Also **in Black Box—severe exacerbation of hepatitis B on stopping drug reported—monitor clinical/labs for several months after stopping in pts with hepB.** Anti-HBV rx may be warranted if FTC stopped.
Lamivudine (3TC) (Epivir)	Well tolerated. Headache 35%, nausea 33%, diarrhea 18%, abdominal pain 9%, insomnia 11% (all in combination with ZDV). Pancreatitis more common in pediatrics (15%).	**Black Box warning.** Make sure to use HIV dosage, not Hep B dosage. **Exacerbation of hepatitis B on stopping drug. Patients with hepB who stop lamivudine require close clinical/lab monitoring for several months.** Anti-HBV rx may be warranted if 3TC stopped.
Stavudine (d4T) (Zerit)	Diarrhea, nausea, vomiting, headache	Peripheral neuropathy 15-20%. Pancreatitis 1%. Appears to produce lactic acidosis more commonly than other NRTIs. **Black Box warning—Fatal & nonfatal pancreatitis with d4T + ddI + hydroxyurea. Fatal lactic acidosis/steatosis in pregnant women receiving d4T + ddI.** Motor weakness in the setting of lactic acidosis mimicking the clinical presentation of Guillain-Barre syndrome (including respiratory failure) (rare).
Zidovudine (ZDV, AZT) (Retrovir)	Nausea 50%, anorexia 20%, vomiting 17%, **headache 62%**. Also reported: asthenia, insomnia, myalgias, nail pigmentation. Macrocytosis expected with all dosage regimens.	**Black Box warning—hematologic toxicity, myopathy. Anemia** (<8 gm, 1%), granulocytopenia (<750, 1.8%). Anemia may respond to epoetin alfa if endogenous serum erythropoietin levels are ≤500 milliUnits/mL.
Nucleotide Reverse Transcriptase Inhibitor (NtRTI) (Black Box warning for all nucleoside/nucleotide RTIs: **lactic acidosis/hepatic steatosis, potentially fatal**. Also carry Warnings that fat redistribution has been observed)		
Tenofovir disproxil fumarate (TDF) (Viread)	Diarrhea 11%, nausea 8%, vomiting 5%, flatulence 4% (generally well tolerated)	**Black Box Warning—Severe exacerbations of hepatitis B reported in pts who stop tenofovir.** Monitor carefully if drug is stopped; anti-HBV rx may be warranted if TDF stopped. Possible ↑ bone demineralization. Reports of Fanconi syndrome & **renal injury induced by tenofovir** (CID 37:e174, 2003; JAIDS 35:269, 2004; CID 42:283, 2006). Modest decline in Ccr with TDF may be greater than with other NRTIs (CID 40:1194, 2005). Monitor creatinine clearance, especially carefully in those with pre-existing renal dysfunction. **Dose reduce to every 48 hrs if CrCl<50 cc/min.** Decline in renal function may be more rapid in pts receiving TDF with a PI vs. TDF with an NNRTI (JID 197:102, 2008).

TABLE 6B (2)

DRUG NAME(S): GENERIC (TRADE)	MOST COMMON ADVERSE EFFECTS	MOST SIGNIFICANT ADVERSE EFFECTS
Non-Nucleoside Reverse Transcriptase Inhibitors (NNRTI)		
Delavirdine (Rescriptor)	Nausea, diarrhea, vomiting, headache	**Skin rash** has occurred in 18%; can continue or restart drug in most cases. Stevens-Johnson syndrome & erythema multiforme have been reported rarely. ↑ in liver enzymes in <5% of patients.
Efavirenz (Sustiva)	**CNS side-effects 52%;** symptoms include dizziness, insomnia, somnolence, impaired concentration, psychiatric sx, & abnormal dreams; symptoms are worse after 1st or 2nd dose & improve over 2–4 weeks; discontinuation rate 2.6%. Rash 26% (vs. 17% in comparitors); often improves wit oral antihistamines; discontinuation rate 1.7%. Can cause false-positive urine test results for cannabinoid with CEDIA DAU multi-level THC assay.	Serious neuropsychiatric symptoms reported, including severe depression (2.4%) & suicidal ideation (0.7%). Elevation in liver enzymes. **Teratogenicity reported in primates; pregnancy category D—may cause fetal harm, avoid in pregnant women or those who might become pregnant** (see *Table 8A*). NOTE: No single method of contraception is 100% reliable. Contraindicated with certain drugs metabolized by CYP3A4. Slow metabolism in those homozygous for the CYP-2B6 G516T allele resulting in exaggerated toxicity and intolerance. This allele much more common in blacks and women (*CID 42:408, 2006*).
Etravirine (Intelence)	Rash 9%, generally mild to moderate and spontaneously resolving; 2% dc clinical trials for rash. More common in women. Nausea 5%.	Hypersensitivity or severe rash (erythema multiforme or Stevens-Johnson) <0.1%. Potential for CYP-mediated drug interactions.
Nevirapine (Viramune)	**Rash 37%:** usually occurs during 1st 6 wks of therapy. Follow recommendations for 14-day lead-in period to ↓ risk of rash (*see Table 6A*). Women experience 7-fold ↑ in risk of severe rash (*CID 32:124, 2001*). 50% resolve within 2 wks of dc drug & 80% by 1 month. 6.7% discontinuation rate.	**Black Box warning—Severe life-threatening skin reactions reported:** Stevens-Johnson syndrome, toxic epidermal necrolysis, & hypersensitivity reaction or drug rash with eosinophilia & systemic symptoms (DRESS) (*ArIM 161:2501, 2001*). For severe rashes, dc drug immediately & do not restart. In a clinical trial, the use of prednisone ↑ the risk of rash. **Black Box warning—Life-threatening hepatotoxicity reported,** 2/3 during the first 12 wks of rx. Overall 1% develop hepatitis. Pts with pre-existing ↑ in ALT or AST &/or history of chronic Hep B or C ↑ susceptible (*Hepatol 35:182, 2002*). Women with CD4 >250, including pregnant women, at ↑ risk. Avoid in this group unless no other option. Men with CD4 >400 also at ↑ risk. Monitor pts intensively (clinical & LFTs), esp. during the first 12 wks of rx. If clinical hepatotoxicity, severe skin or hypersensitivity reactions occur, dc drug & never rechallenge.

Protease inhibitors (PI)
Abnormalities in glucose metabolism, dyslipidemias, fat redistribution syndromes are potential problems. Pts taking PI may be at increased risk for developing osteopenia/osteoporosis. (See *Table 6C*). Spontaneous bleeding episodes have been reported in HIV+ pts with hemophilia being treated with PI. Rheumatoid complications have been reported with use of PIs (*An Rheum Dis 61:82, 2002*). Potential of some PIs for QTc prolongation has been suggested (*Lancet 365:682, 2005*). **Caution for all PIs**—Coadministration with certain drugs dependent on CYP3A for elimination & for which ↑ levels can cause serious toxicity may be contraindicated.

Atazanavir (Reyataz)	Asymptomatic unconjugated hyperbilirubinemia in up to 60% of pts, jaundice in 7–9% (especially wit Gilbert syndrome (*JID 192: 1381, 2005*). Moderate to severe events: Diarrhea 1–3%, nausea 6–14%, abdominal pain 4%, headache 6%, rash 5–7%.	Prolongation of PR interval (1st degree AV block) reported; rarely 2° AV block. QTc increase and torsades reported (*CID 44:e67, 2007*). Acute interstitial nephritis (*Am J Kid Dis 44:E81, 2004*) and urolithiasis (atazanavir stones) reported (*AIDS 20:2131, 2006; NEJM 355:2158, 2006*).
Darunavir (Prezista)	With background regimens, headache 15%, nausea 18%, diarrhea 20%, ↑ amylase 17%. Rash in 17% cf treated; 0.3% discontinuation.	Hepatitis in 0.5%, some with fatal outcome Use caution in pts with HBV or HCV co-infections or other hepatic dysfunction. Monitor for clinical symptoms and LFTs. Stevens-Johnson syndrome, erythema multiforme. Potential for major drug interactions. May cause failure of hormonal contraceptives.
Fosamprenavir (Lexiva)	Skin rash ~20% (moderate or worse in 3–8%), nausea, headache, diarrhea.	Rarely Stevens-Johnson syndrome, hemolytic anemia. Pro-drug of amprenavir. Contains sulfa moiety.

39

TABLE 6B (3)

DRUG NAME(S): GENERIC (TRADE)	MOST COMMON ADVERSE EFFECTS	MOST SIGNIFICANT ADVERSE EFFECTS
Protease inhibitors (continued)		
Indinavir (Crixivan)	↑ in indirect bilirubin 10–15% (≥2.5 mg/dl), with overt jaundice especially likely in those with Gilbert syndrome (JID 192: 1381, 2005). Nausea 12%, vomiting 4%, diarrhea 5%. Paronychia of big toe reported (CID 32:140, 2001).	**Kidney stones.** Due to indinavir crystals in collecting system. Nephrolithiasis in 12% of adults, higher in pediatrics. Minimize risk with good hydration (at least 48 oz. water/day) (AAC 42:332, 1998). Tubulointerstitial nephritis/renal cortical atrophy reported in association with asymptomatic ↑ urine WBC. Severe hepatitis reported in 3 cases (Ln 349:924, 1997). Hemolytic anemia reported.
Lopinavir/Ritonavir (Kaletra)	GI: **diarrhea** 14–24%, nausea 2–16%. More diarrhea with q24h dosing.	Lipid abnormalities in up to 20–40%. Hepatitis, with hepatic decompensation; caution especially in those with pre-existing liver disease. Pancreatitis. Inflammatory edema of legs (AIDS 16:673, 2002)
Nelfinavir (Viracept)	Mild to moderate **diarrhea** 20%. Oat bran tabs, calcium, or oral anti-diarrheal agents (e.g., loperamide, diphenoxylate/ atropine sulfate) can be used to manage diarrhea.	Potential for drug interactions.
Ritonavir (Norvir) (With rare exceptions, only use is to enhance levels of other anti-retrovirals, because of ↑toxicity/ interactions with full-dose ritonavir)	GI: bitter aftertaste ↓ by taking with chocolate milk, Ensure, or Advera; nausea 23%. ↓ by initial dose esc (titration) regimen; vomiting 13%; diarrhea 15%. Circumoral paresthesias 5–6%. ↑ dose >100mg bid assoc. with ↑ GI side-effects & ↑ in lipid abnormalities.	Hepatic failure (AnIM 129:670, 1998). Black Box warning relates to many important drug-drug interactions—inhibits P450 CYP3A & CYP2D6 system—may be life-threatening (see Table 16A). Rarely Stevens-Johnson syndrome, anaphylaxis.
Saquinavir (Invirase: hard cap, tablet)	**Diarrhea**, abdominal discomfort, nausea, headache	**Black Box Warning—Use Invirase only with ritonavir.** Avoid garlic capsules (may reduce SQV levels) and use cautiously with proton-pump inhibitors (increased SQV levels significant; may lead to increased GI sx, triglycerides, DVT).
Tipranavir (Aptivus)	Nausea & vomiting, diarrhea, abdominal pain. Rash in 8–14%, more common in women, & 33% in women taking ethinyl estradiol. Diarrhea 32%, nausea 23%, fatigue 20%.	**Black Box Warning—associated with hepatitis & fatal hepatic failure.** Risk of hepatotoxicity increased in hepB or hepC co-infection. **Associated with fatal/nonfatal intracranial hemorrhage (can inhibit platelet aggregation).** Caution in those with bleeding risks. Potential for major drug interactions. Contains sulfa moiety.
Fusion Inhibitor		
Enfuvirtide (T20, Fuzeon)	Local injection site reactions (98% at least 1 local ISR, 4% dc because of ISR) (pain & discomfort, induration, erythema, nodules & cysts, pruritus, & ecchymosis). Diarrhea 32%, nausea 23%, fatigue 20%.	↑ Rate of bacterial pneumonia (6.7 pneumonia events/100 pt yrs). **hypersensitivity reactions** ≤1% (rash, fever, nausea & vomiting, chills, rigors, hypotension, & ↑ serum liver transaminases); can occur with reexposure.
CCR5 Co-receptor Antagonists		
Maraviroc (Selzentry)	With ARV background: cough 13%, fever 12%, rash 10%, abdominal pain 8%. Also, dizziness, myalgia, arthralgias. ↑ Risk of URI, HSV infection.	**Black box warning-Hepatotoxicity.** May be preceded by allergic features. No hepatoxicity was noted in clinical trials. Black box inserted owing to concern about potential CCR5 class effect. Use with caution in pt with HepB or C. Cardiac ischemia/infarction in 1.3%. May cause ↓BP, syncope. Significant interactions with CYP3A inducers/inhibitors. Long-term risk of malignancy unknown.
Integrase Inhibitors		
Raltegravir (Isentress)	Diarrhea, headache, nausea. LFT ↑ may be more common in pts co-infected with HBV or HCV.	Hypersensitivity can occur. ↑CK with myopathy or rhabdomyolysis reported, with unclear relationship to drug.

TABLE 6C: DRUG ADVERSE EFFECTS BY CLINICAL PRESENTATION[1]

Clinical Presentation	Implicated Drug Class or Drug(s)	Onset; Clinical Signs & Symptoms (S&S)	Estimated Frequency	Risk Factors	Prevention/ Monitoring	Clinical Management
LIFE THREATENING ADVERSE EFFECTS (in alphabetical order)						
Drug-induced hepatitis	Nevirapine (Viramune)	Onset: Any time 1st few wks S&S: nausea/vomiting/icterus. Skin rash in 50%	2.5–11% in clinical trials	Females with CD4 >250; men with CD4 >400	Monitor ALT/AST q2wks x1mo, then every month x3, then q3mos.	DC all antiretrovirals + other potential hepatotoxic drugs
Lactic acidosis/ hepatic steatosis ± pancreatitis (Mitochondrial toxicity: JAC 61:8, 2008)	Nucleoside reverse transcriptase inhibitors: stavudine (Zerit), didanosine (Videx), zidovudine (Retrovir)	Onset: Months after starting therapy. S&S: Nausea, vomiting, fatigue, dyspnea, icterus. Lab: Metabolic acidosis with anion gap and elevated lactate	Rare: 0.85 cases/1000 pt yrs, mortality up to 50%	Didanosine + stavudine. Female, pregnancy, obesity.	Lactic acid levels if suggestive symptoms and low serum HCO$_3$ and/or high anion gap. Routine lactate levels **not** recommended	DC all antiretrovirals. IV thiamine &/or riboflavin reported helpful. If needed, use NRTIs[2] with low potential for mitochondrial toxicity: i.e., abacavir, tenofovir, lamivudine, emtricitabine
Lactic acidosis/rapid progressive ascending neuromuscular weakness	Stavudine (Zerit)	Onset: After months S&S: Rapid progressive ascending polyneuropathy that mimics Guillain-Barre. Lab: Metabolic acidosis with arion gap & elevated lactate + high CPK	Rare	Prolonged stavudine use	Early recognition	DC all antiretrovirals, mechanical ventilation. Unclear benefit from plasmapheresis, IVIG, corticosteroids, carnitine. **Do not rechallenge with stavudinne.**
Stevens-Johnson syndrome/toxic epidermal necrosis (see drug-induced hepatitis above)	Non-nucleoside reverse transcriptase inhibitors. Rare case reports other classes	Onset: 1st few days to weeks S&S: Skin eruption with mucosal ulcers ± epidermal detachment	Nevirapine (Viramune) 0.3–1% Efavirenz (Sustiva) & delavirdine (Rescriptor) 0.1%	Nevirapine— female, black, Asian, Hispanic	Educate pts for early recognition	DC all antiretrovirals + other possible drug etiology, e.g., TMP/SMX. Usually requires ICU care.
Systemic hypersensitivity reaction	Abacavir (Ziagen) DO NOT rechallenge with abacavir.	Onset: Median 9 days; 90% within 1st 6 wks. S&S: Fever, diffuse rash, nausea/ vomiting/diarrhea/arthralgia, dypsnea, cough, or pharyngitis	8% in clinical trials (range 2–9%)	HLA-B 5701 or HLA-DR7 positive.	Educate pts for early recognition	DC all antiretrovirals; Resolution within 48 hrs.
	Nevirapine (Viramune)	Severe skin reactions	2%		Do not restart	

[1] Adapted from Table 18, Guidelines for use of antiretroviral agents in HIV-1 infected adults and adolescents, DHHS, 01/29/2008
[2] **NRTI** = nucleoside reverse transcriptase inhibitor

TABLE 6C (2)

Clinical Presentation	Implicated Drug Class or Drug(s)	Onset; Clinical Signs & Symptoms (S&S)	Estimated Frequency	Risk Factors	Prevention/ Monitoring	Clinical Management
SERIOUS ADVERSE EFFECTS (in alphabetical order)						
Bleeding events:						
Hemophiliac patients	Protease inhibitors	Spontaneous bleeding	Unknown	Protease inhibitor use	Try to avoid PIs	Increased use of Factor VIII
Intracranial hemorrhage	Ritonavir boosted tipranavir (TPR/R)	Median time to hemorrhage: 525 days	13 cases with 8 deaths in 2006	CNS disease, injury or surgery, anti-coagulants	Avoid TPR/R in at-risk patients	
Bone marrow suppression	Zidovudine (Retrovir)	Onset: Weeks to months S&S: Fatigue Lab: Anemia &/or neutropenia	Anemia 1.1–4% Neutropenia 1.8–8%	AIDS; high dose concomitant marrow-suppressive drug(s)	Avoid marrow suppressive drugs. CBC & differential at least q3 mos.	If severe, could use G-CSF &/or erythropoietin
Hepatotoxicity	All NNRTIs, all PIs, most NRTIs, maraviroc	PIs: clinical hepatitis reported with TPR/r Onset: variable NNRTI: Asym ↑ed AST/ALT + lactic acidosis (ZDV, ddI, d4T)	Variable	Co-infection: Hep B, Hep C, alcoholism, other hepatotoxic drugs	Nevirapine: monitor LFTs frequently. TPR/R: avoid in pts with hepatic insufficiency	Test for Hep B&C. If symptomatic, discontinue all retroviral drugs
Nephrolithiasis/ urolithiasis/ crystalluria	Indinavir (Crixivan) most often, rarely atazanavir	Onset: Any time S&S: Flank pain & dysuria Lab: Hematuria, crystalluria, pyuria	Range in clinical trials: 4.7–34.4%	Dehydration; history of nephrolithiasis	Intake of 1.5–2 liters water/day	Hydration
Nephrotoxicity— tenofovir (CID 42:283, 2006)	Indinavir (Crixivan) crystalluria (see above) & tenofovir (Viread) tubular injury	Onset: Tenofovir—weeks to months S&S: Tenofovir—nephrogenic diabetes insipidus, **Fanconi syndrome** Lab: Non-anion gap metabolic acidosis, glycosuria, hypokalemia, hypophosphatemia	Unknown but severe toxicity is rare	Other nephrotoxic drugs; other anti-HIV drugs handled by proximal tubular cells; report of predisposing human genetic variant (JID 194:1471 & 1481, 2006).	Monitor serum creatinine. Theoretic drug-drug interactions with ritonavir & atazanavir. Decrease dosing frequency of tenofovir if est. CrCl <50 cc/min.	**Stop offending drug if possible.** Renal injury is reversible. Tenofovir (TDF): Fall in CrCl greater with TDF + PI vs. TDF + NNRTI (JID 197:102, 2008).
Pancreatitis	Didanosine (Videx); didanosine + stavudine (Zerit); lamivudine (Epivir) in children; ddI + ribavirin or tenofovir.	Onset: Weeks to months S&S: Abd./back pain, nausea/vomiting Lab: ↑ amylase/lipase	Didanosine alone 1–7%. Lamivudine in children—range in clinical trials <1–15%	High serum/cell didanosine levels; alcoholism; hypertriglyceridemia. Failure to ↓ dose of didanosine if given with tenofovir	No didanosine if history of pancreatitis. Adjust dose of didanosine if tenofovir used. Avoid use of ddI with d4T, tenofovir or ribavirin.	Discontinue antiretrovirals

TABLE 6C (3)

ADVERSE EFFECTS WITH LONG-TERM COMPLICATIONS (in alphabetical order): at least, in part, due to HIV replication

Clinical Presentation	Implicated Drug Class or Drug(s)	Onset; Clinical Signs & Symptoms (S&S)	Estimated Frequency	Risk Factors	Prevention/Monitoring	Clinical Management
Atherosclerotic cardiovascular disease potential Ref. *NEJM* 356:1723 & 1773, 2007	**All protease inhibitors (PIs) except atazanavir (Reyataz); maybe efavirenz, stavudine, abacavir & ddI**	Onset: Months to years S&S: Premature or accelerated atherosclerotic vascular disease (e.g., MI, stroke)	Incidence of MI: 3–6/1000 pt yrs on protease inhibitor. RR increase of MI while on ABC (1.9-fold) or ddI (1.5-fold). DAD study: Ln 371:1417, 2008.	Tobacco use, age, hyperlipidemia (see below), hypertension, diabetes	Address risk factors	Manage risk factors; may have to avoid protease inhibitors, except atazanavir. Ref. *JAC* 61:238, 2008.
Hyperlipidemia Ref. *LnID* 7:787, 2007.	All protease inhibitors (PIs) except atazanavir (Reyataz); stavudine (Zerit); efavirenz (Sustiva)	Onset: Weeks to months Lab: ↑ LDL & total cholesterol & triglycerides; ↓ HDL d4T: Increase in triglycerides Efavirenz: Increase in HDL	1.7–2.3 fold increase with PIs other than atazanavir	PIs: ritonavir boosted lopinavir NNRTI: Efavirenz NRTI: Stavudine	Use non-PI, non-stavudine regimen; if need PI, use ritonavir-boosted atazanavir. Lipid profile baseline & then at 3–6 months of therapy	Lifestyle modification. For ↑ total cholesterol, LDL, triglycerides 200–500, pravastatin, atorvastatin or fluvastatin. For triglycerides >500 mg/dl, gemfibrozil or fenofibrate.
Insulin resistance/ diabetes mellitus Ref. *JAC* 61:238, 2008	Protease inhibitors (PIs); atazanavir has minimal effect.	Onset: Weeks to months S&S: Polydipsia, polyuria, polyphagia	3–5% of pts	Underlying hyperglycemia, family history	Non-PI regimen. Ideally, monitor fasting blood glucose levels.	Diet & exercise, metformin, "glitazones," sulfonylureas, insulin
Osteonecrosis	All protease inhibitors (PIs)	Onset: Insidious S&S: Periarticular pain. 85% involve one or both femoral heads	Symptomatic 0.08–1.3% Asymptomatic by MRI 4%	Diabetes; prior steroid use; alcohol use; hyperlipidemia	No steroids. Periodic MRIs to assess disease progression.	Remove risk factors; less weight-bearing; some require total joint arthroplasty

ADVERSE EFFECTS THAT INFLUENCE QUALITY OF LIFE

Fat Maldistribution (*JAC* 61:238, 2008)

Clinical Presentation	Implicated Drug Class or Drug(s)	Onset; Clinical Signs & Symptoms (S&S)	Estimated Frequency	Risk Factors	Prevention/Monitoring	Clinical Management
Lipoatrophy	NRTIs, especially Stavudine > zidovudine. Protease inhibitors	Loss of subcutaneous fat on face, buttocks & extremities	Precise frequency unknown	Low nadir CD4 count, older age. Low baseline body mass index.	If possible, avoid stavudine and zidovudine. Another possible treatment: tesamorelin 2 mg sc daily x 52 wks effective (*NEJM* 357:2359, 2007).	Substitute abacavir or tenofovir for stavudine. Perhaps some benefit from a thiazolidinedione: e.g., proglitazone, 30 mg once daily. Dermal fillers approved: polylactic-2-acid & radiesse (Ca^{++} hydroxyapatite) but limited efficacy.
Fat Accumulation		Excess adipose tissue in abdominal viscera, breast size, dorsocervical fat pad	Precise frequency unknown	Obeseity prior to HIV infection; low CD4 count prior to therapy; older age	If overweight; diet & exercise	Metformin 1500 mg daily in patients with insulin resistance; growth hormone 4–6 mg SQ daily (can cause glucose intolerance). Switching from PI no help

43

TABLE 6C (4)

Clinical Presentation	Implicated Drug Class or Drug(s)	Onset; Clinical Signs & Symptoms (S&S)	Estimated Frequency	Risk Factors	Prevention/ Monitoring	Clinical Management
ADVERSE EFFECTS THAT INFLUENCE QUALITY OF LIFE *(continued)*						
Gastrointestinal— Diarrhea	All protease inhibitors (PIs), didanosine (Videx)	Onset: 1st dose Symptoms: Perhaps worst with lopinavir/ritonavir, nelfinavir, & buffered didanosine	Varies	All patients	Antidiarrheals	For diarrhea, consider: loperamide, diphenoxylate/ atropine, calcium tabs, psyllium products, pancreatic enzymes
Peripheral neuropathy	Didanosine (Videx), stavudine (Zerit), zalcitabine (HIVID)	Onset: Weeks to months S&S: Usually legs. Numbness & paresthesias. Often irreversible even if drug(s) stopped	Didanosine 12–34% Stavudine 52% Zalcitabine 22–35%	Pre-existing neuropathy; advanced HIV; concomitant drugs that ↑ intracellular didanosine, e.g., ribavirin, hydroxyurea	Avoid use, esp. in combination	If painful can try gabapentin or tricyclic antidepressants; high concentration capsaicin dermal patch.

TABLE 6D: Overlapping Toxicities Between Antiretrovirals and Other Drugs Commonly Used in HIV Patients* (Anti-HIV Drugs are BOLD)

Bone Marrow Suppression	Peripheral Neuropathy	Pancreatitis	Nephrotoxicity	Hepatotoxicity	Rash	Diarrhea	Ocular Effects
Amphotericin B	**Didanosine**	Cotrimoxazole	Acyclovir (IV, HD)	Azithromycin	**Abacavir**	Atovaquone	Cidofovir
Cidofovir	Isoniazid	**Didanosine**	Adefovir	Clarithromycin	**Atazanavir**	Clindamycin	**Didanosine**
Cotrimoxazole	Linezolid	**Lamivudine** (child)	Aminoglycosides	**Darunavir**	Atovaquone	**Darunavir**	Ethambutol
Cytotoxic chemotherapy	**Stavudine**	Pentamidine	Amphotericin B	**Delavirdine**	Cotrimoxazole	**Fosamprenavir**	Linezolid
Dapsone		**Ritonavir**	Cidofovir	**Efavirenz**	Dapsone	**Lopinavir/ritonavir**	Rifabutin
Flucytosine		**Stavudine**	Foscarnet	Fluconazole	**Darunavir**	**Nelfinavir**	Voriconazole
Ganciclovir			**Indinavir**	Isoniazid	**Delavirdine**	**Ritonavir**	
Hydroxyurea			Pentamidine	Itraconazole	**Efavirenz**	**Tipranavir**	
Interferon-alpha			**Tenofovir**	Ketoconazole	**Fosamprenavir**		
Linezolid				**Maraviroc**	**Maraviroc**		
Peg-interferon alpha				**Nevirapine**	**Nevirapine**		
Primaquine				**Didanosine** (hepatic steatosis)	Sulfadiazine		
Pyrimethamine				**PIs** (esp. tipranavir)	**Tipranavir**		
Ribavirin				Rifabutin	Voriconazole		
Rifabutin				Rifampin			
Sulfadiazine				Voriconazole			
Trimetrexate							
Valganciclovir							
Zidovudine							

*Adapted from Table 19, Guidelines for use of antiretroviral agents in HIV-1 infected adults and adolescents, DHHS, 1/29/2008 and available at http://aidsinfo.nih.gov

TABLE 6E: ANTI-HIV DRUGS AVAILABLE VIA EXPANDED ACCESS PROGRAMS (www.aidsinfo.nih.gov; 800-448-0440)
No Drugs Available by Expanded Access at the present time

SELECTED DRUGS IN DEVELOPMENT

Drug Name(s), Number, (Manufacturer)	Drug Class (Site of Anti-HIV Activity)	Dose	Comments
Vicriviroc (Schering)	CCR5 antagonist	20 mg daily (dose still being defined)	Recent study (Victor; CROI 2008) good activity when combined with optimized background drugs in salvage regimen. Early studies raised concern about malignancy association; not substantiated yet in later studies.
Rilpivirine (TMC 278)	NNRTI	25 mg daily (Higher doses associated with QTc prolongation)	Studies underway in both naive and experienced patient populations. Drug is active against virus with Y181C/K103N & L100I/K103N mutations in the RT region.
Apricitabine (ATC)	nRTI	600 mg twice daily (dose being finalized in current studies)	3TC-like agent with activity against virus harboring an M184V mutation. Antagonistic against 3TC and FTC; don't use with either of these drugs.
Elvitegravir (GS-9137)	Integrase Inhibitor	125 mg daily Dosing still being determined; Requires ritonavir boosting	Studies are underway; unclear if activity similar to raltegravir or not.
Bevirimat (PA-457)	Maturation Inhibitor	Dose still being determined	Inhibits Gag processing at the CA-Sp1 cleavage site. Initial studies yielded inconsistent results, later found to be due to resistance conferred by mutations at the gag cleavage site (CROI, 2008)

TABLE 6F: MONITORING BLOOD LEVELS OF ANTIRETROVIRAL DRUGS (THERAPEUTIC DRUG MONITORING)
(www.hivpharmacology.com; CID 42:1189 & 1197, 2006)

I. **Purpose - Motivation**
   A. Interpatient variability in drug levels
   B. Correlation between drug concentration and efficacy and/or toxicity

II. **Which anti-retrovirals?**
   A. Concentration response data exist for NNRTIs and PIs
   B. To date, unclear relationship between plasma concentration of NRTIs and effective intracellular concentrations

III. **Which patients? Not recommended in all pts**
   A. Potential drug-drug or drug-food interaction
   B. Impaired function of drug excretion pathway
   C. HIV isolates with reduced drug susceptibility
   D. Pregnancy
   E. Concentration-dependent toxicity
   F. Monitoring for drug use adherence
   G. Unexplained inadequate virological response

IV. **Limitations**
   A. No prospective study that documents improved outcome
   B. Incomplete knowledge of therapeutic or toxic ranges
   C. Considerable intraindividual variability in levels (CID 42:1189, 2006)
   D. Only a few qualified labs

V. **Suggested trough blood concentrations for PIs and efavirenz for infections caused by wild-type HIV-1[1] (from www.aidsinfo.nih.gov)**

Drug: Generic Name (Brand)	Target Trough Concentration (ng/ml)
Atazanavir (Reyataz)	150
Fosamprenavir (Lexiva)	400[2]
Indinavir (Crixivan)	100
Lopinavir/Ritonavir (Kaletra)	1000
Nelfinavir (Viracept)	800[3]
Saquinavir (Invirase)	100-250
Efavirenz (Sustiva)	1000

[1] Check levels in steady-state. Target concentrations my be higher for virus that is not fully drug-susceptible
[2] Measured as amprenavir
[3] Active metabolite

TABLE 6G: Antiretrovirals approved or tentatively approved by FDA for INTERNATIONAL AIDS RELIEF (from www.fda.gov/oia/pepfar.htm)

As a requirement of the President's Emergency Plan for AIDS Relief (PEPFAR), the US FDA reviews international marketing applications for individual antiretroviral agents, fixed dose combinations & co-packaged ARVs, & grants *approval* (A) or *tentative* (T) approval (when products continue to have marketing protection) status to products that meet efficacy, safety & manufacturing standards for marketing in the US.

Generic name	Pharmaceutical Prep.	Supplier	Status
Single agents:			
Abacavir sulfate	300 mg tabs, 20 mg/mL oral solution	Aurobindo Pharma, Ltd	T
	300 mg (base) tabs	Cipla, Ltd	T
	300 mg (base) tabs	Matrix Laboratories, Ltd	T
Didanosine	200 mg, 250 mg, 400 mg delayed release caps	Barr Laboratories, Inc.	A
	100 mg, 150 mg, 200 mg tablets	Aurobindo Pharma, Ltd	T
	10 mg/mL oral solution	Aurobindo Pharma, Ltd	A
Zidovudine (ZDV)	300 mg tabs	Ranbaxy Laboratories, Ltd	A
	100 mg caps, 300 mg tabs, 50 mg/5 mL oral solution	Aurobindo Pharma, Ltd	A
	100 mg caps	Cipla, Ltd	A
	300 mg tabs	Matrix Laboratories, Ltd	A
Lamivudine (3TC)	150 mg tabs	Ranbaxy Laboratories, Ltd	T
	150 mg tabs	Matrix Laboratories, Ltd	T
	150 mg, 300 mg tabs	Aurobindo Pharma, Ltd	T
	10 mg/mL oral solution	Cipla, Ltd	T
	150 mg, 300 mg tabs	Hetero Drugs, Ltd	T
Stavudine (d4T)	15 mg, 20 mg, 30 mg, 40 mg caps	Aurobindo Pharma, Ltd	T
	1 mg/mL oral solution	Strides Arcolab, Ltd	T
	30 mg, 40 mg caps	Matrix Laboratories, Ltd	T
	30 mg, 40 mg caps	Cipla, Ltd	T
	1 mg/mL oral solution	Hetero Drugs, Ltd	T
	15 mg, 20 mg, 30 mg, 40 mg caps		T
Tenofovir Disoproxil Fumarate	300 mg tabs	Matrix Laboratories, Ltd	T
Nevirapine	200 mg tabs	Ranbaxy Laboratories, Ltd	T
	200 mg tabs	Cipla, Ltd	T
Nevirapine (con'td)	200 mg tabs	Strides Arcolab, Ltd	T
	200 mg tabs	Aurobindo Pharma, Ltd	T
	50 mg/5mL oral suspension	Huahai US, Inc	T
	200 mg tabs	Hetero Drugs, Ltd	T
	200 mg tabs	Emcure Pharmaceuticals, Ltd	T
Efavirenz	600 mg tabs	Aurobindo Pharma, Ltd	T
	600 mg tabs	Cipla, Ltd	T
	600 mg tabs	Strides Arcolab, Ltd	T
	600 mg tabs	Matrix Laboratories, Ltd	T
	600 mg tabs	Emcure Pharmaceuticals, Ltd	T
	600 mg tabs	Hetero Drugs, Ltd	T
	50 mg, 100 mg, 200 mg caps	Aurobindo Pharma, Ltd	T
Atazanavir sulfate	100 mg, 150 mg, 200 mg caps	Emcure Pharmaceuticals, Ltd	T
Combinations and/or co-packaged products			
Lamivudine/Zidovudine	Tabs: (150 mg 3TC + 300 mg ZDV)	Aurobindo Pharma, Ltd	T
	Tabs: (150 mg 3TC + 300 mg ZDV)	Pharmacare, Ltd	T
	Tabs: (150 mg 3TC + 300 mg ZDV)	Cipla, Ltd	T
	Tabs: (150 mg 3TC + 300 mg ZDV)	Emcure Pharmaceuticals, Ltd	T
	Tabs: (150 mg 3TC + 300 mg ZDV)	Matrix Laboratories, Ltd	T
Lamivudine/Stavudine	Tabs: (150 mg 3TC + 30 mg d4T)	Cipla, Ltd	T
	Tabs: (150 mg 3TC + 40 mg d4T)		

TABLE 6G (2)

Generic name	Pharmaceutical Prep.	Supplier	Status
Lamivudine/Zidovudine co-packaged with Abacavir sulfate	Tabs: (150 mg 3TC + 300 mg ZDV) with Tabs: 300 mg abacavir sulfate	Aurobindo Pharma, Ltd	T
Lamivudine/Zidovudine co-packaged with Nevirapine	Tabs: (150 mg 3TC + 300 mg ZDV) with Tabs: 200 mg nevirapine	Aspen Pharmacare, Ltd	T
	Tabs: (150 mg 3TC + 300 mg ZDV) with Tabs: 200 mg nevirapine	Strides Arcolab, Ltd	T
Lamivudine/Zidovudine/Nevirapine	Tabs: (150 mg 3TC + 300 mg ZDV + 200 mg nevirapine)	Aurobindo Pharma, Ltd	T
	Tabs: (150 mg 3TC + 300 mg ZDV + 200 mg nevirapine)	Cipla, Ltd	T
Lamivudine/Zidovudine co-packaged with Efavirenz	Tabs: (150 mg 3TC + 300 mg ZDV) with Tabs: 600 mg efavirenz	Aurobindo Pharma, Ltd	T
	Tabs: (150 mg 3TC + 300 mg ZDV) with Tabs: 600 mg efavirenz	Strides Arcolab, Ltd	T

Generic name	Pharmaceutical Prep.	Supplier	Status
Lamivudine/stavudine (cont'd)	Tabs: (150 mg 3TC + 40 mg d4T)	Strides Arcolab, Ltd	T
	Tabs: (150 mg 3TC + 30 mg d4T)	Matrix Laboratories, Ltd	T
	Tabs: (150 mg 3TC + 40 mg d4T)		T
Lamivudine/Stavudine co-packaged with Nevirapine	Tabs: (150 mg 3TC + 40 mg d4T) with Tabs: 200 mg nevirapine	Strides Arcolab, Ltd	T
Lamivudine/Stavudine/Nevirapine	Tabs: (150 mg 3TC + 30 mg d4T + 200 mg nevirapine) Tabs: (150 mg 3TC + 40 mg d4T + 200 mg nevirapine)	Cipla, Ltd	T
	Dispersible tabs: (30 mg 3TC + 6 mg d4T + 50 mg nevirapine) Dispersible tabs: (60 mg 3TC + 12 mg d4T + 100 mg nevirapine)	Cipla, Ltd	T
Lamivudine/Stavudine co-packaged with Efavirenz	Tabs: (150 mg 3TC + 40 mg d4T) with Tabs: 600 mg efavirenz	Strides Arcolab, Ltd	T

TABLE 7: METHODS FOR PENICILLIN DESENSITIZATION

Perform in ICU setting. Discontinue all β-adrenergic antagonists. Have IV line, ECG & spirometer (*Curr Clin Topics Inf Dis 13:131, 1993*). Once desensitized, rx must not lapse or risk of allergic reactions ↑. A history of Stevens-Johnson syndrome, exfoliative dermatitis, erythroderma are nearly absolute contraindications to desensitization (use only as an approach to IgE sensitivity).

Oral Route: If oral prep available & pt has functional GI tract, oral route is preferred. 1/3 pts will develop transient reaction during desensitization or treatment, usually mild.

Step*	1	2	3	4	5	6	7	8	9	10	11	12	13	14
Drug (mg/mL)	0.5	0.5	0.5	0.5	0.5	0.5	0.5	5	5	5	50	50	50	50
Amount (mL)	0.1	0.2	0.4	0.8	1.6	3.2	6.4	1.2	2.4	4.8	1.0	2.0	4.0	8.0

* Interval between doses: 15 min. After Step 14, observe for 30 minutes, then 1 gm IV.

Parenteral Route:

Step**	1	2	3	4	5	6	7	8	9	10	11	12	13	14	15	16	17
Drug (mg/mL)	0.1	0.1	0.1	0.1	1	1	1	10	10	10	100	100	100	100	1000	1000	1000
Amount (mL)	0.1	0.2	0.4	0.8	0.16	0.32	0.64	0.12	0.24	0.48	0.1	0.2	0.4	0.8	0.16	0.32	0.64

** Interval between doses: 15 min. After Step 17, observe for 30 minutes, then 1 gm IV.

[Adapted from Sullivan, TJ, in Allergy: Principles & Practice, Middleton, E., et al, Eds. C.V. Mosby, 1993, p. 1726, with permission]

TABLE 8A: HIV/AIDS IN WOMEN/PREGNANCY*

I. **General Aspects**
   A. Women represent half of persons with HIV/AIDS in the world. Among young people (15–24yrs) in developing countries with HIV/AIDS, 64% are women.
   B. Heterosexual transmission is dominant mode of transmission worldwide. Among new HIV/AIDS diagnoses among women in the U.S. in 2005: 80% heterosexual contact, 18% IDU.
   C. Transmission of HIV from men to women occurs more readily than from women to men. Risk factors for male-to-female transmission: genital ulcers, partner with advanced disease, other STDs, trauma.
   D. Risk after several years of unprotected sex with same infected partner is 10–45%.
   E. Despite these aspects, relatively less is written about women's issues. Only small numbers of women have been included in therapy trials.

II. **Initial Assessment:** *See Table 2*

III. **Clinical Manifestations** *(Adapted from Newman, MD, in Medical Mgmt of AIDS, 6th ed., 1999; J AIDS 9:361, 1995)*
   A. **AIDS-defining diagnoses:**
      - Disease progression similar in women & men *(NEJM 333:751, 1995)*
      - Survival is related to access to care, which may be worse for women
      - Viral load at high CD4 counts tends to be lower in women *(CID 35:313, 2002)*
      - Gender difference narrows as CD4 drops
   B. **Human papillomavirus:**
      - HPV disease incidence increased! Cervical intraepithelial neoplasia (CIN) more prevalent in multiple studies. Prevalence increases with decreasing CD4 *(CID 38:737, 2004)*
      - Aggressive course, with high rate of progression to cancer if immunosuppressed
      - Pap smear recommended for HIV+ women. If initial Pap smear is neg, repeat in 6mos. If both are negative, annual Pap smears adequate (CDC Guidelines). We recommend every 6mos for those with CD4 <200. Colposcopy recommended for any suspicious lesions. There are no contraindications to standard treatment modalities for CIN.
      - Although many women with HIV are already infected with some HPV genotypes, there may be benefit to use of HPV vaccine according to recommendations for HIV negative women
   C. **Recurrent/refractory vaginal candidiasis**
      - May be early manifestation although poorly predictive of HIV infection (CD4 may be >500)
      - HIV diagnosis often missed because testing not offered
   D. **Other conditions**
      - PID may be more severe, 7–17% require hospitalization
      - Menstrual disorders (41% HIV+ women had menstrual abnormalities vs 24% in controls) include irregular periods, heavier or scantier periods, early menopausal symptoms, ↑ in premenstrual symptoms

IV. **Family Planning.** 85% of women with AIDS are in child-bearing years. Contraceptive and pre-conceptonal planning are essential components of care. Certain contraceptives may pose health hazards for HIV+ women *(Zeeman B, Hirschhorn LR, p. 616, in HIV Infection, Libman H, Witzburg RA. 3rd Ed., Little Brown & Co.)*

Method of Contraception	Failure Rate	Risks
Sterilization	0.4	No HIV protection
Oral contraceptive	3	May ↑ disease progression; drug-drug interactions common
IUD	3	↑ risk of PID, not higher for HIV+ vs HIV-
Latex condom	12	
Diaphragm cervical cap	18	Potential vaginal abrasions
Sponge	18–28	Potential vaginal abrasions
Nonoxynol-9	21	Irritation of vaginal mucosa with freq. use; may ↑ HIV transmission

V. **Treatment Issues**
   A. Inadequate gender-specific data!
   B. Theoretical issues
      - Baseline anemia (iron deficiency)
      - Low mean body weight, higher body fat, different hepatic metabolism compared to men
   C. Menstrual dysfunction
      - Amenorrhea should be evaluated; start with pregnancy test
      - Premature menopause occurs frequently; consider short term hormone replacement therapy
   D. Recommended treatment regimens currently identical for men & women
      - Rates of some side effects different in women (↑ rash and hepatitis on nevirapine with CD4 > 250, ↑ GI side-effects on lopinavir/ritonavir)
      - **Efavirenz should be avoided in women who may become pregnant**
      - Lactic acidosis may be more common in women, associated with d4T & ddI

VI. **HIV in Pregnancy: Care of the Mother**
   A. **Pre conception counseling**
      - All HIV + women should be asked if they are or might consider becoming pregnant
      - This may influence decision to start ARV if CD4 > 350 or influence choice of agents (eg include AZT, avoid efavirenz). Achieving stable viral load suppression to <50 copies/mL before conceiving is desirable.
      - Consider folate supplement or multivitamin
   B. **Antepartum Care**
      - **All** pregnant women should be offered HIV testing & counseling **regardless** of risk factors. Inclusion in routine testing with opt-out preferred to opt-in
      - Quantitative measure of **HIV RNA**
      - Obtain CD4 count and percent at outset & each trimester (some ↓ CD4 count in normal pregnancy)
      - **Screening tests** (HBsAg, RPR, chlamydia) as in any pregnancy
      - Discourage illicit drug use, smoking, unprotected sex with multiple partners
   C. **Use of antiviral therapy in pregnancy** *(www.aidsinfo.nih.gov)*. Treatment of HIV in pregnancy requires attention to 2 separate but equal goals:
      - Provide optimal treatment to the woman that does not limit future options
      - Prevent transmission to the infant without drug toxicity

TABLE 8A (2)

1. Risk factors for mother-to-child transmission (MTCT)
   - Maternal viral load (outset & at delivery are independent predictors *(JID 183:539, 2001)*
   - Maternal CD4 count (risk of transmission ↑ 3-fold if CD4 <400)
   - Lack of antiviral therapy (independent of other factors) *(JID 183:539, 2001)*
   - Prolonged rupture of membranes (rate doubled if >4 hours) *(NEJM 334:1617, 1996)*
   - Mode of delivery *(see next page)*
   - Breastfeeding (additional 10–14% transmission) *(JAMA 282:744, 1999)*
2. General principles
   - Preventing MTCT should be integrated with obstetrical & HIV medical care for the mother. The mother should be informed & involved in decisions.
   - Combination antiretroviral therapy ↓ risk of MTCT regardless of viral load
   - ARV is generally safe for the mother (avoid use of ddI with d4T—↑ risk of lactic acidosis and efavirenz)
   - Maximal viral suppression with combination therapy ↓ risk of resistance in mother & loss of future options, & is more effective than 1- or 2-drug regimens. Preferred for all pregnant women
   - Resistance testing recommended before beginning ARV if it is available
   - Longterm safety of ARV for infant exposed in utero is not fully known. Generally safe, although conflicting data on mitochondrial toxicity
   - Some data suggest ↑ rate of prematurity, low birth weight with PI use during pregnancy
   - Optimal dosing in pregnancy has not been adequately studied for all agents
   - PI levels fall in third trimester (nelfinavir, indinavir, lopinavir/ritonavir). Consider obtaining levels.
3. Combination therapy with ZDV, 1 other NRTI, & either nevirapine or potent protease inhibitor recommended:
   a. **For all women for whom ARV therapy is otherwise appropriate**
   b. **For all women with >1000 copies of HIV RNA**
   c. **Should be strongly considered for all pregnant woman**
      - Transmission in cohorts 0.7–2.0% with 3-drug ARV RX
      - ZDV & 3TC preferred nucleosides based on experience, but d4T & 3TC are probably a reasonable choice if they are more readily available through national formulary, although data are limited
      - Tenofovir associated with decreased in growth and bone abnormalities in pregnant monkeys, but likely a reasonable choice
      - WHO recommends ZDV, 3TC & nevirapine or d4T, 3TC & nevirapine for pregnant women who will receive ARV RX
      - While use of ZDV is recommended when possible based on trial data, choice of nucleoside regimen should consider the patient's viral resistance and ability to tolerate ZDV
4. Many trials have demonstrated significant efficacy of more limited regimens. Some may be more affordable or practical in specific settings. *(For detailed overview, see http://womenchildrenhiv.org/wchiv?page=pi-10-02)*
5. Single dose nevirapine should be considered for women without prenatal care. However, emergence of nevirapine resistance can occur in up to 50%. Use of additional drugs, such as ZDV & lamivudine, continued for 3–7 days after delivery has been shown to to ↓ the emergence of resistance.
6. **Efavirenz is contraindicated in pregnancy due to risk of teratogenicity.**
7. **Stavudine & didanosine combination should not be used in pregnancy due to risk of lactic acidosis.**
8. **Severe skin rash, ↑ transaminases & rarely fulminant hepatitis can occur after starting nevirapine. Rates higher in non-pregnant women than in men, esp. with higher CD4 count. Monitor LFTs, instruct mother to seek care for nausea, abdominal pain. Check transaminases in any woman who develops rash. Consider non-nevirapine containing regimens if CD4 count >250 unless benefits clearly outweigh risks.**

D. **Specific situations**
   1. **For pregnant women not on therapy with an indication for ARV therapy:** Evaluate clinical, virologic, social factors, & previous therapy. Obtain resistance testing. Discuss options, risks, & benefits. Begin therapy after 10–14wks gestation & after nausea has resolved, and certainly before 28 weeks, as long as adherence can be assured. See regimens in Table 6A Section D4. Avoid efavirenz.
   2. **For pregnant women not on therapy who do not otherwise require ARV therapy:** As for women who need therapy for their own health, and combination therapy is strongly preferred. Begin ARV's after 1st tri
   3. **For women on antiretroviral therapy when pregnancy is diagnosed:** If pregnancy dx after 1st tri, continue therapy, modify as necessary. Efavirenz & combination stavudine/didanosine must be avoided. If pregnancy dx in 1st tri, most experts would continue therapy to avoid viral rebound. If the decision is made to stop until the 2nd trimester, all drugs should be stopped at once, with attention to ½ lives.
   4. **For women in labor with no prior therapy:** Several options may be considered:
      - Intrapartum IV ZDV & 4–6wks of po ZDV for the infant
      - Intrapartum ZDV & 3TC, followed by 1wk of ZDV & 3TC for the infant
      - 2-part nevirapine regimen with intrapartum po nevirapine (200mg) and zidovudine followed by single dose for the infant (2mg/kg). High risk of nevirapine resistance. Consider following option
      - Intrapartum nevirapine combined with ZDV & 3TC, followed by po nevirapine for the infant & 4–6wks po ZDV. Strongly consider 1wk of ZDV & 3TC for mother to reduce nevirapine resistance in the mother.
      - C-section is likely to provide additional benefit if membranes have not ruptured. There is no evidence of benefit in preventing MTCT for emergency C-section *(see D.)*
      - Evaluate mother's need for ongoing ARV RX after delivery.
   5. **For infants born to HIV-infected women who did not receive therapy:**
      - Offer po ZDV to the infant begun as soon as possible & continue for 6wks
      - Some experts would use additional agents, e.g., ZDV & 3TC, or ZDV, 3TC & single dose nevirapine
   6. **HIV-infected women who are ARV experienced and not suppressed when becoming pregnant:**
      - Counsel about adherence, address issues contributing to difficulties. Discuss unknown safety and dosing of newer agents in pregnancy.
      - Obtain ARV history and viral resistance testing. Expert consultation recommended. For maternal health, constructing new regimen may be essential, despite uncertainties of new agents in pregnancy
      - If viral load not <1000 copies/mL on new regimen, strongly consider scheduled elective C-section
E. **Elective C-section before the onset of labor** ↓ transmission by 50% for women on no therapy or ZDV monotherapy *(NEJM 340:977, 1999)*. However, in recent cohorts on effective therapy, no apparent additional benefit of C-section was observed.
   - This should be discussed with the woman & she should be involved in the decision.
   - Elective C-section (before 38 weeks) should be considered if:
     - Maternal viral load >1000 at delivery despite ARV RX

TABLE 8A (3)

- Mother received less than 3-drug therapy
- Mother presents late in pregnancy
- Obstetrical indications or maternal preference
- Elective C-section is not cost-effective in resource-poor settings

F. **PCP prophylaxis:** Recommended for women with CD4 count <200 or on prophylaxis. PCP during pregnancy can be more severe.
- **TMP/SMX** may be used, although use in last trimester may be associated with ↑ bilirubin. Risk of kernicterus unknown but very small. TMP/SXZ reduced maternal & infant mortality among mothers with CD4 < 200 in resource poor setting.
- **Dapsone:** no known adverse effects, although experience limited.
- **Aerosolized pentamidine.** Little systemic absorption, although less effective in advanced disease. Effect of ventilation changes due to pregnancy on distribution is unknown.

TABLE 8B: HIV IN THE FETUS & NEWBORN

GENERAL:
- In 2006, fewer than 100, only an est 48 children in the U.S. were diagnosed with AIDS, compared to an est 800,000 children newly infected with HIV worldwide. In the U.S., 1695 children were living with an AIDS diagnosis in 2004 & an additional 3000–3500 are living with HIV. Worldwide, an estimated 2.7 million children are living with HIV.
- In 1995, an est 7,000 HIV-infected women gave birth. This number has ↑substantially, but accurate est. aren't available
- Thus, the success of HIV testing of pregnant women & intrapartum treatment in Western countries dramatically ↓ HIV infection in children. Universal testing & counseling **must be offered to all pregnant women** to improve this.
- At the same time, millions of children are infected in resource-poor settings.
- In the U.S., 73% of children living with AIDS in 2006 were black, 11% Hispanic, & 10% white. Injection drug use identified as a risk factor for a minority of mothers; most due to demonstrated or presumed heterosexual transmission.

TRANSMISSION[1]:
- **Over 90% of HIV+ children in U.S. acquired infection from their mothers perinatally:** in utero, during delivery, or postpartum through breastfeeding. Risk of transmission 13–40% (http://aidsinfo.nih.gov/guidelines).
- **Time of transmission:**
  - In utero: HIV has been identified in fetal tissues as early as 8 weeks. Probably in the majority, in utero transmission occurs late in pregnancy *(Lancet 345:518, 1995)*.
  - Intrapartum: 50–70% of transmissions believed to occur through exposure to mother's blood, cervical secretions or amniotic fluid during delivery.
  - Postpartum acquisition rare in developed countries, important in developing countries. Breast-fed infants have a 10-14% add'l risk of becoming infected. In mothers seroconverting during lactation, risk is 1/3 *(Lancet 342:1437, 1993)*.

DIAGNOSIS: *(See Table 8C, below)*
- HIV can be diagnosed in most infants by 1mo & all infants by 6mos of age by demonstration of virus by viral culture, viral DNA PCR, or viral RNA PCR.
- DNA PCR is currently considered the preferred method because of more supportive data (http://aidsinfo.nih.gov/guidelines), but RNA PCR (e.g., Roche Amplicor) may be more sensitive *(JID 175:707, 1997; J AIDS 32:192, 2003)*. Some experts perform both assays.
- Maternal anti-HIV IgG crosses the placenta & persists until 9–15mos, so infants born to HIV-infected mothers may test positive for up to 15mos regardless of infection. Assays for p24 antigen are less sensitive & less specific than PCR.
- PCR should be performed:
  - By age 48hrs (not on cord blood) (Some clinicians omit this test)
  - At 2–3wks
  - At 4–8wks
  - Repeat at 4–6mos if initial tests negative
- Any pos test should be repeated immediately along with quantitative HIV RNA PCR (viral load) before treatment begun.
- Presumptive evidence of in utero infection is PCR positive in 1st 48 hours of life. Intrapartum infection defined by negative test in 1st 48 hours followed by positive test *(NEJM 275:606, 1995)*.
- If PCR is not available, HIV can be diagnosed by persistence of HIV antibody after 18 months of age.
- HIV infection can be presumptively excluded by 2 negative PCRs; one at > 14 days and one at > 1 month; HIV is definitively excluded (in absence of breast feeding) by at least 2 negative PCR tests; one at >1 month and one at >4 months.

NATURAL HISTORY:
Bimodal distribution. Approximately 20% will be rapid progressors with onset of symptoms by median 8 months & median survival of <2yrs. Median survival, untreated, for non-rapid progressors was 66mos. Survival has greatly ↑ in the era of ARV RX, & many perinatally infected children are reaching adolescence & young adulthood.

---

[1] *From Pediatric AIDS, A. Pavia, Medical Mgmt of AIDS, 6th Ed., Eds. M.A. Sande, P.A. Volberding, W.B. Saunders & Co., 1999.*

TABLE 8C: HIV INFECTION IN CHILDREN

1. HIV-Infected
   - Child <18mos known to be HIV+ or born to HIV+ mother **&** has positive results on 2 separate determinations from one or more: HIV culture, HIV PCR, HIV 24 antigen.
   - Child ≥18mos born to HIV+ mother or infected by blood products, sexual contact who is HIV antibody + by ELISA & Western blot or + HIV culture, PCR or p24 antigen.

2. Perinatally Exposed: A child who does not meet criteria above but
   - is HIV seropositive & <18mos of age
   - unknown antibody status but born to HIV+ mother

3. Seroreverter: (CDC definition): A child born to HIV+ mother: Documented HIV negative (2 or more neg. EIA at 6–18mos, or 1 neg. EIA at >18mos) & no other lab evidence of infection & not had an AIDS-defining condition

4. HIV-uninfected (definitive): Child with 2 or more HIV PCR assays which are neg after 1mo of age & 1 assay negative after 4mos

1994 CDC PEDIATRIC HIV CLASSIFICATION[1]

Immunologic Categories	Clinical Categories (Level of Signs/Symptoms)			
	N: None	A: Mild	B: Moderate	C: Severe
1: No evidence of suppression	N1	A1	B1	C1
2: Evidence of moderate suppression	N2	A2	B2	C2
3: Severe suppression	N3	A3	B3	C3

Immunologic Categories (CD4 counts change with age)

Immunologic Category	Age of Child					
	<12mos		1–5yrs		6–12yrs	
	CD4 μL	(%)	CD4 μL	(%)	CD4 μL	(%)
1: No evidence of suppression	≥1,500	(≥25)	≥1,000	(≥25)	≥500	(≥25)
2: Evidence of moderate suppression	750–1,499	(15–24)	500–999	(15–24)	200–499	(15–24)
3: Severe suppression	<750	(<15)	<500	(<15)	<200	(<15)

WHO STAGING SYSTEM FOR HIV INFECTION & DISEASE IN CHILDREN

Clinical Stage I:
1. Asymptomatic
2. Generalized lymphadenopathy

Clinical Stage II:
3. Chronic diarrhea >30 days duration in absence of known etiology
4. Severe persistent or recurrent candidiasis outside of the neonatal period
5. Weight loss or failure to thrive in absence of known etiology
6. Persistent fever >30 days duration in absence of known etiology
7. Recurrent severe bacterial infections other than septicemia or meningitis, e.g., osteomyelitis, bacterial (non-TB pneumonia, abscesses)

Clinical Stage III:
8. AIDS-defining opportunistic infection
9. Severe failure to thrive in absence of known etiology
10. Progressive encephalopathy
11. Malignancy
12. Recurrent septicemia or meningitis

---

[1] 1994 revised classification system for HIV infection in children less than 13yrs of age [MMWR 43(RR-12):1–10, 1994]

TABLE 8D: INITIATION OF ANTIRETROVIRAL THERAPY, P. CARINII PROPHYLAXIS, & SUPPORTIVE THERAPY [MMWR 47(RR-8):1, 2002. http://aidsinfo.nih.gov/guidelines]

A. P. carinii Prophylaxis—Revised Guidelines

1. In infants with perinatally acquired HIV, PCP occurs most frequently at 3–6mos, often acute in onset with poor prognosis. HIV+ infants <1yr of age at risk even with CD4 ≥1500.
   - Identify infants born to HIV+ mothers promptly (screen mothers during pregnancy), obtain PCR or viral culture as described above.
   - Begin PCP prophylaxis at–6wks in infants born to HIV-infected mothers who are HIV positive or who remain indeterminate.
   - Stop prophylaxis in children found to be HIV-negative (e.g., 2 negative PCRs; one obtained after 14 days and one after 1mo of age)
   - Continued PCP prophylaxis in HIV-infected children depends on immunologic stage (see previous page). Recommended for all children Immunologic Category 3. If CD4 not available, use for WHO Clinical Stages II & III. Some would give to all HIV+ children in resource-poor country.

2. Drug Regimens for PCP Prophylaxis in Children ≥4Wks of Age:
   - **TMP/SMX (150mg TMP/M^2/day)** po divided twice daily 3x/wk on consecutive days (i.e., Mon., Tues., Wed.). Alternatives: same daily dose 1x/day, divided q12h 7 days/wk or q12h on alternate days. Once-daily regimen may be best for adherence.
   - If TMP/SMX not tolerated:
     - **Dapsone 2mg/kg po 1x/day** (not to exceed 100mg) or 4mg/kg po q wk
     - **Aerosolized pentamidine (children ≥5yrs)** 300mg via Respirgard II inhaler monthly
     - **Atovaquone 30mg/kg po q24h** for children 1–3mos old. Atovaquone 45mg/kg po q24h for children 4–24mos.
     - **IV pentamidine 4mg/kg q2 or 4wks** when other options are not available

B. Antiretroviral Therapy

1. **When to start:** This decision is much more complex in children than in adults. Data specific to outcomes in children are limited, & clinical trial data do not address when to start. Natural history studies in children & extrapolation from adult studies are used to derive guidelines. Some factors argue for **early** treatment in children:
   - 25–35% of HIV-infected children will be rapid progressors
   - Viral load & CD4 are associated with rapid progression but cannot accurately identify all rapid progressors in first year of life
   - The CHER study in South Africa demonstrated improved survival in asymptomatic infected infants when therapy was started at < 12 wks compared to waiting for symptoms (4th AIDS Conference on HIV Pathogenesis, Treatment and Prevention 2007 Sydney Abstract LB WES103).
   - Immune control of virus limited in first year of life
   - HIV encephalopathy, other neurological disease & cardiac involvement may occur at young age
   - Some trials of early therapy have shown promising results

   Some factors favor more **delayed** institution of therapy:
   - Slow progressors may maintain good immune function for many years without treatment
   - Limited number of drugs with liquid formulation
   - Highly variable & inadequately understood pharmacokinetics of ARVs in children may lead to inadequate levels & drug failure
   - Metabolic complications, including abnormal lipids, glucose intolerance, fat redistribution & possibly bone mineral abnormalities can occur in children
   - Children may have excellent immune reconstitution even with advanced disease
   - Difficulties with adherence are common & lead to drug failure
   - Children may rapidly run out of treatment options

Three sets of guidelines have been developed. They share several features. In infants who are known to be HIV-infected, they favor starting therapy in all infants, due to the inability to identify rapid progressors. In older children, the guidelines favor treatment when the child reaches a more advanced disease stage. All emphasize the need for education to ensure adherence, & routine monitoring for efficacy & safety:

RECOMMENDATIONS FOR BEGINNING TREATMENT IN INFANTS & CHILDREN

	DHHS	PENTA	WHO
Infants (< 1 yr)	All infants regardless of symptoms or CD4 % **(Recommended)**	<1yr with CDC Category B or C disease or CD4% < 25-35% **(Recommended)**	<18mos, virologically confirmed infection with WHO Pediatric Stage III **(Recommended)**
		Younger than 1yr regardless of symptoms or CD4 % **(Consider)**	<18mos, virologically confirmed infection with WHO Pediatric Stage II (consider using CD4 <20%) **(Recommended)**
			<18mos, virologically confirmed infection with WHO Pediatric Stage I & CD4 <20% **(Recommended)**
			<18mos, HIV seropositive but virologic confirmation not available, WHO Pediatric Stage III & CD4 <20% **(Recommended)**
Children 1-<5 yrs	CDC Category B or C disease **or** CD4 <25% regardless of RNA level **(Recommended)**	CDC Category C disease **or** CD4 <20% if 1-3 or <15% if >4 **(Recommended)**	WHO Pediatric Stage III disease **or** CD4 <15% **(Recommended)**
	CDC Category A or N disease **and** CD4 >25% **and** viral load >5 log **(Consider)**	CDC Category B disease **or** CD4 <20% or viral load >5.3 log **(Consider)**	WHO Pediatric Stage II disease **(Recommended)**. Consider using CD4 <15% as a criterion

TABLE 8D (2)

Children ≥5 yrs	CDC Category B or C disease **or** CD4 <25% regardless of RNA level **(Recommended)** **CD4 count < 350 cells/ µL (Recommended)** CDC Category A or N disease **and** CD4 count > **350 cells/ µL and** viral load >5 log **(Consider)**	As for children 1-<5 yrs	As for children 1-<5 yrs

DHHS = Department of Health & Human Services (U.S.) Working Group updated Mar 13, 2008 (www.aidsinfo.nih.gov)
PENTA = Paediatric European Network for the Treatment of AIDS 2003 (www.pentatrials.org)
WHO = World Health Organization: Scaling up antiretroviral therapy in resource-limited settings (Draft: 2003 revision http://www.who.int/3by5/publications/documents/arv_guidelines/en/)

2. **Recommended therapy**
Combination therapy with at least 3 antiretroviral drugs is recommended for all children started on therapy. Choice of drugs depends on supporting data, age of the patient, local availability, & need for liquid formulation. WHO guidelines emphasize initial use of NNRTI-based regimens because of costs, local availability, & to complement adult guidelines. U.S. & European guidelines recommend either PI-based or NNRTI-based initial regimens, but recognize the risk of NNRTI-resistant virus being transmitted from mother to child (see below).

If available, resistance testing should be obtained for children before starting ARV RX, especially if an NNRTI is being considered. If the local prevalence of resistance is known, it may influence the need for resistance testing.

If abacavir therapy is being considered, HLA B*5701 screening can virtually eliminate risk of hypersensitivity reaction and should be obtained if available.

RECOMMENDED FIRST-LINE THERAPY FOR HIV-INFECTED INFANTS & CHILDREN

	DHHS	PENTA	WHO
Strongly recommended	2 NRTIs[1] **plus** lopinavir/ ritonavir **or** 2 NRTIs[1] **plus** nevirapine (if <3yrs) if >3yrs: 2 NRTIs1 plus efavirenz[3]	2 NRTIs[2] **plus** one PI (lopinavir/ritonavir **or** nelfinavir) 2 NRTIs **plus** 1 NNRTI (efavirenz **or** nevirapine)	If <3yrs **or** <10 kg: (ZDV **or** d4T) **plus** 3TC **plus** nevirapine If >3yrs **or** >10 kg: (ZDV **or** d4T) **plus** 3TC **plus** efavirenz
Alternative regimens	2 NRTIs **plus** fosamprenavir **plus** low dose ritonavir 2 NRTIs plus nevirapine (if >3yrs) 2 NRTIs plus nelfinavir (if >2 yrs) ZDV **plus** 3TC **plus** abacavir 2 NRTIs plus other ritonavir boosted PIs if adolescent who can receive adult dosage	2 NRTIs[2] **plus** abacavir	
Use in special circumstance	Two NRTIs **plus** fosamprenavir (children 2–6years old) Two NRTIsplus low-dose ritonavir **plus** atazanavir **or** indinavir **or** saquinavir in post-pubertal adolescents who weigh enough to receive adult doses Zidovudine plus lamivudine **plus** abacavir		
Insufficient data to recommend for initial therapy	Dual or boosted PIs, with the exception of lopinavir/ ritonavir and fosamprenavir/ritonavir NRTI **plus** NNRTI **plus** PI Tenofovir-containing regimens Tanner 1-3 Enfuvirtide (T-20)-containing regimens Darunavir-containing regimens Tipranavir-containing regimens Maraviroc-contaning regimens Raltegravir-containing regimens Etravirine-containing regimens		

[1] DHHS preferred NRTI combinations (alphabetical): ABC + (3TC or FTC); ddI + FTC; Tenofovir (Tanner 4 or 5 only) + (3TC or FTC); ZDV + (3TC or FTC)
DHHS alternative NRTI combinations: ABC+ ZDV; ddI + ZDV.
DHHS special circumstances: D4T + (3TC or FTC).
DHHS describes tenofovir-containing regimens as having inadequate data to recommend in pre-adolescents. Evidence of decreased bone mineralization in pediatric trials but clinical significance is unclear.
[2] PENTA acceptable NRTI combinations: ZDV + ddI; ZDV + 3TC; ZDV + ABC; 3TC + ABC; ddI + 3TC
[3] Must be able to swallow capsules

TABLE 8D (3)

AVOID: monotherapy, dual NRTI alone, d4T + ZDV, use of ddC. 3TC + FTC, **Adjust ddI dose if used with tenofovir.** d4T + ddI is effective **but** associated with a higher rate of side effects including lactic acidosis & lipoatrophy. Tenofovir +ABC + 3TC or Tenofovir + ddI + 3TC triple NRTI therapy associated with high rates of early failure. Nelfinavir not recommend for initial regimens until further notice because of ethyl methane sulfonate levels.

3. **Monitoring of children on antiretroviral therapy**
   Children should be monitored at 1-2 weeks after beginning a new antiretroviral regimen to check for adherence and adverse effects. When nevirapine is started, serum transaminases should be monitored at 2 and 4 weeks and then monthly for 3 months.
   Children on antiretroviral therapy should be followed at regular intervals, usually every 3mos.
   Clinical parameters:
   - Weight & height growth
   - Nutritional status
   - Developmental milestones & neurological symptoms
   - Adherence & side effects
   - No consensus on bone mineral density testing by DEXA but considered by some experts

   Laboratory monitoring should include: CBC with differential, CD4 % & count. If available, viral load, liver enzymes, creatinine, glucose, electrolytes, & total cholesterol should be monitored.

4. **Therapeutic drug monitoring**
   Age-related changes in drug metabolism & wide interpatient variability of drug levels along with generally low success rates suggest that therapeutic drug monitoring may be very useful for PIs & NNRTIs. In some European countries, therapeutic drug monitoring has become routine. Information on laboratories & on laboratory participation in quality assurance programs is available at www.hivpharmacology.com. Target minimum trough concentrations in table 6f and in the DHHS Guidelines for the Use Antiretroviral Agents at www.aidsinfo.nih.gov.

5. **When to change antiretroviral therapy**
   Deciding on when to change therapy can be a complex process that takes into account the remaining options, the level of adherence, the social situation & the clinical status. The goal of initial therapy is to suppress viral load to the lowest level possible, usually below the limits of quantification, & to allow the immune system to reconstitute. Ongoing viral replication permits the selection of resistant mutants, & will lead to increasing drug resistance. When initial therapy "fails," good treatment options are usually available. With subsequent treatment regimens, the number of remaining options becomes progressively limited.

   Ideally, the goal of subsequent regimens is to re-establish maximal viral suppression. With the availability of enfuvirtide, tipranavir, darunavir, raltegravir, maraviroc and etravirine, it has become possible to construct regimens for many treatment experienced adults that will control viral load to below the level of quantification. However, many of these agents are not yet available in formulations for children, and have limited data on appropriated dosing. It may be very difficult to address adherence issues in a timely manner.

   Many children with multiply drug-resistant virus who develop breakthrough viremia will still have stable or rising CD4 counts. Often the viral load remains significantly below the pretreatment baseline. In this situation, many experts weigh the option of continuing the current therapy as long as clinical & immune status are stable against the option of creating a new regimen that might exhaust remaining regimens. This may allow time to develop adequate data for use of newer agents, or allow the child or adolescent to become better able to succeed with the next regimen. The decision will depend on remaining options, clinical status, family preference, & family situation.

   Considerations on when to change are divided into virologic, immunologic, & clinical. These are not absolute. Clinical changes, however, are the clearest & most non-controversial indications for change of therapy:

Virologic considerations	• **Incomplete response:** Less than a minimally acceptable virologic response after 8–12wks of therapy (defined as a <10-fold (1.0 $\log_{10}$) decrease from baseline HIV RNA levels • HIV RNA not suppressed to undetectable levels after 4–6mos of antiretroviral therapy • **Viral Rebound:** Repeated detection of HIV RNA in children who initially had undetectable levels in response to antiretroviral therapy. Consider observation if rebound is to low level (<500 copies) • A reproducible ↑ in HIV RNA copy number among children who have had a substantial HIV RNA response but still have low levels of detectable HIV RNA. Such an ↑ would warrant change in therapy if, after achieving a virologic nadir, a >3-fold (>0.5 $\log_{10}$) ↑ in copy number for children aged >2yrs & >5-fold (>0.7 log10) ↑ is observed for children aged <2yrs
Immunologic considerations	• **Incomplete immunologic response to therapy:** Failure of a child with severe immune suppression (CD4 percentage <15%) to ↑ CD4 % by at least 5 points above baseline or, if > 5 years, ↑ CD4 cell count by at least 50 cells/mL above baseline over first year • **Immunologic decline:** Persistent ↓ of 5 percentagepoints in CD4 % or ↓ to below pre-therapy baseline in CD4 cell count > 5 yrs at baseline
Clinical considerations	• Progressive neurodevelopmental deterioration* • Growth failure: persistent decline in weight-growth velocity despite adequate nutritional support & without other explanation* • Severe or recurrent infection or illness – Recurrence or persistence of AIDS-defining conditions or other serious infections*
Toxicity	• It may be desirable to control some side effects (e.g., diarrhea) rather than changing therapy. If a single drug can be associated with the toxicity, it is acceptable to change the offending agent

* Criteria marked with asterisk are from WHO guidelines (& may overlap with DHHS recommendations). These may be particularly helpful in the resource-limited setting.

TABLE 8D (4)

6. **What to use as alternate therapy**
   There are limited data on sequencing antiviral therapy in HIV-infected children. Several general principles are useful:
   a. When treatment failure occurs, always assess adherence to the treatment
   b. Try to address adherence problems before changing regimens
   c. If adherence has been good, assume viral resistance has developed, but it may not have developed to all agents. Viral resistance testing, if available, should be performed. If possible, obtain viral resistance testing while on failing regimen. Without testing, all 3 drugs should be changed if possible.
   d. Take into account predicted cross-resistance
   e. Avoid dose reduction for toxicity unless levels can be measured
   f. Treatment failure may occur due to inadequate absorption or drug levels
   g. **The use of at least 2 new active drugs with non-overalapping resistance best predicts responsee. Never add a single drug to a regimen that is clearly failing**
   h. **Consider likelihood of availability of (or ability to use) new drugs in near future and try and construct regimen with 2-3 active drugs**

First-Line Regimen	Suggested Options
ZDV + 3TC	ABC + 3TC or FTC Tenofovir + 3TC or FTC Some would consider ZDV + (3TC or emtricitabine) + tenofovir
d4T + 3TC	ABC + 3TC or FTC Tenofovir + 3TC or FTC Some would consider ZDV + 3TC + tenofovir
NNRTI	Protease inhibitor: • Lopinavir/ritonavir • Fosamprenavir/ritonavir **Consider:** • **Atazanavir with ritonavir** • Saquinavir/ritonavir
Nelfinavir	NNRTI or boosted PI • Lopinavir/ritonavir • Fosamprenavir/ritonavir • Atazanavir + ritonavir • Consider darunavir or tipranavir + ritonavir
Ritonavir	NNRTI or boosted PI • Lopinavir/ritonavir (cross resistance likely) • **Fosamprenavir/ritonavir** • Atazanavir + ritonavir • Consider darunavir or tipranavir + ritonavir
Lopinavir/ritonavir	• NNRTI • Consider tipranavir or darunavir + ritonavir • Consider raltegravir • Consider maraviroc

Enfuvirtide (T-20) can be used in children as part of a salvage regimen, but should be used with 1 or 2 additional active drugs.

C. **Supportive Treatment & Prophylaxis**

1. Intravenous gamma globulin (IVIG)
   a. Not routinely used. Recommended for infants & children with evidence of humoral immune defects (hypogammaglobulinemia or documented failure to form specific antibody responses) IVIG 400mg/kg q28 days is recommended.
   b. Thrombocytopenia (<20,000/mm³) on antiretroviral therapy: IVIG 0.5–1gm/kg/dose x3–5 days *(See Table 22 for Winrho®)*
2. Immunization: *See Table 19*
3. Pneumocystis carinii: *See above, Section A*
4. Mycobacterium avium complex: prophylaxis recommended *[MMWR 46(RR-12), 1997]*. Begin if CD4 <50 for children ≥6yrs; for children 2–6yrs, begin if CD4 <75; for 1–2yrs if CD4 <500; <1yr CD4 <750. Clarithromycin 7.5mg/kg po q12h or azithromycin 20mg/kg po once weekly is preferred. Rifabutin now used as 3rd-line, 5mg/kg po once daily (only for children ≥6yrs). Dose of rifabutin should not exceed 300mg/day.
5. Psychosocial support *(see Am Acad Pediatrics, Red Book, 1994)*: School attendance, child/foster care, adolescent education

TABLE 8E: CLINICAL SYNDROMES, OPPORTUNISTIC INFECTIONS, IN INFANTS & CHILDREN, WHICH DIFFER FROM ADULTS*

In HIV-infected infants & children, disease progression is manifest by decrements in growth & delayed neurodevelopment as well as opportunistic infections as occur in adults
(J Ped 128:58, 1996)

CLINICAL SYNDROME	INFANT/CHILD	ADULT	CLINICAL FEATURES (in children)/COMMENTS
Central Nervous System Encephalopathy			General: HIV encephalopathy is a syndrome that includes motor & cognitive dysfunction seen in pts with advanced HIV. Administration of ARV therapy has been shown to be beneficial in treating children with HIV encephalopathy.
Static course	Common	0	25% children show cognitive & motor deficits. Most have head circumference in 10–25th percentile. Problems with verbal expression, attention deficits, hyperactivity. Mild ↑ reflexes in legs to spastic diplegia. IQ stable.
Plateau course	Uncommon	0	Infant's or child's gain of cognitive or motor skills plateaus. Motor deficits are common. IQ usually only 50–79.
Subacute progressive course	Uncommon	AIDS dementia common	Gradual progressive decline in motor, language, adaptive function. Early, child is alert, wide-eyed, with a paucity of facial movements. Endstage: mute, dull-eyed, quadriparetic. CSF: mild pleocytosis, ↑ protein, may be + for HIV antibody & virus. CT: atrophy, progressive calcification in basal ganglia (most common in infants & young children).
Focal brain diseases: seizures, focal neurologic deficits			
Infections Toxoplasmosis	V. rare	Common	Toxo is uncommon in infants & children since it is most often due to reactivation.
Progressive multifocal leuko-encephalopathy (JC virus)	V. rare	Common	PML is uncommon in infants & children since it is most often due to reactivation.
Endocrine Failure to thrive & growth retardation	Common	Wasting syndrome common	33/36 HIV+ children showed failure to thrive, not purely related to diarrhea & malnutrition. Known causes of growth failure are growth hormone deficiency, hypothyroidism, & glucocorticoid excess. 1/3 of HIV+ children have abnormal thyroid function (↑ thyrotropin, ↑ TBG) which correlates with disease progression (J Ped 128:70, 1996).
Eye Cytomegalovirus retinitis	Uncommon	Common	CMV chorioretinitis in 1.6% children vs 10–20% in adults (Arch Ophthal 107:978, 1989). In children it usually occurs with generalized CMV infection, viremia & multiple organ involvement. When present, ocular lesions are same as in adults, Table 11A, page 110.
Retinal depigmentation, on ZDV	~5%	0	Asymptomatic peripheral retinal depigmentation (dosages >300 mg/M²/day)
HIV-associated "cotton wool" spots	Rare	Common	Seen only in children >8–10yrs, while seen in 60–70% of adults.
Gastrointestinal Tract Mouth Kaposi's sarcoma	V. rare	Common	More prevalent in HIV+ children in areas of Africa.
Esophagus Dysphagia, odynophagia	Uncommon	Common	When pain/difficulty occur, children more likely to refuse to eat. CMV—odynophagia, Candida—dysphagia.
Diarrhea	Common	Common	Most common agents: rotavirus 24% (more common in inpatient setting), salmonella (19%), campylobacter (8%) (more common in outpatients). Presence of blood &/or WBC in stool has high positive predictive value for salmonella or campylobacter (PIDJ 15:876, 1996).

TABLE 8E (2)

CLINICAL SYNDROME	INFANT/CHILD	ADULT	CLINICAL FEATURES (in children)/COMMENTS
Heart			
Cardiomyopathy	Common	Common	Abnormal ECG changes (ventricular hypertrophy & non-specific ST-T changes) in 55–93% HIV+ children.
	Common	Uncommon	Left ventricular dysfunction 29–74% (most important cardiac change). 20% transient or chronic congestive failure. Unexpected cardiorespiratory arrests in 8/81 (JAMA 269:2869, 1993). Pericardial effusions & tamponade have been noted frequently in children (PIDJ 15:819, 1996).
Hematologic			
Hypergammaglobulinemia	Common	Uncommon	By age 6mos, almost all HIV+ children have ↑ gamma-globulins.
Protein S (coagulation inhibitor)	Common	Common	19/26 children had ↓ levels, but risk of thrombosis low (Ped IDJ 15:106, 1996). Adults, ↑ protein S in 27–73%, thrombotic complications in 12%.
Hepatobiliary	Rare	Common	Very few reports relating to children. Etiologies such as AIDS cholangiopathy, peliosis hepatis (bacillary angiomatosis) not reported. 2 cases of fatal hepatic necrosis associated with adenovirus reported (Rev Inf Dis 12:303, 1990).
Lung			
Tuberculosis	Uncommon	Common	Virtually all are primary infections. Clinical: fever, cough. X-ray: often focal infiltrates with hilar adenopathy, cavitation uncommon.
Lymphocytic interstitial pneumonitis (LIP)	Common	V. rare	LIP occurs in 40% of children with perinatally acquired HIV. HIV & EBV antigens have been demonstrated in lung tissue. Usually diagnosed in children >1yr as compared with PCP which is most common in first year. LIP has better prognosis than PCP. Median survival is ~5x shorter in children diagnosed with PCP than in children with LIP (Lancet 348:866, 1996). Clinical: slowly progressive tachypnea, cough, wheezing, hypoxemia. Rales are infrequent. Clubbing of digits is characteristic. Generalized lymphadenopathy, hepatosplenomegaly & parotid swelling. X-ray: diffuse reticulonodular infiltrates associated with hilar lymphadenopathy. Bacterial superinfection is common. Diagnosis by lung biopsy. Rx: steroids may be of some benefit.
Cryptococcosis	Uncommon	Common	Disseminated infection or localized process of the lungs. Intermittent fever is most common presenting manifestation. All pts have low CD4, history of previous OIs, & onset of cryptococcosis most commonly in 2nd decade of life (PIDJ 15: 796, 1996).
Congestive heart failure	Common	Uncommon	See Heart, above
Leiomyosarcoma	Rare (but ↑)	V. rare	EBV demonstrated by PCR in tumors (NEJM 332:12, 1995)
Renal			
Nephropathy	Common	Rare	Nephropathy observed in 29% children with perinatal AIDS (Kidney 31:1167, 1987). In children may present with nephrotic syndrome with a course of 12–18mos (NEJM 321:625, 1989). Steroid rx may be of value.
"Sepsis"	Common	Uncommon	25% of symptomatic HIV+ children will have bacteremic episodes, most due to bacteremic pneumonia or bacteremia without a focus (Pediatric AIDS, Eds. P.A. Pizzo, C.M. Wilfert, Ch. 13, page 199, 1991).
Fungemia (a nosocomially-acquired infection)			Risk factors: central venous catheter (>90 days), prior antibiotic therapy (>3 different antibiotics, parenteral ↑ risk), parenteral hyperalimentation, hemodialysis, prolonged neutropenia, colonization by Candida species (CID 23:515, 1996)
Skin			
Impetigo	Common	Uncommon	Due to Staph. aureus or Group A strep. Clinical: areas of erythema with "honey crusting." May be widespread & evolve into "cellulitis." Increasing incidence of MRSA skin & soft tissue infections

TABLE 8F: SELECTED DRUGS COMMONLY USED IN CHILDREN WITH HIV INFECTION

INDICATION/DRUG	DOSAGE	FORMULATIONS	COMMENTS
Antifungal Drugs			
Amphotericin B	0.5–1 mg/kg/day IV (same as adult, see Table 12, pages 135)	Same as adult	
Ampho B lipid complex	5 mg/kg/day IV as for adults		
Caspofungin	75 mg/M² IV q24h loading dose then 50 mg/M² IV q24h	Same as adult	
Fluconazole			**Adult Dose** / **Pediatric Equivalent**
Oral/esophageal candidiasis	6–12 mg/kg/day	Oral suspension (orange-flavored), 50 mg/5ml (teaspoon)	100 mg / 3 mg/kg
Systemic candidiasis	12 mg/kg/day po		200 mg / 6 mg/kg
Cryptococcal meningitis			400 mg / 12 mg/kg (not to exceed 600 mg/day)
Treatment	12 mg/kg po 1st day, then 6 (to 12) mg/kg/day po		
Suppression	6 mg/kg/day po		
Itraconazole	3 mg/kg po q24h (capsules) 5 mg/kg po q24h (suspension)	Oral suspension 10 mg/ml	Efficacy & safety not established. Extensive drug-drug interactions Bioavailability of capsules is low & variable Administer suspension on empty stomach with 4-6 oz of Coca-Cola.
Voriconazole	6 mg/kg q12h x2 then 4 mg/kg q 12h	Capsules 50 mg, 200 mg Oral suspension 40 mg/mL	Extensive drug-drug interactions Reversible visual disturbance in 20%
Anti-HIV Drugs[1]			
Nucleoside analogue reverse transcriptase inhibitors (NRTIs)			
Abacavir (Ziagen)	8 mg/kg 2x/daily not to exceed 300mg Neonatal dose unknown Adolescent/adult dose 300mg 2x/day or 600mg 1x/day	Solution 20 mg/ml 300 mg tablets Fixed combination 600 mg with 300 mg lamivudine (Epzicom) Fixed combination 300 mg with 300 mg zidovudine & 150 mg lamivudine (Trizivir)	Hypersensitivity reaction in ~5%, may be difficult to recognize. Rechallenge may be fatal. Hypersensitivity associated with HLA B*5701. Screening for HLA B*5701 virtually eliminates hypersensitivity reactions and should be considered if available

[1] Adolescents ≥ Tanner 4 should be dosed according to adult dosing (see Table 6B)

TABLE 8F (2)

INDICATION/DRUG	DOSAGE	FORMULATIONS	COMMENTS
Anti-HIV Drugs/Nucleoside analogue reverse transcriptase inhibitors (NRTIs) *(continued)*			
Didanosine (ddI, Videx)	120 mg/M² q12h not to exceed 200mg per dose. 240 mg/M² q24h not to exceed 400mg per dose if > 3 and treatment naive Body weight 40-60kg: Videx EC 250mg once daily Body weight >60kg: Videx EC 400mg once daily Videx EC 240 mg/M² appropriate in small PK study *(Antivir Ther 7:267, 2002)* Neonatal dose (2 weeks-8 months): 100 mg/M² q12h	Pediatric powder (when reconstituted with antacid): 10 mg/ml Delayed-release capsules (enteric-coated beadlets): Videx EC 125, 200, 250, 400 mg Generic delayed-release capsules 200, 250, 400 mg	Dose on empty stomach. Reduce didanosine dose if combined with tenofovir. Do not administer with ribavirin
Emtricitabine (Emtriva)	Consider using 50 mg/M² q12h if <4 months 6 mg/kg 1x/day 3 months of age to 17 years or 33kg 200 mg 1x/day if > 33kg Small study in neonates < 3months used 3 mg/kg 1x/day (CROI 2006 Abstr 568) Adolescent/adult dose 200 mg 1x/day	Solution 10 mg/mL Tablet 200 mg Fixed combination 200 mg with 300 mg tenofovir (Truvada) Fixed combination 200 mg with 300 mg tenofovir, 600 mg efavirenz (Atriplia)	24-wk data on emtricitabine, didanosine & efavirenz once daily showed good response in children *(11th CROI, 2004, Abst. 936)*. Efavirenz AUC slightly ↓ than target. Emtricitabine, stavudine, & lopinavir/ritonavir was well tolerated & very effective in pediatric trials *(Intl AIDS Conf, 2004, Abst Tu PeB 4431)*.

Lamivudine (3TC, Epivir)	4 mg/kg 2x/day
	Neonatal dose (<30 days): 2 mg/kg 2x/day
	Wt based recommendations for tablet
	Body weight 14-21kg: 75 mg po 2x/day
	  21-30kg: 75 mg AM/150 mg PM
	  >30kg: 150 mg po 2x/day
	Adolescent/adult dose (weight >30kg) 150 mg 2x/day or 300 mg once daily
		Solution 10 mg/ml (Epivir) 5 mg/mL (Epivir HBV)
		Tablets 100 mg, 150 (scored), 300 mg
		Fixed combination 150 mg with 300 mg ZDV (Combivir)
		Fixed combination 150 mg with 300 mg ZDV, 300mg abacavir (Trizivir)
		Fixed combination 300 mg with 600 mg Abacavir (Epzicom)	

Stavudine (d4T, Zerit)	Body weight <30kg: 1 mg/kg 2x/day
	  30-60kg: 30 mg 2x/day
	  >60kg: 40 mg 2x/day
	Neonatal dose birth to 13 days 0 mg/kg 2x/day
		Solution 1 mg/ml
		Capsules 15, 20, 30, 40 mg
			Better tolerated than zidovudine but more strongly associated with lipoatrophy, peripheral neuropathy. Combination with ddI associated with increased risk of lactic acidosis

Zidovudine (ZDV, AZT, Retrovir)	160 mg/M² q8h or 180-240 mg/M² q12h Adolescent/adult dose 300 mg 2x/day Neonatal dose (age <6wks) 2 mg/kg po q6h; 1.5 mg/kg IV q6h. Premature infant 1.5 mg/kg IV or 2 mg/kg po q 12h. Increase to q 8h at 2wks (>30wks EGA or at 4wks <30wks EGA)	Syrup 10 mg/ml Capsules 100 mg Tablets 300 mg Generic syrup 10 mg/mL & tablets 300 mg 10 mg/ml IV Fixed combination 300 mg with 150 mg 3TC (Combivir) Fixed combination 300 mg with 150 mg 3TC, 300mg abacavir (Trizivir)	

TABLE 8F (3)

INDICATION/DRUG	DOSAGE	FORMULATIONS	COMMENTS
Anti-HIV Drugs *(continued)*			
Nucleotide reverse transcriptase inhibitor (NtRTI)			
Tenofovir (Viread)	Pediatric dose currently under study, not yet approved. 8 mg/kg once daily for children age 2–8 Median dose in concentration controlled Phase III study 210 mg/M² target dose. Neonatal dose unknown Adult dose 300 mg 1x/day	Tablets 300 mg Tablets 75 mg (investigational) Tablets dissolve in water, orange or grape juice Powder formulation under development Fixed combination 300 mg with 200 mg emtricitabine (Truvada) Fixed combination 300 mg with 200 mg emtricitabine and 600 mg efavirenz (Atriplia)	↓ bone mineral density observed in young animals. ↓ BMD was prevalent in HIV-infected children before treatment; small ↓ in BMD in 5/15 at 1yr in 1 study (*Pediatrics* 116:e846,2005). No change compared to controls at 1yr in another (*JAIDS* 40:448, 2005). Use with caution & decrease dose if any renal impairment. Decrease ddl dose if used with tenofovir
Non-nucleoside reverse transcriptase inhibitors (NNRTIs)			
Delaviridine (Rescriptor)	Pediatric dose not established Neonatal dose unknown Adolescent/adult dose 600 mg 2x/day or 400 mg 3x/day	Tablets 100, 200 mg	Not approved for children, limited clinical use
Efavirenz (Sustiva)	**10–15kg, 200 mg; 15–20kg, 250 mg; 20–25kg, 300 mg; 25–32.5kg, 350 mg; 32.5–40kg, 400 mg; >40kg, 600 mg—all 1x/day** Neonatal dose unknown/not approved for infants Adult dose 600 mg 1x/day	Capsules 50, 100, 200 mg Tablets 600 mg Fixed combination 600 mg with Tenofovir 300 mg/Emtricitabine 200 mg (Atriplia) Liquid preparation used in PACTG 382 (contact BMS to check on availability)	Give at night to reduce CNS side-effects. Capsules can be opened & added to food or liquid but contents have peppery taste. Atriplia should be administered on an empty stomach. Minimum weight for Atriplia 40 kg. Lowers concentration of unboosted PIs and LPV/ritonavir. Pregnancy Class D. Avoid if possibility of pregnancy
Etravirine (Intelence)	Not approved in children. No PK data available for children <5 years. In children 6-17 years, 4 mg/kg 2x/day with food yielded exposure similar to adult dosing. Higher dose (5.2 mg/kg2x/day with food) under study. CROI 2008 abstr 578	Tablets 100 mg Tablet 25 mg used in research	Administer with food. Tablets disperse in water. Glass should be rinsed with water and the rinses swallowed to ensure consuming the entire dose
Nevirapine (Viramune)	Adolescent/adult dose 200 mg 2x/day with food <8yrs of age, 7 mg/kg 2x/day or 200 mg/M² >8yrs of age, 4 mg/kg 2x/day or 150 mg/M² **Note:** Initiate dosing once daily x14d; if no rash, ↑ to 2x/day. **Dosing by M² preferred** Neonatal dose 5 mg/kg or 120 mg/M² 1x/day x14d, then 120 mg/M² 2x/day x14d, then 200 mg/M² 2x/day Adolescent/adult dose 200 mg 1x/day x14d then 200 mg 2x/day	Suspension 10 mg/ml Tablets 200 mg	Do not dose-escalate in presence of rash. If rash is associated with fever, oral lesions, conjunctivitis, blistering, or hepatitis, stop medication immediately. Severe cholestatic hepatitis & Stevens-Johnson syndrome are rare but life-threatening complications that may occur in the 1st 6wks. In adults, risk of severe toxicity increased in women with CD4 > 250 & men with CD4 > 400 Lowers concentration of LPV/ritonavir

TABLE 8F (4)

INDICATION/DRUG	DOSAGE	FORMULATIONS	COMMENTS
Anti-HIV Drugs *(continued)*			
Protease Inhibitors			
Atazanavir (Reyataz)	PACTG 1020a demonstrated boosting with ritonavir is necessary in children. Preliminary recommendations from PACTG 1020b (CROI 2007 Abstr 715): 3m-13 yrs ATV powder 310 mg/M² 1x/day + ritonavir 100 mg/M² >6 yrs ATV capsules 205 mg/M² 1x/day + ritonavir 100 mg/M² Neonatal use not recommended Adolescent/adult dose 400 mg 1x/day or 300 mg + 100mg ritonavir both 1x/day	Capsules 100, 150, 200 mg, 300 mg	Administer with food. Wide variability in levels in children with unboosted atazanavir. Ritonavir-boosted atazanavir may give more consistent levels. Avoid in infants due to ↑ bilirubin. Do not co-administer with proton pump inhibitors. Boost with ritonavir if co-administered with tenofovir or efavirenz.
Darunavir (Prezista)	Not approved in children, data available for children > 5 years. Must be given with ritonavir. Preliminary recommendation from DELPHI (CROI 2008 Abstr 78LB 20-29kg: darunavir 375mg + ritonavir 50mg 2x/day 30-39kg: durunavir 450mg + ritonavir 60mg 2x/day >40kg: Adult dose Adult/adolescent dose 600mg + ritonavir 100mg 2x/day	Tablets 300 mg 600 mg Tablets 75 mg used in research	Active against many strains with extensive protease inhibitor resistance. Potential for many drug-drug interactions. Review other medications. Drug exposure in DELPHI similar to adult

Fosamprenavir (Lexiva)	2-5 yrs naïve only: 30 mg/kg 2x/day (not to exceed adult dose of 1400 mg 2x/day)
	6-11 naïve or experienced: 18mg/kg + ritonavir 3 mg/kg 2x/day (not to exceed adult dose of 700 mg + 100 mg ritonavir 2x/day)
	Neonatal use not recommended
	Adolescent/adult dose:
	Antiretroviral naïve:
	  1400 mg 2x/day
	  700 mg + 100 mg ritonavir 2x/day
	  1400 mg + 100 or 200 mg ritonavir 1x/day
	Antiretroviral experienced: 700mg + 100mg ritonavir 2x/day
		Tablet 700 mg (equivalent to 600mg amprenavir)
		Oral suspension 50 mg/mL
			Administer with or without food
			Data are not adequate to recommend a dose of antiretroviral experience children 2-5 years

Indinavir (Crixivan)	500mg/M² q8h (not approved) Adolescent/adult dose 800mg q8h or 800 mg + ritonavir 100 or 200m g 2x/day	Capsules 200, 400 mg	Response associated with C_{min} (AAC 44:1029, 2000). Consider measuring C_{min} if available & adjusting dose. Nephrolithiasis in 20% of children

TABLE 8F (5)

INDICATION/DRUG	DOSAGE	FORMULATIONS	COMMENTS
Anti-HIV Drugs/Protease Inhibitors (continued)			
Lopinavir/ritonavir (Kaletra)	230 mg/M^2 lopinavir/57.5 mg/M^2 ritonavir 2x/day with food if not taking nevirapine, efavirenz or fosamprenavir or weight based dosing: 7–15kg: 12 mg/kg lopinavir; 15–40kg: 10 mg/kg lopinavir Alternate: 7–1 kg 1.25 mL >10–<15kg 1.75 mL 15–20kg 2.25 mL or 100/25 mg tab 2x/day >20–25kg 2.75 mL or 100/25 mg tab 2x/day >25–30kg 3.5 mL or 100/25 mg tab 3/day >30–35kg 4 mL or 100/25 mg tab 3/day >35–40kg 4.75 mL or 200/50 mg tab 2x/day >40kg 5 mL or 200/50 mg tab 2x/day 300mg/ M^2 lopinavir/75mg/M^2 ritonavir with nevirapine, efavirenz or fosamprenavir or weight-based dosing: 7–15kg: 13mg/kg; 15–50kg: 11mg/kg Neonatal dose investigational 300 mg/75 mg/M^2 2x/day (yields good exposure and virologic response (AIDS 11:249 2008) Adolescent/adult dose 400 mg lopinavir/100 mg ritonavir 2x/day or 600 mg lopinavir/150 mg ritonavir 2x/day if co-administered with efavirenz, nevirapine, amprenavir, or nelfinavir	**Pediatric solution 80mg lopinavir/20mg ritonavir per ml.** Tablets 100 mg lopinavir/25 mg ritonavir 200 mg lopinavir/50 mg ritonavir	Administer tablets with or without food. Do not split or crush. Oral solution should be administered with food. Oral solution should be refrigerated. New tablet formulation has decreased diarrhea. For adults who are treatment naïve, tablets can be dosed as 400 mg/100mg once daily in naïve PI naïve patients; this has not been evaluated in adolescents who might have more rapid clearance Higher doses (eg 300 mg/M^2 or 600mg/ 140 mg 2x/day should be considered in treatment experienced patients with PI resistance mutations. Standard dose of 230 mg/M^2 gives trough lower than target associated with response in treatment experienced adults (5.7 mcg/mL. CROI 2008 abstr 574)
Nelfinavir (Viracept)	45–55 mg/kg q12h (8th CROI, 2001, Abst. 250). Approved dose of 30mg/kg q8h may lead to inadequate levels. Neonatal dose 40 mg/kg q12h was inadequate. 50–60 mg/kg under investigation Adolescent/adult dose 1250 mg q12h	Powder for oral suspension 50 mg/level scoop Tablets 250, 625 mg	Take with meal to ↑ absorption. Large variability in levels. Crushed or dissolved tablets more reliably absorbed. Consider measuring C$_{min}$ if available & adjusting dose. Maintaining Ctrough > 0.8mcg/mL associated with improved response in one study.

TABLE 8F (6)

INDICATION/DRUG	DOSAGE	FORMULATIONS	COMMENTS
Anti-HIV Drugs/Protease Inhibitors *(continued)*			
Ritonavir (Norvir)	350-400 mg/M² 2x/day Neonatal dose not established; 450 mg/M² 2x/day led to lower exposure than target in adults Adolescent/adult dose 600 mg 2x/day	Solution 80 mg/ml Capsules 100 mg	Dose should be escalated over 1st 7 days to ↓ side effects. Use lower dose as pharmacokinetic enhancer. Solution is unpleasant tasting. High levels of side effects in older children and adults relative to other PI's
Saquinavir (Invirase) Note: Soft-gel capsules no longer available.	Under study: Not approved in infants or children Adolescent/adult dose: 1000 mg + 100 mg ritonavir 2x/day With Lopinavir/ritonavir: Saquinavir 1000 mg + Lopinavir/ritonavir 400mg/100mg both 2x/day	Hard-gel capsules 200 mg Film-coated tablets 500 mg	Consider measuring C_{min} if available & adjusting dose. (C_{min} >100ng/ml associated with response.) Should only be used with ritonavir enhancement
Tipranavir (Aptivus)	Not approved in children. 375 mg/M² + ritonavir 150 mg/M² 2x/day used in PACTG1051 with good clinical response Adolescent/Adult dose: 500 mg with 200 mg ritonavir 2x/day	Capsule 250 mg	Administer with food. Active against many virus strains with extensive PI resistance, & used only in patients with extensive prior experience. Most effective when given with other active agents, such as enfuvirtide. Activity and tolerability in PACTG1051 similar to adult trials (*Int AIDS Conf 2006 Abstr WEAB0301*) Induces metabolism of other PIs & should not be co-administered with them Possible association with intracranial hemorrhage
Fusion Inhibitors			
Enfuvirtide (Fuzeon)	6-16yrs 2 mg/kg 2x/day, maximum dose 90 mg (1ml) injected subcutaneously <6yrs not approved Adolescent/adult dose 90 mg (1 ml) 2x/day injected subcutaneously	Injection: lyophilized powder for injection 108mg of enfuvirtide, when reconstituted with 1.1ml sterile water to deliver 90mg/ml	Most effective when started with 1-2 new drugs to which virus is sensitive. Must be reconstituted & used within 24hrs. Inject in upper arm, abdomen, anterior thigh—rotate site. Common injection site reactions include tender itchy nodules.
CCR5 Inhibitors			
Maraviroc (Selzentry)	Not approved in children Adolescent/adult doses: 150 mg 2x/day when given with strong CYP3A inhibitors (with or without CYP3A inducers) including all PIs (except tipranavir/ritonavir) 300 mg twice daily when given with NRTIs, enfuvirtide, tipranavir/ritonavir, nevirapine 600 mg twice daily when given with CYP3A inducers, including efavirenz, rifampin, phenobarbital, phenytoine, etc. (without a CYP3A inhibitor)	Tablets 150 mg, 300 mg	Tropism assay should be used before prescribing to exclude X4/dual tropic virus. Cytochrome P450 substrate.

TABLE 8F (7)

INDICATION/DRUG	DOSAGE	FORMULATIONS	COMMENTS
Anti-HIV Drugs (continued)			
Integrase Inhibitors			
Raltegravir (Isentress)	Not approved in children; under study in IMPAACT P1066 Adolescent/adult dose 400 mg 2x/day	Tablets 400 mg	Give with or without food
Antimycobacterial Drugs			
M. tuberculosis			
Ethambutol	15–25 mg/kg/day po	No pediatric formulation	Not approved in children <13 yrs but can be given. Monitor for closely for visual change
Isoniazid	Neonates: 10 mg/kg po q24h. Infants/Children: 10–20 mg/kg po q24h (maximum 300 mg/day)	50 mg/5 ml syrup	Can give IM
Pyrazinamide	20–40 mg/kg po q24h as 1 or more doses (maximum 2 gm/day)	No pediatric formulation	
Rifampin	10–20 mg/kg po q24h (maximum 600mg/day)	No pediatric formulation. Ad hoc solution can be made by pharmacy	Can give po or IV. Do not use with protease inhibitors. Reduced dose rifabutin can be substituted
Streptomycin	10–20 mg IM q12h (max. 1gm/day)		
MAC—Mycobacterium avium-intracellulare complex			
Azithromycin	5 mg/kg/day for treatment 20 mg/kg once weekly, not to exceed 1200 mg	Oral suspension 100 or 200 mg/5 ml	
Clarithromycin	15 mg/kg/day divided q12h po (not to exceed 500 mg po q12h)	Granules for oral suspension (125 or 250 mg/5 ml) (DO NOT refrigerate suspension)	
Clofazimine	1–2 mg/kg/day po to max. of 100 mg/day	No pediatric formulation	
Rifabutin	10–20 mg/kg/day po (max 300 mg/day)	No pediatric formulation	↓ dose with protease inhibitors, inc with NNRTI's
Antiparasitic Drugs			
P. carinii			
Prophylaxis (See Table 8D—after 4wks of age)			
TMP/SMX OR	150 mg/M² TMP component po divided q12h on 3 consecutive days (M, T, W) each week. Abbreviated schedules: Table 8D	Oral suspension (cherry or grape flavored), 40 mg TMP/ 200 mg SMX/5 ml (teaspoon)	Breakthrough episodes of PCP: TMP/ SMX 3%, dapsone 15% or higher, aerosol pentamidine 15%, IV pentamidine 25% (*J Ped* 122:163, 1993)
Dapsone OR	2 mg/kg/day po (not to exceed 100 mg)	No pediatric formulation	

TABLE 8F (8)

INDICATION/DRUG	DOSAGE	FORMULATIONS	COMMENTS
Antiparasitic Drugs *(continued)*			
Aerosolized pentamidine—only if ≥5 yrs old	300 mg with Respirgard II inhaler 1x monthly		Used as young as 8 mos (*PIDJ 12:958, 1991*)
Treatment			
Atovaquone suspension	30–40 mg/kg po q24h. Dosing interval not established	Not FDA-approved for pediatric use	Efficacy in children not established. CNS levels <1%.
Pentamidine isethionate	4 mg/kg/day IV or IM x12–14days		Start with IV in all but mildest cases
TMP/SMX	Children >2 mos 20 mg TMP/100 mg SMX/kg/day divided q6h po or IV in same dose q6–8h		
Antiviral Drugs—other than anti-HIV			
Cytomegalovirus			
Cidofovir	No studies in children.	IV solution only	Must follow guidelines for hydration & probenecid. Dose adjust for renal disease
Induction	5 mg/kg once a week for two doses		
Maintenance	5 mg/kg every 14 days		
Foscarnet			No studies reported in children. Deposited in teeth & bone of growing animals. Dose adjust for renal disease
Induction	180 mg/kg/day divided q8h		
Maintenance	90–120 mg/kg IV q24h		
Valganciclovir		No pediatric formulation	For adolescents who can take adult dose only. Dose adjust for renal diseases
Induction	900 mg po 2x/day for 21 days		
Maintenance	900 mg po q day		
Ganciclovir		Adult capsule or IV solution	Has potential carcinogenicity Dose adjust for renal disease
Induction	5 mg/kg IV q12h		
Maintenance	5 mg/kg IV q24h		
Herpes simplex virus			
Acyclovir	250–500 mg/M² IV q8h. Infuse over 1 hr	200 mg/5ml oral suspension (banana flavored) available if appropriate	Daily urine output should be 1 ml/1.3mg of acyclovir
Varicella zoster (<2yrs old)			
Acyclovir	500 mg/M² IV q8h		

For additional data on drugs for pain &/or nutritional management, see www.aidsinfo.nih.gov/guidelines, Supplements to Pediatric Guidelines Mar 2008.

TABLE 8G: PROPHYLAXIS FOR FIRST EPISODE OF OPPORTUNISTIC DISEASE IN HIV-INFECTED INFANTS & CHILDREN

PATHOGEN	INDICATION	PREVENTIVE REGIMENS*	
		FIRST CHOICE	ALTERNATIVES
Pneumocystis jiroveci	HIV-infected or HIV-indeterminate infants aged 1–12mos HIV-infected children aged 1–5yrs with CD4 count <500 or CD4 percent <15%	TMP/SMX 150/750 mg/M²/day in 2 div. doses po 3x/wk on consecutive days (A2) Acceptable alternative dosage schedules: (A2) Single dose po 3x/wk on consecutive days	Aerosolized pentamidine (children aged ≥5yrs) 300 mg 1x monthly via Respirgard II nebulizer (C3); dapsone (children aged ≥1 mo.) 2 mg/kg (max 100mg) po q24h (C3); Atovaquone 30mg/kg po q24h for 1–3mos old & >24mos old; 45mg/kg po q24h for 4–24mos old; IV pentamidine 4mg/kg every 2–4wks if other options are unavailable (C3)
	HIV-infected children aged 6–12yrs with CD4 <200 or CD4 percent <15%	2 div. doses po q24h; 2 div. doses po 3x/wk on alternate days	
Mycobacterium tuberculosis Isoniazid-sensitive	TST reaction ≥5mm OR prior positive TST result without treatment OR contact with case of active tuberculosis	Isoniazid 10–20 mg/kg (max. 300 mg) po q24h x9mos. (A1) OR 20–40 mg/kg (max. 900 mg) po 2x/wk x9mos. (B3)	Rifampin 10–20 mg/kg (max. 600mg) po or IV q24h x12mos. (B2) (Rifampin duration of rx is 4–6mos. according to 1999 USPHS guidelines.)
Isoniazid-resistant	Same as above; high probability of exposure to isoniazid-resistant tuberculosis	Rifampin 10–20 mg/kg (max. 600 mg) po or IV q24h x12mos. (B2)	Uncertain
Multidrug (isoniazid & rifampin)-resistant	Same as above; high probability of exposure to multidrug-resistant tuberculosis	Choice of drug requires consultation with public health authorities	None
Mycobacterium avium complex	For children aged ≥6yrs, CD4 <50; 2–6yrs, CD4 <75; 1–2yrs, CD4 <500; <1yr, CD4 <750	Clarithromycin 7.5 mg/kg (max. 500 mg) po q12h (A2) OR azithromycin 20 mg/kg (max. 1200 mg) po 1x/wk (A2)	Children aged ≥6yrs, rifabutin 300 mg po q24h (B1); <6yrs, 5 mg/kg po q24h when suspension becomes available (B1); azithromycin 5 mg/kg (max. 250 mg) po q24h (A2)
Varicella zoster virus	HIV-infected children who are asymptomatic & not immunosuppressed	Varicella zoster vaccine	
	Significant exposure to varicella with no history of chickenpox, shingles, or varicella vaccine	Varicella zoster immune globulin (VZIG), 1 vial (1.25 ml)/10kg (max. 5 vials) IM, administered ≤96hrs after exposure, ideally within 48hrs (A2)	None

* See Table 4A for HIV classification

TABLE 9: MANAGEMENT OF EXPOSURE TO HIV-1 & HEPATITIS B/C

OCCUPATIONAL EXPOSURE TO BLOOD, PENILE/VAGINAL SECRETIONS OR OTHER POTENTIALLY INFECTIOUS BODY FLUIDS OR TISSUES WITH RISK OF TRANSMISSION OF HEPATITIS B/C &/OR HIV-1 (E.G., NEEDLESTICK INJURY) [Adapted from *MMWR 50(RR-11):1, 2001; NEJM 348:826, 2003; MMWR 54(RR-9), 2005; MMWR 55(RR-11), 2006 (available at www.cdc.gov/mmwr)*].

Free consultation for occupational exposures: call (PEPline) 1-888-448-4911.

General steps in management:
1. Wash clean wounds/flush mucous membranes immediately (use of caustic agents or squeezing the wound is discouraged; data lacking regarding antiseptics).
2. Assess risk by doing the following: (a) Characterize exposure; (b) Determine/evaluate source of exposure by medical history, risk behavior, & testing for hepatitis B/C, HIV; (c) Evaluate & test exposed individual for hepatitis B/C & HIV

Hepatitis B Occupational Exposure [Adapted from CDC recommendations: *MMWR 50(RR-11), 2001*]

Exposed Person*	Exposure Source		
	HBs Ag+	HBs Ag–	Status Unknown or Source Unavailable for Testing†
Unvaccinated	Give HBIG 0.06 mL per kg IM & initiate HB vaccine	Initiate HB vaccine	Initiate HB vaccine
Vaccinated (antibody status unknown)	Do anti-HBs on exposed person: If titer ≥10 milli-International units per mL, no rx If titer <10 milli-International units per mL, give HBIG 1 month apart as if source were HBsAG positive.	No rx necessary	Do anti-HBs on exposed person: If titer ≥10 milli-International units per mL, no rx If titer <10 milli-International units per mL, give 1 dose of HB vaccine**

* Persons previously with HBV are immune to reinfection and do not require postexposure prophylaxis. For known vaccine series responder (titer ≥10 milli-International units per mL), monitoring of levels or booster doses not currently recommended. Known non-responder (<10 milli-International units per mL) to 1° series HB vaccine & exposed to either HBsAg+ source or suspected high-risk source—rx with HBIG & re-initiate vaccine series or give 2 doses HBIG 1 month apart. For non-responders after a 2nd vaccine series, 2 doses HBIG 1 month apart is preferred approach to new exposure [*MMWR 40(RR-13):21, 2001*].

† If known high risk source, treat as if source were HBsAG positive.

** Follow-up to assess vaccine response or address completion of vaccine series.

Hepatitis B Non-Occupational Exposure [Adapted from CDC recommendations; *MMWR 55(RR-11), 2006 and MMWR 55(RR-16), 2006*]
Post-exposure prophylaxis is recommended for persons with discrete nonoccupational exposure to blood or body fluids. Exposures include percutaneous (e.g., bite, needlestick or mucous membrane exposure to HBsAG-positive blood or sterile body fluids, sexual or needle-sharing contact of an HBsAG-positive person, or a victim of sexual assault or sexual abuse by a perpetrator who is HBsAg-positive. If immunoprophylaxis is indicated, it should be initiated ideally within the first 24h of exposure. Postexposure prophylaxis is unlikely to be effective if administered more than 7 days after a parenteral exposure or 14 days after a sexual exposure. The hepatitis B vaccine series should be completed regardless. The same guidelines for management of occupational exposures can also be used for nonoccupational exposures. For a previously vaccinated person (i.e., written documentation of being vaccinated) and no documentation of postvaccination titers with a discrete exposure to a HBsAG-positive source, it also is acceptable to administer a booster dose of hepatitis B vaccine without checking titers. No treatment is required for a vaccinated person exposed to a source of unknown HBsAG status.

Hepatitis C Exposure
Determine antibody to hepatitis C for both exposed person &, if possible, exposure source. If source + or unknown and exposed person negative, follow-up HCV testing for HCV RNA (detectable in blood in 1-3 weeks and HCV antibody (90% who seroconvert will do so by 3 months) is advised. **No recommended prophylaxis**; immune serum globulin not effective. Monitor for early infection, as therapy may ↓ risk of progression to chronic hepatitis. Persons who remain viremic 3-12 weeks after exposure should be treated with a course of pegylated interferon (*Gastro 130:632, 2006 and Hpt 43:923,2006*). See *Table 12*. Case-control study suggested risk factors for occupational HCV transmission include percutaneous exposure to needle that had been in artery or vein, deep injury, male sex of HCW, & was more likely when source VL >6 log10 copies/mL (*CID 41: 1423, 2005*).

HIV: OCCUPATIONAL EXPOSURE MANAGEMENT [adapted from *MMWR 54(RR-9), 2C05 (available at **www.cdc.gov/mmwr**)*]

- The decision to initiate post-exposure prophylaxis (PEP) for HIV is a clinical judgment that should be made in concert with the exposed healthcare worker (HCW). It is based on:
  1. Likelihood of the source patient having HIV infection: ↑ with history of high-risk activity—injection drug use, sexual activity with known HIV+ person, unprotected sex with multiple partners (either hetero- or homosexual), receipt of blood products 1978–1985. ↑ with clinical signs suggestive of advanced HIV (unexplained wasting, night sweats, thrush, seborrheic dermatitis, etc.).
  2. Type of exposure (approx. 1 in 300–400 needlesticks from infected source will transmit HIV).
  3. Limited data regarding efficacy of PEP (*Cochrane Database Syst Rev. Jan 24;(1):CD002835, 2007*).
  4. Significant adverse effects of PEP drugs & potential for drug interactions.

TABLE 9 (2)

- Substances considered potentially infectious include: blood, tissues, semen, vaginal secretions, CSF, synovial, pleural, peritoneal, pericardial, & amniotic fluids; & other visibly bloody fluids. Fluids that are normally low-risk for transmission, unless they are visibly bloody, include: urine, vomitus, stool, sweat, saliva, nasal secretions, tears & sputum (*MMWR 54(RR-9), 2005*)
- If source person is **known positive for HIV** or **likely to be infected & status of exposure warrants PEP**, antiretroviral drugs should be started **immediately** (ASAP or within hours). If source person is HIV antibody negative, drugs can be stopped **unless source is suspected of having acute HIV infection**. The HCW should be re-tested at **3–4wks, 3 & 6mos whether PEP is used or not** (the vast majority of seroconversions will occur by 3mos; delayed conversions after 6mos are exceedingly rare). Testing up to 12 mos is recommended if HCW becomes infected with HCV from co-infected source. Advise HCW to take precautions to avoid secondary transmission during this period of monitoring following exposure to known or suspected HIV+ source. Tests for HIV RNA should not be used for dx of HIV infection because of false-positives (esp. at low titers) & these tests are only approved for established HIV infection [exception is if pt develops signs of acute HIV (monomucleosis-like) syndrome within the 1st 4–6wks of exposure when antibody tests might still be negative.]
- PEP for HIV is usually given for 4wks & monitoring of adverse effects recommended: baseline **complete blood count, renal & hepatic panel** to be **repeated at 2wks**. 50–75% of HCW on PEP demonstrate mild side-effects (nausea, diarrhea, myalgias, headache, etc.) but in up to 50% severe enough to discontinue PEP (*Antivir Ther 3:195, 2000*). Consultation with infectious diseases/ HIV specialist valuable when questions regarding PEP arise. **Seek expert help in special situations, such as pregnancy, renal impairment, treatment-experienced source.**

3 Steps to HIV Post-Exposure Prophylaxis (PEP) After Occupational Exposure:
[For latest CDC recommendations, see *MMWR 54(RR-9), 2005* (available at www.aidsinfo.nih.gov)]

Step 1: Determine the exposure code (EC)

Is source material blood, bloody fluid, semen/vaginal fluid or other normally sterile fluid or tissue (see above)?

- → No → No PEP
- → Yes → What type of exposure occurred?
  - → Intact skin → No PEP*
  - → Mucous membrane or skin integrity compromised (e.g., dermatitis, open wound) → Volume
    - → Small: Few drops → EC1
    - → Large: Major splash &/or long duration → EC2
  - → Percutaneous exposure → Severity
    - → Less severe: Solid needle, scratch → EC2
    - → More severe: Large-bore hollow needle, deep puncture, visible blood, needle used in blood vessel of source → EC3

* Exceptions can be considered when there has been prolonged, high-volume contact

Step 2: Determine the HIV Status Code (HIV SC) for Exposure Source

What is the HIV status of the exposure source?

- → HIV negative → No PEP
- → HIV positive
  - → Low titer exposure: asymptomatic & high CD4 count, low VL (<1500 copies per mL) → HIV SC 1
  - → High titer exposure: advanced AIDS, primary HIV, high viral load or low CD4 count → HIV SC 2
- → Status unknown → HIV SC unknown
- → Source unknown → HIV SC unknown

TABLE 9 (3)

Step 3: Determine Post-Exposure Prophylaxis (PEP) Recommendation

EC	HIV SC	PEP
1	1	Consider basic regimen[1a]
1	2	Recommend basic regimen[1a, b]
2	1	Recommend basic regimen[1b]
2	2	Recommend expanded regimen[1]
3	1 or 2	Recommend expanded regimen[1]
1, 2, 3	Unknown	If exposure setting suggests risks of HIV exposure, consider basic regimen[1c]

[a] Based on estimates of ↓ risk of infection after mucous membrane exposure in occupational setting compared with needlestick.

Modification of CDC recommendations:
[b] Or, consider expanded regimen[1].
[c] In high risk circumstances, consider expanded regimen[1] on case-by-case basis.

**Around the clock, urgent expert consultation available from:
National Clinicians' Post-Exposure Prophylaxis Hotline
(PEPline) at 1-888-448-4911 (1-888-HIV-4911)**

[1] **Regimens:** (Treat for 4 weeks; monitor for drug side-effects every 2 weeks)
Basic regimen: (ZDV + 3TC), or **(FTC + TDF)**; or as alternative d4T + 3TC
Expanded regimen: Basic regimen + one of the following: lopinavir/ritonavir (preferred); or (as alternatives) atazanavir/ritonavir, or, fosamprenavir/ritonavir. Efavirenz can be considered (except in pregnancy or potential for pregnancy—**Pregnancy Category D**), but CNS symptoms might be problematic. [**Do not use nevirapine;** serious adverse reactions including hepatic necrosis reported in healthcare workers (*MMWR 49:1153, 2001*).]
Other regimens can be designed. If possible, use 2 antiretroviral drugs for which resistance is unlikely based on susceptibility data or treatment history of source pt (if known). Seek expert consultation if ARV-experienced source or in pregnancy or potential for pregnancy.

NOTE: Some authorities feel that an expanded regimen should be employed whenever PEP is indicated (*NEJM 349:1091, 2003; Eur J Epidemiol 19:577, 2004*) Expanded regimens are likely to be advantageous with ↑ numbers of ART-experienced source pts or when there is doubt about exact extent of exposures in decision algorithm. Mathematical model suggests that under some conditions, completion of full course basic regimen is better than prematurely discontinued expanded regimen (*CID 39:395, 2004*). However, while expanded PEP regimens have ↑ adverse effects, there is not necessarily ↑ discontinuation (*CID 40:205, 2005*).

POST-EXPOSURE PROPHYLAXIS FOR NON-OCCUPATIONAL EXPOSURES TO HIV From *MMWR 54(RR-2):1, 2005—DHHS recommendations*

Because the risk of transmission of HIV via sexual contact or sharing needles by injection drug users may reach or exceed that of occupational needlestick exposure, it is reasonable to consider PEP in persons who have had a non-occupational exposure to blood or other potentially infected fluids (e.g., genital/rectal secretions, breast milk) from an HIV+ source. Risk of HIV acquisition per exposure varies with the act (for needle sharing & receptive anal intercourse, ≥0.5%; approximately 10-fold lower with insertive vaginal or anal intercourse, 0.05–0.07%). Overt or occult traumatic lesions may ↑ risk in survivors of sexual assault.

For pts at risk of HIV acquisition through non-occupational exposure to HIV+ source material having occurred ≤72 hours before evaluation, DHHS recommendation is to treat for 28 days with an antiretroviral **expanded regimen**, using preferred regimens [efavirenz *(not in pregnancy or pregnancy risk*—**Pregnancy Category D**) + (3TC or FTC) + (ZDV or TDF)] **or** [lopinavir/ritonavir + (3TC or FTC) + ZDV] or one of several alternative regimens *[see Table 6A Section B & MMWR 54(RR-2):1, 2005]*. Prophylaxis failures have been reported, and may be associated with longer intervals from exposure to start of PEP (*CID 41:1507, 2005*); this supports prompt initiation of PEP if it is to be used.

Areas of uncertainty: (1) expanded regimens are not proven to be superior to 2-drug regimens, (2) while PEP not routinely recommended for exposures >72hrs before evaluation, it may possibly be effective in some cases, (3) when HIV status of source patient is unknown, decision to treat & regimen selection must be individualized based on assessment of specific circumstances.

Evaluate for exposures to Hep B, Hep C (*see Occupational PEP above*), & bacterial sexually-transmitted diseases [*see Sanford Guide to Antimicrobial Therapy Table 15A, & MMWR 55(RR-11), 2006*] & treat as indicated. DHHS recommendations for sexual exposures to viral and bacterial pathogens are available in MMWR 55(RR-11), 2006. Persons who are unvaccinated with or who have not responded to full HepB vaccine series should receive HBIG (hepatitis B immune gobulin) preferably within 24 hrs of percutaneous or mucosal exposure to blood/body fluids of an HBsAg-positive person, along with HepB vaccine, with follow-up to complete vaccine series. Unvaccinated or not fully vaccinated persons exposed to a source with unknown HBsAG status should receive vaccine and complete vaccine series. For details and recommendations in other circumstances see *MMWR 55(RR-11), 2006*.

TABLE 10: PRIMARY PROPHYLACTIC ANTIMICROBIAL AGENTS AGAINST OPPORTUNISTIC PATHOGENS IN ADOLESCENTS & ADULTS

Prevention of First Episode of Disease (for 2nd, see *Table 12*). [For 2004 USPHS/IDSA Guidelines for Prevention of OIs in HIV, see *MMWR 53:RR-15, 2004*] See *Figure 2*.

Lowest CD4 Count	Pathogen	Preventive Regimens Primary	Preventive Regimens Alternative	Comments
All patients regardless of CD4 level See also *Table 12, page 126* [See AnIM 137(Suppl.5, part 2), 2002; JID 196:S35, 2007]	**Mycobacterium tuberculosis:** TST[1] ≥5 mm or prior untreated pos. TST or contact with case of active TB	[**INH** 5 mg/kg/day po, maximum 300 mg po + **pyridoxine** 50 mg po q24h x9mos.] or [**INH** 900 mg po + **pyridoxine** 100 mg po 2x/wk x9mos.]	**RIF**** 600 mg po q24h or **RFB**** 300 mg po q24h x4 mos.[2]	See *Table 11A, page 103*. No longer called "prophylaxis", but now termed treatment of latent infection with M. tuberculosis (LTBI) *(AJRCCM 161:S221, 2000)*. 2 mo. rx with RIF + PZA as effective as 12mos. of INH in HIV+ pts *(JAMA 283: 1445, 2000)*. **However, there are reports of severe & fatal hepatitis in pts on RIF + PZA** *(MMWR 50:289, 2001)*. Therefore, this regimen is no longer recommended by CDC for LTBI *(MMWR 52:735, 2003)*. Not all agree with CDC recommendations and recent study suggests short course therapy is safe with monitoring and more likely to be completed than longer Rx *(CID 43:271, 2006)*.
	As above but high probability of exposure to INH-resistant TB	**RIF**** 600 mg po q24h or **RFB**** 300 mg po q24h x4mos.		
	Exposure to multi-drug resistant TB	Consultation recommended		
CD4 <200/mm³ REF: *CID 40 (Suppl.3), 2005*	**Pneumocystis jiroveci (formerly carinii)** (See *Table 11A page 106*) **DC prophylaxis when CD4 count >200 for >12 wks in response to ARV RX** [*MMWR 51(RR-8):4, 2002*]. Restart if CD4 drops <200/mm³.	**Trimethoprim/ sulfamethoxazole (TMP/SMX)-DS:** one tab po q24h or 3x/week or **TMP/SMX-SS** one tab po q24h or **Dapsone** 100 mg po q24h	**Aerosolized pentamidine** 300 mg q month via Respigard II nebulizer (if toxo pos., see below) OR [**Dapsone** 100 mg po q24h + **pyrimethamine** 50mg po q wk + **leucovorin** 25 mg po q wk (also effective for toxo prophylaxis)] OR [Dapsone 200 mg po + pyrimethamine 75mg po + leucovorin 25 mg po], all 1x/week] OR [Dapsone 50 mg po q12h or 100 mg po q24h] OR [TMP/SMX-DS 3x/wk po] OR [Atovaquone suspension 1500 mg po q24h]	TMP/SMX superior to other rx in actual practice (incidence of failure 0.0002/100 person yrs) vs dapsone or inhaled pentamidine or atovaquone (0.001/100 person yrs) & odds ratio for failure 4.5, 5.8 & 6.7, respectively vs TMP/ SMX *(J AIDS & HR 19:182, 1998)*. Atovaquone = pentamidine but had ↑ rx-limiting adverse events *(JID 180:369, 1999)*. ATS/IDSA Consensus Statement: *AJRCCM 175:367, 2007*.

[1] TST = tuberculin skin test (Mantoux).
[2] Interaction with protease inhibitors to be considered; see *Table 12, pg 126*.
** See *Table 12, pg 126*, for options regarding concurrent use of protease inhibitors & RIF or RFB.

TABLE 10 (2)

Lowest CD4 Count	Pathogen	Preventive Regimens Primary	Preventive Regimens Alternative	Comments
CD4 <100/mm³ REF: *CID 40 (Suppl.3), 2005*	**Toxoplasma gondii** (in pts with + IgG toxo, antibody titer). DC primary prophylaxis in toxo Ab+ pts with CD4 >200 for >12wks in response to ARV RX.	**TMP/SMX-DS** one po q24h.	**Dapsone** 50 mg po q24h + **pyrimethamine** 50 mg pc q week + **leucovorin** (folinic acid) 25 mg po q week	Another option: Atovaquone 750 mg po q6–12h + pyrimethamine 25 mg q24h + leucovorin 10 mg po q24h
	Histoplasmosis Not routinely recommended. Can be considered for patients at high risk because of occupational exposure or who live in a hyperendemic region for histoplasmosis (≥10 cases/100 patient-years).	**Itraconazole 200 mg twice daily**		
CD4 <50/mm³	**Mycobacterium avium-intracellulare**[1] (See Table 11A, page 110). DC prophylaxis when CD4 count >100 sustained for 3 mos. in response to ARV RX *[NEJM 342:1085, 2000; AnIM 133:493, 2000; MMWR 51(RR-8):10, 2002; CID 41:549, 2005]*. Restart if CD4 drops <50–100/mm³.	[**Clarithromycin** 500 mg po q12h or **azithromycin** 1200 mg po weekly (both assoc. with emergence of resistant respiratory flora)] *(HIV Clin Trials 2:453, 2001)*.	**Rifabutin** 300 mg po q24h[2] OR (**azithromycin** 1200 mg po weekly + **rifabutin** 300 mg po q24h)	*See Table 12, page 127.* Rifabutin reduced cryptosporidium-associated diarrhea *(AIDS 14:2889, 2000)*. Single daily dose of 500 mg of clarithro better than rifabutin but no direct comparison available between std. q12h dosage *(AIDS 13:1367, 1999; ATS/IDSA Consensus Statement: AJRCCM 175:367, 2007)*.
	Cytomegalovirus (See Table 12, page 150) Authors feel it is reasonable to observe pts closely, rx active CMV infection. Preemptive rx of pts with CMV viremia without evidence of organ involvement generally not recommended. **May safely dc chronic suppression when CD4 count >100–150 for ≥6mos.** *[MMWR 51(RR-8):19, 2002]*. Restart if CD4 drops ≤100–150/mm³	Chronic suppression: **Valganciclovir** 900 mg po q24h (see Comment)	Oral **ganciclovir** 1 gm po q8h	*See Table 12, page 150, primary prophylaxis.* Prophylaxis decision should include risk group: gay males 35% vs IVDA 4.7% risk of CMV during life. If plasma PCR for CMV pos, 43% risk of disease (↓ to 26% on oral ganciclovir); if PCR neg, 14% (↓ to 1% on oral ganciclovir). Therefore, some use prophylaxis in gay males when PCR pos.
	Candida species, cryptococcus Not routinely recommended prior to 1st fungal infection *[MMWR 51(RR-8):15, 2002]*			

---

[1] Authors think it reasonable to observe pts closely, rx strongly suspected or active MAC, then institute chronic suppression *(see Table 12, page 126.)*
[2] Interaction with protease inhibitors to be considered; *see Table 12, page 127.*

TABLE 11A:[1] **DIAGNOSIS & DIFFERENTIAL DIAGNOSIS OF CLINICAL SYNDROMES, OPPORTUNISTIC INFECTIONS & NEOPLASMS** (For Treatment, see Table 12)

CLINICAL SYNDROME, ETIOLOGY, EPIDEMIOLOGY	CLINICAL PRESENTATION, DIAGNOSTIC TESTS, COURSE
Acute retroviral (HIV) syndrome (symptomatic primary HIV infection): Differential diagnosis includes: EBV mononucleosis, CMV mononucleosis, toxoplasmosis, rubella, viral hepatitis, syphilis, primary HSV, drug reactions Many new infections in US may now occur in adolescents. **Think acute HIV when mononucleosis suspected but serological tests for mono negative.** NOTE: During acute retroviral syndrome, individuals have very high plasma & genital secretion viral titers (AIDS 21:1723, 2007) & **are highly infectious both from sexual activity & needle sticks** (JID 191:1403, 2005). 25–60% of all HIV infections may be transmitted during this period of acute infection. Depending on frequency of coitus, 7–24% of ♀ partners would be expected to become infected over 2 months of acute HI. Drug-resistant virus commonly isolated in acute retroviral syndrome (J Acquir Defic Syndr 38:545,2005). Some mutations (M184V) may transmit less effectively. Genotyping recommended of initial viral isolate and before initiation of treatment (Panel for Antiretroviral Guidelines for Adults and Adolescents. DHHS. Jan 29, 2008). Massive depletion of CD4 memory T cells, including lymphocyte reservoirs in the GI tract, occurs within days to weeks of HIV infection (Clin Exp Immunol 149:211, 2007).	**Symptoms:** Occur in 50–90%, others have asymptomatic seroconversion; diagnosis made in <10% Time from exposure to sx usually 2–6wks. | Symptoms | Frequency (%) | Symptoms | Frequency (%) | Lab Abnormalities | Freq (%) | |---|---|---|---|---|---| | Fever | >95 | Headache | 33 | ↑ ALT, AST | 50 | | Adenopathy | 75 | Hepatosplenomegaly | 15 | ↓ platelets | 45 | | Pharyngitis | 75 | Neuropathy | 6 | ↓ lymphs (CD4) | 35 | | Macular or papular rash | 70 | Oral/genital ulcers | <5 | Atypical lymphs (↑ CD8) | 35 | | Myalgias/arthralgias | 80 | Esophageal ulcers | <5 | | | | N, V, or diarrhea | 30–60 | Palpable purpura | <5 | | | | | | Conjunctivitis | <5 | | | Up to 50% have neurological manifestations from severe headache to signs of meningitis or encephalitis. Those with acute neurologic syndromes have 10x higher CSF viral loads than those without neurologic symptoms. OIs are rare. **Laboratory:** thrombocytopenia 45%, lymphopenia, (neutropenia reported & may be severe, Eur J Intern Med 16:120,2005) followed by lymphocytosis (↓ CD4, ↑ CD8, **often atypical lymphs**), ↑ hepatic enzymes 21%. **Viral burden: high-level HIV viremia (10^5–10^8 copies/ml plasma)**, high p24 antigen [75–89% sensitive, 100% specific (AnIM 134:25, 2001; JID 195:416, 2007)], standard HIV antibody tests usually neg., **false-positive viral RNA in low titers reported.** HIV RNA testing now dx test of choice where available and recommended when epidemiology suggests ↑ likelihood of infection (STD, contact with HIV+, etc.)(J Acquir Immune Def Syndr 42:75, 2006). All tests may be negative in "window" within week or so following infection (CID 44:459, 2007). **Course/Prognosis:** symptoms usually resolve in 1–2wks & rarely up to 10wks. The occurrence of the acute retroviral syndrome, a short incubation period to symptoms (fever, fatigue, myalgias), & duration of illness >14 days correlate with more rapid progression to AIDS. See Table 6A. Effective anti-HIV CTL activity assoc. with ↑ rate of viral clearance & lower setpoint which is assoc. with ↓ rate of progression to AIDS. Treatment of acute HIV not known to confer long-term virologic, immunologic, or clinical benefit and remains optional (Panel for Antiretroviral Guidelines for Adults and Adolescents. DHHS. Jan 29, 2008).

---

[1] These summaries initially used the 6th Edition of *The Medical Mgmt of AIDS*, edited by Merle A. Sande & Paul A. Volberding, W.B. Saunders & Co., 1999. See Table 12 for details of treatment/disease entity.

TABLE 11A (2)

CLINICAL SYNDROME, ETIOLOGY, EPIDEMIOLOGY	CLINICAL PRESENTATION, DIAGNOSTIC TESTS, COURSE
Central Nervous System CNS invasion occurs early in HIV infection. ARV RX produced 95% ↓ CNS AIDS- defining events but other CNS conditions may be increasing (immune reconstitution leukoencephalitis, chronic "burnout" VZV encephalitis, toxoplasma or PML). In Thailand the incidence of crypto meningitis (18), toxo (14.8), & CMV encephalitis (7/100 person yrs). ↓ in the era of ARV RX compared to pre-ARV RX but incidence of primary CNS lymphoma & stroke increased (*Eur J Neurol* 13:233, 2006).	
Cognitive Disorders, Diffuse Brain Dysfunction	
Declining mental acuity with preservation of alertness **HIV-1 associated dementia (HAD or HIVD), also known as AIDS dementia complex (ADC)**, multinucleated giant cell encephalitis, or HIV-1-associated cognitive/motor complex. Frequency:1/3 of adults, ½ children with AIDS. Most common cause of dementia worldwide in adults < 40 years of age (*J Neuroimmune Pharmacol* 1:138, 2006). Stage 0: normal Stage 1: mild, can work Stage 2: moderate but cannot work Stage 3: severe, cannot work, major intellectual disability Stage 4: vegetative **(In AIDS dementia complex, a "vegetative" patient can be aroused to a level of alertness. This is an important distinction between AIDS dementia complex & many other potential etiologies.)** HIVD may not have declined as dramatically as other CNS OIs, 4.4% of initial AIDS-defining illness before ARV RX, but 6.5% during ARV RX era **Pathogenesis:** (*J Neuroimmune Pharmacol* 1:138, 2006; *Microbes & Infection* 8:1347, 2006). HIV appears to produce **infection of brain macrophages/microglia** (but not of neurons or macroglia). HIV infects brain macrophages directly via CCR5 β-chemokine receptor; pts heterozygous for the CCR5 Δ32 mutation are less likely to develop HIVD. ↑ frequency of apoptotic & HIV-infected astrocytes assoc. with ↑ severity of HIVD. **β-chemokines** (MIP-1α, MIP-1β & RANTES) themselves are ↑ in HIVD, likely indicating ongoing macrophage activation. Macrophages may be newly recruited/trafficked into the CNS late in disease accounting for the demonstrated benefit from ARV RX. CD8 T cells found in CSF express adhesion molecules & chemokine receptors which appear to play an important role in trafficking through the blood-brain barrier & to inflammatory sites in CNS. The final pathway by which the cells destroy neurons is not known, but HIV-infected brain macrophages do over-respond to 2° stimuli with release of neurotoxic substances (glutamate-like neurotoxins, free radicals, arachidonic acid, l-cysteine, or so-called virotoxins). These toxins and tat overstimulate N-methyl-D-aspartate (NMDA) receptors, resulting in ↑ levels of neuronal calcium ion (similar to injury in stroke, trauma).	These pts usually present with impaired short-term memory, ↓ **concentration, clumsiness, slowness, apathy, irritability, & personality changes.** Process is slowly progressive, weeks to months (usually occurs after AIDS defining diagnosis) **& CD4 count usually <200/mm³.** Degree of intellectual impairment & stage of ADC correlates with CSF HIV RNA. Higher levels of HIV RNA in CSF predict progression of neuropsychological impairment & postmortem evidence of HIV encephalitis. **Neuro exam: non-focal** |	Early	Late
---	---	---
Cognition	Inattention ↓ concentration Forgetfulness, slowing of thought processing	Global dementia
Motor	Slowed movements Clumsiness Ataxia	Paraplegia
Behavior	Apathy Blunting of personality Agitation	Mutism	 **CSF:** Normal 30–50%, ↑ WBC (monos) 5–10% [CSF abnormalities: pleocytosis, ↑ protein or ↑ immunoglobulin levels reported in 30% asymptomatic HIV+ individuals] **MRI scan:** Early is typically normal. **Cerebral atrophy, occ. with diffuse fluff ("spilled milk"), edema of antral white matter & basal ganglii, best seen on T-2 weighted imaging.** No mass effect. Normal gadolinium rules out most cases of primary brain lymphoma & toxo but does not rule out other infections (neurosyphilis, cryptococcal meningitis, MAC encephalitis).

TABLE 11A (3)

CLINICAL SYNDROME, ETIOLOGY, EPIDEMIOLOGY	CLINICAL PRESENTATION, DIAGNOSTIC TESTS, COURSE
Central Nervous System/Cognitive Disorders, Diffuse Brain Dysfunction/Declining Mental Acuity (continued)	
The **tat gene product alters the blood brain barrier, activates glial cells, and is directly neurotoxic** (*Microbes & Infection 8:1347, 2006*). Tat activates astrocytes to trigger neuronal cell apoptosis, likely through endonuclease G but also ↑ chemokine expression & mediators of inflammation. The **Vpr gene product** may also directly damage neuronal cells by forming ion channels &/or apoptosis by ↑ caspase-8 activity of both mature neurons & neuro precursor cells. **gp120**, a critical surface glycoprotein which initiates attachment of HIV to T lymphocytes via its coreceptor CXCR4 also appears to attach to neuroprogenitor cells via the same chemokine receptor & inhibit activation & proliferation of neuroprogenitor cells in vitro & hippocampal slices. gp120 when injected into the lateral ventricles of rat brains activates caspase-3 on neuro cells directly leading to apoptosis. Both gp120 & tat can induce oxidative stress leading to disruption of the blood brain barrier in vitro (*Brain Res. 1045:57, 2005*).	Pts receiving highly active antiretroviral therapy (ARV RX) have fewer cognitive abnormalities than untreated pts, & when impaired may show marked improvement with rx. Symptoms of acute meningoencephalitis may reflect failure of ARV RX with ↑ CSF HIV viral load & may respond to change in ARV RX. Survival in AIDS pts has dramatically improved: 11.9mos to 48.2mos. Some pts may develop sustained subclinical psychomotor slowing on ARV RX. Improvement in neuropsychological testing correlated with ↓ in CSF HIV-1 RNA after initiation of ARV RX. Progressive HIV encephalopathy responded to ARV RX in a cohort of 126 children (*J Pediatr 146:402,2005*) & another with 146 (*Arch Ped Adol Med 159:651,2005*). In the era of ARV RX the course of ADC has changed: subtypes have been proposed (*The AIDS Reader 16:615, 2006*).
CSF **TNFα levels** also ↑ with ↑ severity of HAD & TNF inhibitors reduce neuronal injury in a murine model of HAD. TNF may kill neurons by recruiting caspases, an apoptotic effect which appears to be blocked by insulin-like growth factor 1 receptor (IGF-1R). TNF related apoptosis-inducing ligand (TRAIL) may also play a role (*Cell Mol Immunol. 2:113, 2005*). A unique human protein, FLJ21908, secreted by HIV-infected macrophages, also induces apoptosis via activation of caspases 9 & 3. The exact mechanism by which activated macrophages kill neuronal cells is an unsolved mystery (*Mol Immunol 42:213, 2005*). Interestingly, HIV-infected macrophages are themselves protected from apoptosis, perhaps contributing to a long-lived CNS viral reservoir. Virus isolated from brain tissue from HIVD appears to express unique neurotropic genotypic features (*PNAS 103:15160, 2006; Acta Neurol Scand 117:108,2008*).	1. Subacute progressive dementia; severe progressive dementia similar to pre-ARV RX era; usually in patients not receiving ARV RX. 2. Chronic active dementia; persons on ARV RX with poor adherence & viral resistance—at risk for neurologic progression. 3. Chronic inactive dementia; effective ARV RX with some recovery neuronal injury & remain neurologically stable. 4. Reversible dementia; effective ARV RX and continued improvement in ADC towards normal. A particularly severe form of demyelinating leukoencephalopathy has been described in pts failing ARV RX. While the impact of ARV RX on AIDS-associated dementia appears from most studies to be beneficial, but dementia eventually affects 10% of adults and remains a problem in late-stage disease. Presence of diabetes was an independent predictor of dementia in the Hawaii Ageing with HIV Cohort (*JAIDS 38;31, 2005*).
Progressive multifocal leukoencephalopathy (PML) in early-stage disease (see page 79)	Dementia is rare, occurs only late
Depression An underdiagnosed & undertreated manifestation of HIV infection that affects quality of life & response to ARV RX especially in women (*J. Neurovirol 11:138,2005*) & orphans in Africa (*Soc.Sci Med 61:555, 2005*)	Depression among the most common neuropsychiatric disorders in HIV-infected individuals, ~ 59% of **HIV-infected persons** & may slow improvement of neurocognitive function response to ARV RX (*HIV Med 7:112, 2006*). Non-adherence to ARV RX correlates with ↑ severity of depression. *Depression itself may impact response to ARV RX* (*Psychosom Med 67:1013, 2005*) and treating depression can improve response to ARV RX. ARV RX also may cause depression (*CID 41:1648, 2005*). Psychotropic therapy can also significantly improve quality of life.
Declining mental acuity with concomitant depression of alertness (without focal findings)	Depression of alertness occurs only in advanced disease.
AIDS dementia complex (ADC) (as above, Stage 3 or 4)	Late stage
Cryptococcal disease (see *meningitis, page 60; Eye, page 58*)	Often assoc. with ↑ CSF pressure
Toxoplasmic encephalitis	Usually focal findings
Progressive multifocal leukoencephalopathy (PML) (see *page 79*)	**Pts usually alert in early stages of disease; can become depressed later**
Primary CNS lymphoma (see *page 78*)	Rare without focal findings, occurs when deep structures in brain involved

TABLE 11A (4)

CLINICAL SYNDROME, ETIOLOGY, EPIDEMIOLOGY	CLINICAL PRESENTATION, DIAGNOSTIC TESTS, COURSE
Central Nervous System/Cognitive Disorders/ Declining mental acuity with concomitant depression of alertness (without focal findings) *(continued)*	
Cytomegalovirus (CMV) encephalitis (CD4 $<50/mm^3$) Frequency not well defined. Overall CMV ~20%, clinical encephalitis occurs in ~1% of CMV cases. **Diagnosis made by detection of CMV DNA by PCR in CSF.** Response to rx variable. CMV can cause apoptosis of neuronal, glial, & endothelial cells of the CNS (*J. Clin Viro 32:218,2005*). Certain CMV genotypes appear to selectively cause CNS infection (*AIDS 19:273, 2005*).	
Encephalitis	Onset subacute: delirium/confusion 90%, apathy & withdrawal 60%, focal neurologic signs 50%. Antecedent CMV disease is common. Metabolic abnormalities, hyponatremia, hyperkalemia, hypo-osmolality, hypernatremia secondary to dehydration. **Non-specific CSF:** no cells or mildly ↑ **cells, ↑ protein, mild ↓ glucose.** Typical neuropathologic feature is ventriculoencephalitis with periventricular necrotic lesions. Micronodular encephalitis with microglial nodules involving parenchyma, cerebellum, spinal cord also occurs; meninges may be involved. **MRI with contrast: meningeal enhancement, focal ring-enhancing lesions, or periventricular enhancement with gadolinium; lacks sensitivity and may be normal despite advanced CMV disease. PCR for CMV DNA ~90% sensitive & 90% specific.**
Polyradiculomyelitis	Sacral pain, urinary retention, and lower extremity weakness progressing to flaccid paralysis. CSF may show low glucose, elevated protein and polymorphonuclear pleocytosis.
Tuberculosis. See *meningitis, page 60*	Always consider in 3rd World (esp. Africa) or immigrant from a region with a high prevalence of TB with symptoms of altered mental status, headache, lethargy or coma.
Neurosyphilis (general paresis, meningovascular)	Serum VDRL & FTA/ABS + in >90%. Diagnosis established by presence of CSF lymphocytic pleocytosis, high protein or positive CSF serology in presence of compatible clinical syndrome and/or + FTA-ABS in serum. CSF FTA-ABS highly sensitive in HIV- cases (>95%), with CSF VDRL sensitivity ranges from 10–89%. MRI: cortical infarcts. (*Clin Radiol 61:393, 2006*). Indications for CSF examination: neurologic, ophthalmic, or otologic symptoms; evidence of acute tertiary syphilis; treatment failure (4-fold increase in nontreponemal serology after treatment or lack of 4-fold decrease within 12 mo. after treatment); late latent syphilis or syphilis of unknown duration (*CID 44:1222, 2007*); serum RPR of 1:32 or higher dilution (*Sex Transm Dis 34:141, 2007*).
Herpes simplex virus (HSV) encephalitis Frequency & role still undefined but probably no more common than in non-AIDS population (*Clin Raiolo 61:393, 2006*).	Clinical presentation: confusion, fever & headache, anxiety & depression, memory loss, aphasia. CSF: virus seldom cultured from CSF. Definitive dx requires brain biopsy or CSF PCR test for HSV DNA [98% sensitive during 1st wk of disease). HSV2 encephalitis also reported (*AIDS Reader 17:67, 2007*)
Causes not directly related to HIV: Drugs: sedative/hypnotic, alcohol, "street drugs"; hypoxemia; sepsis; Metabolic: hypothyroidism, vitamin B_{12} deficiency, electrolyte imbalance	Associated clinical features may suggest etiology but may be subtle, esp. in advanced HIV.
Focal brain dysfunction: seizures &/or focal neurologic findings (hemiparesis, cerebrovascular abnormalities, blindness)	R sk of focal brain lesions ↓ with ARV RX but most dramatic ↓ with primary CNS lymphoma & toxo, PML slight ↑.
Abrupt onset Cerebrovascular events: transient ischemic attack (TIA), cerebrovascular accident (stroke, CVA); risk of ischemic/hemorrhagic stroke may be increasing in ARV RX era (*Eur J Neurol 113:233, 2006; AIDS Care 19:492, 2007*).	Causes of ischemic events include atherosclerosis, embolism, vasculitis, hypercoagulable state (*Neurol 17:1257, 2007*). Exclude meningovascular syphilis, VZV, lymphoma, cryptomeningitis, cocaine use with vasospasm ischemic events. ↑ life expectancy & metabolic side effects leading to atherosclerosis from ARV RX; expect ↑ incidence of strokes.

TABLE 11A (5)

CLINICAL SYNDROME, ETIOLOGY, EPIDEMIOLOGY	CLINICAL PRESENTATION, DIAGNOSTIC TESTS, COURSE
Central Nervous System/Cognitive Disorders/Focal brain dysfunction *(continued)*	
Subacute course (days)	
Toxoplasmic encephalitis (TE). First or second most common neurologic disorder in untreated AIDS and frequent AIDS-defining illness, even during ARV RX era *(Clin Microbiol Infect 13:510, 2007)*. Frequency ↓ with use of TMP/SMX prophylaxis vs *P. jiroveci* and ARV RX. Seroprevalence varies widely among countries: from 10–20% to 50% or higher, especially in African countries. **With such high seroprevalences, HIV pts with unexplained headache, altered mental status, focal neurological findings & CD4 <100/mm³ should be considered for antitoxo rx. *(J Neurovirol 11 s-1;17, 2005)***	Symptoms: Headache 50–70%, altered mental status 70%, hemiparesis &/or other focal signs 60%, seizures 30%. Fever, confusion, coma also seen. Symptoms may recur with immune reconstitution from ARV RX even with successful rx for toxo. **Lab: CD4 <100/mm³ in 80%.** Toxoplasma serum IgG is + in essentially all pts who develop TE (frequency 85–99%) & titer predictive of development of disease: Relative risk ↑ with >150 intl units/ml IgG and CD4 <200. Specific prophylaxis is protective. Scan: MRI more sensitive than CT. MRI not always necessary if multiple lesions seen on CT. **Multiple spherical ring-enhancing lesions,** corticomedullary junction, basal ganglia, thalamus often involved and mass effect common. Lesions often identified even without concomitant neurologic findings. **Course:** >85% will respond to specific anti-toxo treatment *(Cochrane Database System Rev Jul19:CD005420, 2006)*, most within 7 days. **If no improvement after 7–10 days of rx—biopsy.** Primary CNS lymphoma common in "non-responsive" cases. Brain biopsy indicated earlier (in <7 days) in patients with CD4 >100 or if negative toxo antibody titer, single lesion & progression of symptoms on antitoxo rx. If improvement, biopsy not required. Neurologic deficits often persist *(Clin Microbiol Infect 13:510, 2007)*.
Primary CNS lymphoma ↓ incidence from 8.0/1000 person-years pre-ARV RX to 2.3/1000 person-yrs post-ARV RX. Epstein-Barr virus DNA present in nearly all.	Symptoms: Usually afebrile; headache, confusion, focal neurologic deficits, seizures. Often alert, but with mass effect may have more global mental dysfunction. **Lab:** CSF: Normal 30–50%, protein 10–150mg/dl, cells (monos) 0–40/mm³, cytology + in <5%. PCR for detection of **EBV DNA has sensitivity >90%, but lacks specificity and may have a poor positive predictive value** *(CID 38:1629, 2004)*. Scan: White matter more often involved than gray matter. One or a few weakly enhancing irregular lesions, typically in periventricular region with mass effect. Biopsy necessary for definitive diagnosis: stereotactic biopsy effective. **Course:** median survival time poor (< 3 mo); improved survival with ARV RX.
Tuberculous brain abscess (see meningitis, page 60)-tuberculoma	Uncommon.
Cryptococcoma *(see meningitis, page 60)* May coexist or be confused with toxo encephalitis	Usually concomitant with cryptococcal meningitis, CRAG of CSF & serum positive, but with an isolated cryptococcoma, CRAG (serum & CSF) may be negative.
Varicella zoster virus (VZV) encephalitis *(AIDS Reader 17:64, 2007)* Less common complication of dermatomal zoster with ARV RX.	Often associated with dermatomal zoster. Signs and symptoms: headache, altered mental status, seizures, seizures, cranial nerve palsies. May mimic CNS lymphoma clinically & cytologically. CSF: 0-300 WBCs, predom. lymphs, mild ↑ in protein. **PCR detection of VZV DNA sensitive & specific.** Scan: nonspecific with multifocal white matter lesions. >50% recovery with antiviral therapy.
Cytomegalovirus (CMV) infection	See above.
Aspergillosis • ↑ in pts with ↓ WBC & rx with corticosteroids • Direct extension from sinuses or orbits—also from lung	Nonspecific neuro symptoms including headache, cranial or somatic nerve weakness or paresthesias, altered mental status & seizures. High mortality; medical rx usually unsuccessful. Scan—CT reveals hypodense lesions
Herpes simplex virus (HSV) encephalitis	See page 77.
Bartonella henselae, with neurologic complications	Encephalitis, dementia. Scan: Contrast-enhancing mass lesion.
Chagas' Disease (*Trypanosoma cruzi*) *(Ann Trop Med Parasitol 101:31, 2007)*.	Reactivation in 20%, chronic Chagas in 28%.
Nocardia brain abscess	Rare; can be confused with tuberculosis.

78

TABLE 11A (6)

CLINICAL SYNDROME, ETIOLOGY, EPIDEMIOLOGY	CLINICAL PRESENTATION, DIAGNOSTIC TESTS, COURSE
Central Nervous System, Cognitive Disorders/Focal Brain Dysfunction *(continued)*	
Chronic course (weeks)	
Progressive multifocal leukoencephalopathy (PML) Frequency 4–7% of AIDS patients. Caused by JC virus (a papovavirus), which infects oligodendrocytes, the myelin-producing cells of the CNS. JC virus may affect expression of the myelin basic protein gene leading to disruption of myelin sheaths; co-infection & activation of HHV-6 may be associated with demyelinative lesions. CD4 usually ≤100/mm^3. Prolonged survival & remission reported with highly effective antiretroviral rx but not consistently. Although typically non-inflammatory, inflammatory lesions from immune reconstitution syndrome upon institution of ARV RX may worsen and lead to a fatal outcome (*Acta Neuropathol 109:449, 2005; Scand J Infect Dis 39:347, 2007*).	**Symptoms: Develops insidiously with a single focus** (limb weakness 1/3, ataxia 13%, visual defects 1/3, altered mental status 1/3) but afebrile & arousable (preservation of alertness until late into disease course). W th progression, multiple foci occur. Seizures found in 20% in one series. **Lab**: CSF: Normal (pleocytosis in 20%, ↑ protein 30%). **JC IgM antibody & PCR of CSF for JCV 82% sensitive, 100% specific**. JC viral load in CSF predictive of disease state & progression but not in patients R$_x$ with ARV RX (*CID 40:738, 2005*). **MRI Scan: Multiple fluffy or diffuse hypodense non-contrast enhancing lesions in subcortical white matter, no mass effect.** High signal intensity on T-2 images in hemispheric white matter, ill-defined margins (CT/MRI—clinical dissociation, images worse than pt. symptoms). May become contrast-enhancing with immune reconstitution assoc. with ARV RX. Occ. inflammation present without ARV RX. Brain biopsy is definitive diagnostic procedure (demyelination, JCV on electron microscopy), sensitivity 40–96%, but not required if MRI is characteristic & JC PCR positive. **Course**: Death usual within 6 mos but spontaneous sustained remissions occur in 5–10. **Immune reconstitution with ARV RX may have serious consequences due to ↑ inflammatory changes in area of PML lesion. No clear consensus on management of PML currently exists.**
Seizures *(See causes of focal brain dysfunction)* Cerebral mass lesions (32%) Encephalopathy (24%) Meningitis (16%) Other or undetermined cause (28%)	Considerations are CNS toxo, lymphoma, Toxoplasma, PML, other cerebral infections common (*Seizure 17:27, 2008*). CNS lymphoma also important. cryptomeningitis, tuberculoma, PML, HIV dementia
Headaches	
New headache	<1wk duration: think crypto meningitis, sinusitis, toxo encephalitis, tubercular meningitis, aseptic or pyogenic meningitis, primary CNS lymphoma.
Chronic (*see Focal brain dysfunction, pages 77–79*)	
HIV-associated, early disease	May be a presenting symptom. Not AIDS dementia complex or HIV-associated aseptic meningitis, CSF: 0 pleocytosis but ↑ HIV viral load in CSF.
Nucleoside therapy	ZDV 50–60% in controlled trial, 3% in open study; ddI 1–7%, ddC 2–12%, stavudine 95% in controlled trial, 3% in parallel track program

TABLE 11A (7)

CLINICAL SYNDROME, ETIOLOGY, EPIDEMIOLOGY	CLINICAL PRESENTATION, DIAGNOSTIC TESTS, COURSE
Central Nervous System, Cognitive Disorders *(continued)*	
Meningitis (headache, fever, lethargy with or without nuchal rigidity)	
Cryptococcal meningitis (CD4 usually ≤100/mm^3). Fluconazole use & esp. ARV RX have markedly reduced incidence in developed regions. Still a common AIDS-defining diagnosis in developing countries. More common cause of chronic meningitis than tuberculosis in Thailand in HIV + (*Neuroepidemology 26:37, 2005*)	See *Br Med Bull 72:99, 2005* for description of current dx & therapeutic challenges. **Symptoms: Stiff neck in only ¼ of pts.** May proceed rapidly to coma & death (*Eur J Neurol 11:1468, 2005*). Extraneural disease in 20–60%. Skin lesions resembling Molluscum contagiosum in 3–10%, respiratory sx preceding headache common (78%). **Lab: CRAG* (serum) >99% positive—excellent screening test** but of no value for following early response to rx. Cryptococcal antigenemia preceded symptoms of meningitis by median of weeks to months. CSF: LP opening pressure > 200 in 60% pts. Often non-inflammatory. Median of 4 lymphs/mm^3, glucose normal to low, protein normal to ↑. India ink prep 75% sensitive. **CSF CRAG >90% sensitive. Increased intracranial pressure associated with blindness & ↑ mortality. If opening pressure >250 mmH$_2$O, urgently rx with CSF drainage** (10–20 ml CSF). Control of ↑ CSF pressure (reduction of >10 mm or no change) assoc. with improved outcome/survival vs those whose pressure ↑ >10 mm, p <0.001. Selective placement of lumbar-peritoneal shunts or temporary lumbar drains has also been effectively used to control persistent ↑ CSF pressure. Dexamethasone or mannitol of no value. **Acetazolamide use associated with ↑ serious adverse events—do not use!** If intracerebral mass lesion, think co-infection with toxo. Patients on ARV RX concurrent with or soon after dx of cryptococcosis may develop **immune reconstitution phenomena (IRIS) accompanied by CSF pleocytosis, ↑ ICP, but with neg. fungal cultures. See *Table 11B*.
Bacterial meningitis (occurs at any CD4 level). HIV+ have 20–150x ↑ risk vs HIV-neg. pts. Recent study in Malawi Of 6426 patients with suspected Streptococcus pneumoniae 59% bacterial meningitis in Malawi, Neisseria meningitidis 4% 10% had crypto meningitis; 7.2%, Gram-negatives 5% bacterial meningitis; and 4.4% (*N Eng J Med 357:2441, 2007*) had tuberculous meningitis. Listeria monocytogenes	Presentation similar to non-HIV+ population. CSF Gram-stain frequently positive. Overall mortality approx. 50% in Malawi; steroids of no benefit (*N Eng J Med 357:2441, 2007*). Incidence of listeriosis (meningitis & bacteremia) 65–145X more common than in general population. HIV+ persons should avoid soft cheeses, undercooked chicken.
Tuberculous meningitis (Mycobacterium tuberculosis) (*NEJM 351:1719, 2004*). Occurs at any CD4 level but ↑ incidence in HIV+ pts: 235x ↑ in U.S. stud). Rare in developed world but common cause of meningitis in 3rd World: approx. 5–15%.	**HIV+ at ↑ risk but clinical manifestations are similar to HIV- patients** except intracerebral mass lesions more common and extrapulmonary disease is more common. 9-mo mortality rate significantly increased in HIV +: relative risk 2.9 for HIV+ versus HIV- with 65% mortality in one study from Vietnam (*JID 192:2134; 2005*). Benefit of steroids uncertain (*NEJM 351:1719, 2004; Cochrane Database Syst Rev. 2008 Jan 23;(1):CD002244*). CSF: Lymphocytic pleocytosis (average of ~100/mm^3, 90% lymphocytes); glucose ↓ (mean < 30% of blood value); protein ↑ (mean of 130 mg/dL). Direct AFB smear of CSF 5–20% sensitive; culture 42% sensitive. Conventional PCR sensivity of 54.5%, specificity of 87.5%; RT-PCR sensivity/specificity 70.5%/87.5% (*Int J Infect Dis 11:348, 2007*).
Fungal meningitis (coccidioidal & histoplasmal) CD4 usually <100/mm^3	Consider in endemic areas (*see page 109*)
HIV aseptic meningitis Occurs at any CD4 level	May occur during acute HIV infection or relapsing throughout course. CSF: Mild lymphocytic pleocytosis, modest ↑ protein. These findings may be present in asymptomatic patient but ↑ HIV viral load in CSF.

TABLE 11A (8)

CLINICAL SYNDROME, ETIOLOGY, EPIDEMIOLOGY	CLINICAL PRESENTATION, DIAGNOSTIC TESTS, COURSE
Central Nervous System/Cognitive Disorders/Meningitis *(continued)*	
Meningovascular syphilis: syphilitic meningitis. Occurs usually within first 12 months of infection; incidence of symptomatic early neurosyphilis is 1.7% among HIV+ MSM *(MMWR 56:625, 2007)*.	Cranial nerve dysfunction most common syndrome with ocular and/or auditory sympotoms in 65%, other cranial nerve involvement in 4%; acute, aseptic meningitis, 12%; stroke, 4%; headache or altered mental status, 14%. Lab: Positive serological test for syphilis plus positive CSF VDRL (82%) or negative CSF VDRL plus otherwise unexplained ↑ CSF protein or CSF pleocytosis and clinical signs or symptoms compatible with neurosyphilis (18%). LP should be performed on all cases of syphilis with neurological manifestations and/or RPR of 1:32 or higher dilution in serum *(Sex Transm Dis 34:141, 2007)*.
Candidal meningitis	May mimic crypto or tuberculous meningitis; CD4 < 200/mm³. Rare.
Movement disorders Occur in 3% of HIV+ pts & up to 50% of those with advanced AIDS. Usually present with other clinical features: peripheral neuropathy, seizures, myelopathy, & dementia.	**Most common clinical features:** tremor, Parkinsonism, hemiballism, hemichorea. **Less common:** dystonia, chorea, myoclonus, tics, & dyskinesis. Often associated with OIs, particularly toxo & crypto, & may improve with specific treatment plus ARV RX.
Most Common Peripheral Nerve Syndromes in HIV Disease by Stage: The following are organized according to stage of HIV infection & relative prevalence *(see table on page 83)*. Peripheral neuropathies are common (6–13%) in HIV/AIDS. They most commonly affect the sensory nerves & are caused by either HIV, opportunistic infections, drugs or are idiopathic. They present as part of several discrete syndromes & vary according to stage of disease.	
Acute retroviral syndrome: Neuropathy (6–8%)	See *Acute retroviral syndrome, page 74.* Headache/retro-orbital pain, often ↑ with eye movement (30%), photophobia. Myelopathy, peripheral neuropathy, brachial neuritis, facial palsy, cauda equina & Guillain-Barre syndrome. Course: Usually self-limited, but persistence reported.
Early (asymptomatic HIV) **Inflammatory demyelinating polyneuropathy (IDP)** (occurs <5%) *(see below)* Subacute (Guillain-Barre syndrome) or acute inflammatory demyelinating polyradiculoneuropathy (AIDP).	Ascending paralysis with preservation of sensory function—global limb weakness. Probably represents autoimmune phenomenon. Nerve conduction studies show demyelinating features. One pt with CMV-associated Guillain-Barre responded to ganciclovir + ARV RX. May be associated with immune reconstitution.
Chronic (chronic inflammatory demyelinating polyneuropathy) (CIDP or IDP) (may also occur late)	Progressive weakness in arms & legs, paresthesias with minor sensory loss, may be asymmetrical, absent DTRs Demyelinating polyneuropathy, CSF ↑↑ protein, mild to moderate lymphocytic pleocytosis (10–50cells/mm³), EMG shows demyelination.
Mononeuritis, multiplex (MM) (also occurs late) (rare)	Facial weakness, foot or wrist drop EMG, multifocal axonal neuropathy, multifocal cranial & peripheral neuropathies, thought to be immune mediated or vasculitis
Multiple sclerosis-like syndrome (rare) *(Neurologist 13:154, 2007)*.	Waxing & waning course, multifocal defect, may rarely represent immune reconstitution inflammatory syndrome (IRIS).

TABLE 11A (9)

CLINICAL SYNDROME, ETIOLOGY, EPIDEMIOLOGY	CLINICAL PRESENTATION, DIAGNOSTIC TESTS, COURSE
Central Nervous System/Movement disorders *(continued)*	
Late (symptomatic HIV), CD4 <200/mm^3 **Weakness/spasticity:**	
Vacuolar myelopathy (occurs in as many as 40% of patients at autopsy) & is the most common form of spinal cord disease in HIV-infected individuals; under-recognized clinically. Other infectious causes of myelopathies: HTLV-1, herpesviruses (VZV, HSV2, CMV), enteroviruses, *T. pallidum*, TB, various fungi, & parasites.	Progressive painless gait disturbance with ataxia & spasticity. Also rarely occurring in upper extremities, + Babinski, may involve bowel & bladder. CSF normal or ↑ protein, 5–10cells/mm^3. Imaging usually normal. Use of somatosensory-evoked potentials in pts with absent ankle DTRs valuable dx tool in differential dx of myelopathy from neuropathy; abnormalities in tibial central conduction time correlated with myelopathy.
Progressive polyradiculopathy: CMV lumbosacral polyradiculopathy/ myelitis (also VZV, syphilis, spinal lymphoma) (occurs <5%) (cauda equina syndrome) *(see below)*	Subacute onset. Back & radicular pain, ascending weakness, areflexia, bladder & sphincter dysfunction, variable sensory loss but may produce "saddle anesthesia." May progress rapidly to flaccid paralysis. Myelitis + radiculitis can also be caused by varicella zoster.
Mononeuritis multiplex due to CMV	Multifocal sensory & motor deficits in major peripheral or cranial nerves (esp. laryngeal nerves & upper > lower extremities—acute onset over 1mo), usually painful. CD4 <50 Rx: *See Table 13, page 167*
Numbness/burning: Distal sensory loss with neuropathic pain (most common neuropathy). Symptoms: pain (often described as excruciating unremitting pain), paresthesias, numbness (although ¼ asymptomatic); signs: ↓ ankle reflexes, ↓ vibratory or pinprick sensation.	
Distal predominantly sensory symmetrical polyneuropathy (DSP) *(see table on the next page)* (occurs in up to 50% of pts with late-stage HIV) *(Neurology 66:1679, 2006)*. Risk factors include age >40 (OR 1.17), diabetes (OR 1.79), white race (OR 1.33), nadir CD4 <50 (OR 1.64) & 50–199 (OR 1.40), VL >10,000 copies/ml at 1st measurement (OR 1.44) plus ETOH abuse, drugs (vincristine, INH & thalidomide, used to rx aphthous ulcers), & ribavirin *(CID 40:148, 2005; Neurology 66:1679, 2006)*. ↓ incidence with ARV RX *(CID 40:148, 2005)*.	Hyperesthesia, **burning feet**, painful, may affect walking, distal numbness with ↓ ankle DTR, stocking/glove sensory loss. Severity of symptoms (pain) correlates with plasma HIV-1 RNA levels. Suppression of HIV may improve symptoms. Tricyclic antidepressants not effective in HIV-related neuropathies according to Cochrane Database Syst Rev. Oct 17;(4):CD005454, 2007.
Toxic neuropathy from antiretroviral drugs (TNA) *(also see Table 6C)* (ddI > d4T > 3TC) (occurs >5%) but has been reported to occur in up to 30% of pts on ddI. Frequency usually associated with dose & duration of exposure: for d4T, 13% for <24 mo. rx vs 29% for >24mos., although risk ↓ over time as immunity improves. Others have found that d4T alone or in combination with ddI doubles risk. FDA warning for ribavirin + ddI ± d4T assoc. with mitochondrial toxicity. Disease progression & host factors (mitochondrial haplogroup & age) all predispose individuals to neurotoxic effects of antiretroviral drugs *(CID 40: 148, 2005, AIDS 19:1341, 2005)*. Protease inhibitors may also potentiate neuronal damage & toxic neuropathy *(Ann Neurol 59:816, 2006)*. Etiology appears to be associated with NRTI selective inhibition of γ-DNA polymerase leading to depletion of mitochondrial DNA & degeneration of mitochondria of neurons & Schwann cells.	**Aching feeling of feet, burning sensation.** ↑ serum lactate levels discriminated d4T neuropathy from DSP neuropathy (90% sensitivity, 90% specificity). **EMG**: axonal neuropathy; symptoms (pain) may worsen for up to 4wks after discontinuation of rx. Many are able to continue drugs with full or reduced dose & in most neuropathy improves or resolves. Substantial portion of pts continue to experience debilitating pain. **Lamotrigine** (an anticonvulsant drug) ↓ pain vs placebo in 227 pts. Rash a common side effect. Results confirmed in 92 pts receiving antiretroviral rx but no difference from placebo in 135 pts with DSP without ART. Coenzyme Q actually ↑ pain. Rx with acetyl-l-carnitine (1500mg q12h po) up to 33mos. assoc. with ↓ symptoms & peripheral nerve regeneration in 21 HIV+ pts with TNA *(HIV Clin Trials 6:344, 2005)*. Capsaicin was ineffective in relieving pain *(Cochrane Database Syst Rev CD003937, 2005)*
Weakness/myalgias:	
Myopathy: HIV, zidovudine [ZDV + ddC > ZDV + ddI]	Weakness without sensory finding, DTRs intact with myalgias. EMG: irritative myopathy, ↑ CPK, muscle biopsy, myofibril degeneration + inflammation

TABLE 11A (10)

DIRECT COMPARISON OF THE 4 MAJOR HIV-ASSOCIATED NEUROPATHIES WITH RX SUGGESTIONS

	DISTAL SYMMETRIC POLYNEUROPATHY (DSP)/TOXIC NEUROPATHY FROM ANTIRETROVIRAL DRUGS (TNA)	INFLAMMATORY DEMYELINATING POLYNEUROPATHY	PROGRESSIVE POLYRADICULOPATHY	MONONEURITIS COMPLEX
Distribution:	Stocking/glove	Extremities—ascending	Cauda equina distribution	Cranial nerve + multiple peripheral nerves
Symptoms:	Hyperesthesia, pain, paresthesia with contact, "burning feet"	Muscle weakness; few if any sensory complaints	Radiating pain in distribution of cauda equina; leg weakness. Bladder/bowel dysfunction (urinary retention)	Cranial & peripheral nerve complaints; motor & sensory
Findings:	↓ response to pain, temperature, vibration; ↓ ankle DTRs; normal strength	Facial nerve paresis; ascending weakness; generalized ↓ in DTRs	Flaccid paraparesis; mild sensory loss; absent leg DTRs, anal wink	Typical nerves involved: facial, median, lateral cutaneous femoral, ulnar, peroneal
Possible etiology(ies):	Toxic; metabolic; nutritional; drugs: nucleoside reverse transcriptase inhibitors	Idiopathic; CMV implicated; CSF—lymphocytic pleocytosis; ↑ protein	CMV—PMNs in CSF Lymphoma—monos in CSF	Can be due to CMV or idiopathic (vasculitis)
Treatment:	Symptomatic (e.g., analgesics, anti-inflammatory agents, anticonvulsants, gabapentin). If receiving NRTIs, dc. If not, start ARV RX; ↓ viral load may ↓ symptoms (see above for experimental treatments)	Similar to Guillain-Barré: corticosteroids, plasmapheresis, IVIG	For CMV—ganciclovir, valganciclovir For lymphoma—chemotherapy	Ganciclovir if CMV

CLINICAL SYNDROME, ETIOLOGY, EPIDEMIOLOGY | CLINICAL PRESENTATION, DIAGNOSTIC TESTS, COURSE

Electrolyte & Metabolic Abnormalities

Hyponatremia
Volume depletion 2° to diarrhea
Cardiac, renal, or liver disease
Syndrome of inappropriate secretion of antidiuretic hormone (SIADH) (2° to pulmonary or CNS infections)
Adrenal insufficiency, primary
Hyporeninemic hypoaldosteronism
Nephrotoxic drugs: pentamidine, amphotericin B, foscarnet,
Nephrogenic diabetes insipidus: ganciclovir

About 20% of ambulatory & 50% of hospitalized patients have serum Na of <135mmol/L. On admission ½ due to GI loss & hypovolemia. During hospitalization ½ due to SIADH (PCP, bacterial pneumonias, CNS infection); patients are edema-free, with hypertonic urine with low serum osmolality & high urinary sodium.

Hyperkalemia
Trimethoprim
Hypoaldosteronism-ketoconazole
Adrenal insufficiency

20–53% pts on TMP/SMX or TMP + dapsone for treatment of PCP develop hyperkalemia. TMP is a sodium channel inhibitor & functions as a K-sparing diuretic agent.

Hypercalcemia
Lymphoma
Granuloma formation associated with immune reconstitution

Lab: ↑ serum 1,25-dihydroxy vitamin D concentrations with ↓ levels of intact parathormone.

Hypocalcemia
Drug-related: Foscarnet,, amphotericin B, aminoglycosides

Neuromuscular irritability, carpal or pedal spasm. Foscarnet forms complex with ionized calcium. Ampho B & aminoglycosides may lead to Mg⁺⁺ wasting with inhibition of parathyroid hormone release & action (*AnIM* 151:1441, 1991).

Lactic acidosis/hepatic steatosis (see Table 6C)
Lipodystrophy (lipoatrophy or lipohypertrophy), or HIV-associated metabolic **syndrome** (see Table 11B & Table 6C)

TABLE 11A (11)

CLINICAL SYNDROME, ETIOLOGY, EPIDEMIOLOGY	CLINICAL PRESENTATION, DIAGNOSTIC TESTS, COURSE
Endocrine System: 7/13 asymptomatic ♀ randomly tested had abnormal endocrine function: pituitary-adrenal, pituitary-thyroid, & pituitary-ovarian axis. 6 had menstrual irregularities (*Gynecol Endocrin* 16:33, 2002).	
Pituitary gland Infectious involvement of anterior pituitary: CMV, P. jiroveci (carinii), Toxoplasma gondii	25% of advanced but non-AIDS HIV+ patients have ↓ pituitary reserve (*AJM Sci* 305:321, 1993). Functional pituitary insufficiency is very uncommon but reported (*AJM* 77:760, 1984). Useful diagnostic tests: Corticotropin-releasing hormone (CRH) test; testing for several hormones simultaneously: insulin + thyrotropin-releasing hormone (TRH) + gonadorelin (GnRH); measure glucose, cortisol, GH, TSH, prolactin, LH, FSH & ACTH.
Thyroid gland (see *CID* 45: 488, 2007 for etiologies and test use) Chronic illness	Lab: ↓ T_3 with reciprocal ↑ rT_3 (reverse T_3), T_4 usually normal. Useful diagnostic tests: T_3, T_4, thyroid-binding globulin, rT_3.
HIV infection	Lab: 16% of 350 HIV-infected French pts tested had hypothyroidism: 2.6% were overtly hypothyroid, 6.6% had subclinical hypothyroidism, & 6.8% had ↓ free T4. In multivariate analysis, d4T rx & ↓ CD4 count associated with hypothyroidism (*CID* 37:579, 2003). 18/52 Italian children (35%) had thyroid abnormalities: 16 isolated ↓ T4; T4 level correlated positively with CD4% & duration of ARV RX (*PIDJ* 23:235, 2004). Similar findings in Thai children: 10/37 (28%) had abnormal thyroid function assoc. with advanced disease *J Ped Endo Metab* 17:33, 2004). In an Italian study 12.6% of 182 HIV+ patients on ARV RX had subclinical hypo thyroidism vs. 0% of 20 naive patients. Stavudine Rx most significant risk factor (*Clin Endocrinol* 64:375, 2006). P. jiroveci may involve the thyroid rarely (*Mycoses* 50: 443, 2007).
Graves' disease—1 report assoc. with immune reconstitution from ARV RX (*AIDS Res Hum Retrovir* 20:157, 2004)	
Adrenal gland (the most commonly affected endocrine gland) Primary adrenal failure; causes include: • CMV adrenalitis (found in 33–88% of AIDS pts at autopsy) • HIV infection of adrenal • Infiltration by Kaposi's sarcoma, lymphoma or infection (MAC, crypto, histo, pneumocystis) • Drug-induced: ketoconazole (impairs steroid synthesis), fluconazole (1 report: 800 mg q24h x68 days, *J Microbiol Immun Inf* 37:250, 2004), rifampin & ritonavir (induce hepatic enzymes which ↑ metabolism of steroids), 6 cases of overt Addison's diseases on withdrawal of inhaled corticosteroids (fluticasone) (*J Clin Endocrinol Metab* 90:4394, 2005), megestrol (prolonged use) (*AnIM* 122:843, 1995) • Pituitary insufficiency (see above)	**Addison's disease: fever, hypotension, abdominal pain, hyponatremia, hyperkalemia.** Overt Addison's disease is uncommon, although blunted responses to ACTH are common (*AJM Sci* 305:321, 1993). Addisonian crisis may be precipitated by excessive stress or ketoconazole. In 28 critically ill HIV+ pts, 6 (21%) had stress cortisol levels & low-dose (1 mcg) corticotropin stimulation test levels of <18 μg/dl & dx of adrenal insufficiency. 21/28 (75%) had adrenal insufficiency if 25 mcg/dl was used as diagnostic threshold (*Crit Care Med* 30:1267, 2002). CMV antigenemia assoc. with adrenal insufficiency. Suboptimal response to ACTH stimulation & ↓ stress cortisol serum levels should receive stress doses of corticosteroids where there is infection, trauma, etc. (*Endocr J* 49:641, 2002). Useful diagnostic tests: AM, PM plasma cortisol levels [AM level <275 μmol/L suggests adrenal insufficiency (*Clin Endo* 45:97, 1996)]; single dose cosyntropin stimulation test [but a single normal response may not rule out adrenal insufficiency (*Am J Med Sci* 321:137, 2001)]; plasma ACTH levels. ↑ basal serum cortisol & ↓ dehydroepiandrosterone is actually more common than in HIV-neg. persons, but rarely assoc. with features of Cushing syndrome (*ArIM* 162:1095, 2004).
Pancreas	
Pancreatitis Drug-associated: pentamidine, didanosine (ddI) 2–6%, zalcitabine (ddC) <1%, stavudine (d4T) 1%, lamivudine (3TC) 1% but 15% in children, ddI/d4T 4.16/100pys clinical and 6.25/100pys clinical + laboratory pancreatitis. Among ARV RX regimens rates highest with Indinavir/ddI/d4T (*J Acquir Immune Defic Syndr* 39:159, 2005). Other drugs implicated, including those used to treat OIs and malignancies.	Typical presentation (nausea, vomiting & abdominal pain). Type I diabetes mellitus may develop.

TABLE 11A (12)

CLINICAL PRESENTATION, DIAGNOSTIC TESTS, COURSE

CLINICAL SYNDROME, ETIOLOGY, EPIDEMIOLOGY	CLINICAL PRESENTATION, DIAGNOSTIC TESTS, COURSE
Endocrine System/Pancreas *(continued)*	
Hyperglycemia: Insulin resistance common in ARV RX; see Table 6C. Drug-induced [especially protease inhibitor 6%, megestrol acetate, & corticosteroids (*J AIDS & Human Retro* 17:46, 1998)]. See Table 6B & Table 6C	Other diabetogenic drugs frequently taken by HIV+ patients: dapsone, rifampin, sulfamethoxazole in patients with renal failure, octreotide, ganciclovir (*AnIM* 118:529, 1993). Protease inhibitors produced symptomatic diabetes mellitus in 6/105 pts (*ICAAC* 1997, LB-8). ddI + tenofovir associated with ↑ frequency of hyperglycemia (33% in 78 pts at 12 months)(*AIDS Res Hum Retroviruses* 22:333, 2006).
Hypoglycemia Drug-induced [Pentamidine (IV), 2%]	During destruction of islets, insulin release may cause hypoglycemic coma. Co-trimoxazole (TXS) associated with severe hypoglycemia resulting from increased insulin levels suggesting a sulfonylurea-like effect: 14 cases reported, renal insufficiency in 93%, most were receiving 2 double-strength tabs twice a day for Rx of PCP (*Lancet ID* 6:178, 2006).
Gonads	
Testes Primary testicular failure (see *CID* 33:857, 2001 & *AIDS Pt Care STDs* 19:655, 2005). Drug-associated: ketoconazole, megestrol (McGale)	↓ libido & impotence common. Gynecomastia found in 1.8% of 2275 HIV+ men; related to hypogonadism; ↓ free testosterone index vs controls (*CID* 39:1514, 2004). Efavirenz also assoc. with gynecomastia in a retrospective case-controlled study in 23 pts (*AIDS Reader* 14:29, 2004). ARV RX itself may ↓ libido in males assoc. with ↑ estradiol serum levels (*Int J STD AIDS* 15:234, 2004). Erectile dysfunction found in 74% of HIV+ urban men (*AIDS Pt Care STDs* 20:75, 2006). Lab: ↓ free testosterone levels, ↑ LH & FSH, normal GnRH response. Approx. 30% of men with HIV infection & 50% with AIDS are hypogonadal; ↑ with late stage disease (*CID* 41:1794, 2005). Testosterone replacement useful & ↑ muscle mass, ↑ mood with ↓ depression symptoms & ↑ bone density (*AIDS Reader* 13:515, 2003). Found to ↑ muscle mass in low-wt HIV-infected men (*AnIM* 164:897, 2004). Others have shown that testosterone rx for depression not different than placebo in a prospective randomized double-blind placebo-controlled trial in 123 men (*J Clin Psychopharm* 24:379, 2004).
Ovaries Menstrual irregularities are common, esp. with advanced HIV/AIDS (CD4 <200/mm³) & wasting. ARV RX use associated with ↓ **rates** of menstrual problems (*J Womans Health* 15:591, 2006).	In 69 HIV-infected women, weight loss >10% max. weight was significant predictor of low free testosterone serum level, thus ↓ androgen level common in women with wasting (*CID* 36:499, 2003). Testosterone replacement (patches 2x/wk) ↑ testosterone levels but had little physiological effect in a randomized double-bind study in 52 women (*JCEM*, Dec. 21, 2004).
Eye: Ocular manifestations occur in up to 75% of HIV infected pts (*Ocul Immunol Inflam* 8:263, 2000, *SADJ* 60:386, 2005) — Up to 10-20% of HIV-infected worldwide will lose vision in 1 or both eyes from CMV (*Bull WHO* 79:181, 2001). ½ of 162 African children with HIV infection had ophthalmic involvement; most common finding was perivasculitis of peripheral retinal vessels (38%) (*Ocul Immunol Inflam* 8:263, 2000). 10% of 1250 HIV+ Ugandan adults screened with Schnellen test had visual impairment (Otiti, personal communication; IDI, Mulago Hospital). Introduction of ARV RX has significantly reduced significance of ocular disease but has introduced immune-recovery uveitis associated with CMV (*Ocul Immunol Inflamm* 13:213, 2005) and lesions related to the metabolic alterations induced by ARV RX: chalazion, diabetic & hypertension retinopathy, lipid arc of the cornea and glaucoma (*Eur J Opth* 16:728, 2006).	
Acute loss of vision	Differential Dx: CMV papillitis, VZV—rapidly progressive retinal necrosis (*AIDS* 16:1045, 2002), syphilis, cryptococcal meningitis, TBc, toxo (*Ophth* 111:716, 2004), endophthalmitis (bacterial or fungal) (*CID* 26:34, 1998).
Anterior Segment Infections (*Review of anterior and extraorbital eye disorders in* Survey Ophthalmol 52:329, 2007)	
Chronic follicular conjunctivitis due to Molluscum contagiosum	Lesions larger, more numerous, more rapid in onset than in immunocompetent individuals. Solitary lesions of molluscum contagiosum may persist after ARV RX (*Br J Ophthal* 87:1427, 2003) but may regress with pronounced injection (IRS) (*Graefes Ar Clin Exp Ophth* 242:951, 2004).
Corneal microsporidiosis (Encephalitozoon hellum) (*J Infect* 27:229, 1993)	Photophobia, dry eyes, foreign body sensation, blurred vision. Punctate keratopathy. Pets, esp. birds, suspected source. Nasal sinus epithelium occasionally involved. Dx: epithelial scrapings (*Am J Ophth* 115:285, 1993).

TABLE 11A (13)

CLINICAL SYNDROME, ETIOLOGY, EPIDEMIOLOGY	CLINICAL PRESENTATION, DIAGNOSTIC TESTS, COURSE
Eye/Anterior Segment Infections (continued)	
Keratitis, candida sp., nocardia (Jpn J Ophth 48:272, 2004)	Often no history of trauma, spontaneous & bilateral ulcers. Dx based on corneal scrapings & culture.
Herpes simplex virus keratitis	Predilection for peripheral rather than central involvement. Lesions take longer to heal & recurrences common. Dx: Fluorescein + epithelial "dendrites" (Ophthalmologica 214:337, 2000)
Varicella zoster virus keratitis	Most pts have H. zoster lesions in trigeminal nerve (1st div.) distribution. 2/3 have keratitis, usually punctate.
Eyelids (Ln 348:525, 1996)	
Herpes zoster ophthalmitis, Kaposi's sarcoma, Molluscum contagiosum	Solitary lesions of molluscum contagiosum may persist after ARV RX (Br J Ophthal 87:1427, 2003) or may regress with pronounced injection (IRS) (Graefes Ar Clin Exp Ophth 242:951, 2004).
Posterior Segment Infections	
At least 12 infectious agents identified as causes of retinal or choroidal disease in HIV+ patients (ID Clin NA 6:909, 1992). Considerations include more common or major entities.	Prompt ophthalmologic consultation indicated, etiologic diagnosis usually dependent on clinical characteristics rather than laboratory findings.
Bacterial retinitis: Mycobacterium avium-intracellulare, Rhodococcus equi, Bartonella (cat scratch/bacillary angiomatosis)	Cat scratch disease (Bartonella sp) presented as subretinal mass of an abnormal vascular network (similar to BA in the skin & liver) in 3 pts in Brazil (Am J Opth 141:400, 2006).
Candidal endophthalmitis Prevalence in HIV+ pts unclear. It is rare with only mucocutaneous candidiasis, but may be associated with candidemia with IV lines & neutropenia.	Well-demarcated yellow to white lesions that protrude into vitreous, not associated with hemorrhage & usually unilateral.
Choroid tubercles (choroidal granulomas) (Found in 2.8% of pts with disseminated tuberculosis & AIDS in Malawi (Br J Ophthal 86:1076, 2002). Choroidal pneumocystosis	Ocular tuberculosis in 15 cases (19 eyes) in India presented as: choroidal granulomas in 53%, subretinal abscesses in 37%, increased panophthalmitis 15% & conjunctival TB in 5% (Am J Ophthalmol 142:413, 2006). Almost all patients have had P. jiroveci (carinii) pneumonia & prophylaxis with aerosolized pentamidine. Creamy to orange choroidal lesions, usually bilateral without vitreous inflammation. Visual acuity usually not affected. Course: Response to systemic rx usually good.
Cryptococcosis: choroiditis, endophthalmitis In one series 9/27 (33%) pts with crypto meningitis had neuro-ophthal. signs (Ophth 96:1092, 1989).	Rapid visual loss with optic nerve involvement. May be due to ↑ intracranial pressure, a medical emergency— rx with CSF drainage. Multifocal white or yellow lesions with optic nerve edema usually without vitreous inflammation seen. (Am J Ophthalmol 142:346, 2006). Dx usually based on systemic &/or meningeal crypto. With rx, progressive optic atrophy may occur.
Cytomegalovirus (CMV) retinopathy: Rx: See Table 12, page 150 Occurs in 20–30% of AIDS patients. Found in 32/191 (17%) pts with AIDS in Malawi (Br J Ophthal 86:1076, 2002). Marked reduction with ARV RX (J AIDS 22:228, 1999; HIV Med 2:255, 2001), but less so with advanced disease (AnIM 135:17, 2001). **ARV RX markedly improves survival & success of anti-CMV rx.** (J AIDS & HR 19:13, 1998; AIDS 12:613, 1998) but vision loss from immune recovery uveitis (epiretinal membrane, cystoid macular edema or cataract) reported in up to 63% (Retina 25:633, 2005) (See Table 11B) but account for <10% of causes of vision loss from CMV (Ophthal 113:1441, 2006). ARV RX reduces visual loss from CMV retinitis by approximately 50% (Ophthal 113:1432, 2006 & 113:684, 2006). Rates of 2nd eye involvement ↓ with ARV RX but not if CD4 stays <50/mm³ (Ophthalmology 111:2232, 2004).	**Peripheral retinitis, CD4 count is <50/mm³.** Course: Usually begins with unilateral "floaters" to ↓ visual acuity to blindness. **Ophthal. exam: Findings are usually initially in the periphery, moving centrally until macula &/or optic disc involved. Lesions are large creamy to white areas with granular borders & perivascular exudates & hemorrhages ("cottage cheese & ketchup" appearance) with little overlying vitreous reaction. If redness or pain of the eye, photophobia or irregular-shaped pupil develops, suspect infection other than CMV retinopathy.** Dx: Based on clinical features, CMV DNA+ in serum; ↓ with effective anti-CMV rx (CID 15:1756, 2001). ↑ CMV-specific CD4 &/or CD8 cells predict prevention of recurrence after ARV RX (AIDS Res Hum Retrovir 17:1749, 2001; JID 184:256, 2001), while failure to ↑ CMV-specific CD4 response assoc. with multiple relapses (JID 183:1285, 2001). Mortality from CMV correlates with CMV DNA in plasma (JCI 101:Y97, 1998). CMV genome not found in aqueous humor by PCR in immune recovery uveitis (Ophthalmologia 218:43, 2004).

TABLE 11A (14)

CLINICAL SYNDROME, ETIOLOGY, EPIDEMIOLOGY	CLINICAL PRESENTATION, DIAGNOSTIC TESTS, COURSE
Eye/Posterior Segment Infections *(continued)*	
Primary CMV papillitis	**Rapid ↓ in visual acuity.** Swelling of optic nerve head, atrophy within 4wks. Consider pulsed systemic steroids + ganciclovir or foscarnet *(Am J Ophth 108:691, 1989)*. Dx & rx: See CMV peripheral retinitis, above, & Table 12, page 151.
Herpes zoster/simplex virus (VZV) retinitis (mean CD4 24) 5/10 pts presenting to eye clinic in Nigeria with HZ ophthalmicus were HIV+ *(West Afr J Med 22:136, 2003)*.	**May not be associated with cutaneous zoster.** 1) **Acute retinal necrosis (ARN) syndrome:** rapidly progressive necrosis of peripheral retina (often 360°) with occlusive vasculopathy, marked vitreous & anterior chamber inflammation, optic neuritis & scleritis. Complete visual loss in involved eye. In ½ pts both eyes involved *(Am J Ophth 112:119, 1991; Am J Ophth 110:341, 1990; Ln 348:525, 1996; CID 26:34, 1998)*. May be associated with retrobulbar optic neuritis *(Am J Neuroradiol 25:1722, 2004)*. 2) Ill-defined areas of peripheral retinal whitening without granular borders, minimal vitreous reaction, no pain or foveal lesions (confused with CMV).
HIV-associated "cotton wool" spots (CWS) CWS occurs in about 50% of patients with non-infectious microvascular retinopathy. Nonspecific findings & seen in many other conditions *(Med 82:187, 2003)*	Usually asymptomatic but occur more in late-stage disease. Ophthal. exam: Small fluffy white lesions with indistinct margins without exudates or hemorrhages. Lesions do not progress & usually regress spontaneously, do not require treatment. CWS may indicate ↑ risk for onset of CMV retinitis.
Iritis secondary to cidofovir *(CID 25:337, 1997; CID 28:156, 1999)*	Common with intravitreal injection but recurrent episodes with IV also reported.
PEG interferon alfa-2b—ribavirin ocular changes	8/23 (35%) receiving PEG INF-Rib for Hep C rx developed visual/ocular abnormalities, including cotton wool spots, cataracts, ↓ color vision *(AIDS 18:1805, 2004)*. Uveitis, vascular occlusions reported *(World J Gastroenterol 13:3137, 2007)*.
Retinal depigmentation	5% of children on didanosine (ddl) usually at >300mg/M²/day developed retinal depigmentation[1]. Asymptomatic.
Retinal deposits of clofazimine	Clofazimine deposits in pigmented tissues. May result in brownish refractile crystals in retina.
Rifabutin-associated uveitis Reported in 1–2% pts on 600 mg/day *(NEJM 330:438, 1994)*. Also rarely on 300mg/day *(AnIM 121:510, 1994)*.	Becoming ↑ common with use of protease inhibitors (↑ rifabutin serum levels) in Western world but rare (1/191) in Africa *(Br J Ophthal 86:1076, 2002)* (see Table 16A, Drug/Drug Interactions). Also in non-HIV infected *(Eye 14:344, 2000)*.
Syphilis: iridocyclitis, vitreitis, optic neuritis, chorioretinitis, or combinations of these. *(Eye June 3, 2005)* **Uveitis in HIV: Think syphilis** *(Int J STD AIDS 12:754, 2001)* Focal anterior scleritis with retinitis caused by syphilis uncovered with immune reconstitution *(Clin Exp Ophthalmol 32:526, 2004)*.	**In HIV+, syphilitic ocular disease is more common, more severe & often bilateral.** Sx may include blurred or ↓ vision, scotomata, redness, pain *(Amer J Med 119:448, 2006)*. **Necrotizing retinitis with hemorrhage may be confused with CMV.** Cream-colored posterior plaques may be seen with mucocutaneous lesions in 2° syphilis. May present as bilateral exudative retinal detachment *(Ocul Immunol Inflamm 13:459, 2005)*. **Rule out neurosyphilis.** 7% of 9 pts with syphilitic uveitis has CSF abn. *(Arch Clin Exp Ophthal 243:863, 20C5)*. Lab: Positive VDRL & FTA/ABS on serum. Course: Rx failures reported with penicillin.
Toxoplasmic chorioretinitis Ocular involvement uncommon in AIDS. Lesions may be single or multifocal, usually discrete, perivascular in location. Found in 15/132 pts with new onset vision impairment in Uganda *(J. Otiti, personal communication)*.	Pre-existing chorioretinal scars usually absent. Hemorrhages are absent or minimal. Vitreitis & iridocyclitis (red, painful eye) are common. May occur without intracranial lesions. Lab: PCR for toxo DNA in vitreous fluid may be of value *(Ophthal 106:1554, 1999; Ophthal 111:716, 2004)*. Course: Response to rx usually good, prolonged suppression required. Oral steroids not used.

---

[1] Adapted from R.W. Price, Chapter 14, *ibid.*

TABLE 11A (15)

CLINICAL SYNDROME, ETIOLOGY, EPIDEMIOLOGY	CLINICAL PRESENTATION, DIAGNOSTIC TESTS, COURSE
Fever of Unknown Origin (FUO) Prolonged fever is a common finding in AIDS pts. The etiology varies with geography (AIDS 16:909, 2002), frequency ↑ with ↓ CD4 counts & ↓ with ARV RX (Eur J Clin Micro Inf Dis 21:137, 2002). **Etiology of FUO in AIDS:** In U.S.: **MAC (31%)**, Pneumocystis jiroveci (carinii) pneumonia (13%), bacterial pneumonia (9%), sinusitis (6%, Rhinol 39:136, 2001), lymphoma (7%), catheter infection (1–10%), drug allergy (2–5%), phenytoin reported (Int J STD AIDS 16:178, 2005), disseminated histoplasmosis (7%), Bartonella [8.5% of 250 bc pos. for B. henselae or B. quintana & 68/382 (18%) AIDS pts in San Francisco had Bartonella infection dx by bc, IFA or PCR (CID 37:559, 2003)], & CMV (11%) unexplained in 15–30%. Immune reactivation (IRIS) & drug fever have ↑ (15%) with ARV RX (Inf Med 21:335, 2004). In Spain, **TBc identified in 42%**, leishmaniasis in 14% (less common with ARV RX—CID 37:973, 2003) & MAC in 14% (CID 20:872, 1996). In Brazil, TBc in 33%. 25% have multiple etiologies. Monocytic ehrlichiosis reported (Braz J Infec Dis 10:7, 2006). In Thailand & Vietnam, TBc, crypto, Penicillium marneffei (Sante 13:149, 2003). **In Africa, TBc most common by far**, crypto, malaria, others include histoplasmosis, salmonella bacteremia, bacterial pneumonia (S. pneumo common isolate from blood cultures), Rhodococcus sp. (J Infect 41:227, 2002). Pts with fever & peripheral adenopathy, think TBc & Burkitt's lymphoma (Int J Cancer 92:687, 2001) **In India**, TBc 63%, crypto 10%, PCP 7%, others include bacterial pneumonia, amebic liver abscess, histoplasmosis, & cerebral toxo (Nat/ Med J India 16:193, 2003; BMC Inf Dis 22:52, 2004). **In areas of high prevalence, malaria should be ruled out**, but HIV+ pts with fever are frequently rx for malaria delaying dx of above. Co-infection with both common; frequency of falciparum malaria fever ↑ with ↓ in CD4 count (JID 192:984, 2005, Ln 362:1008, 2003). Malaria assoc. with ↑ VL (Lancet 365:233, 2005).	In 704 HIV+ pts with fever at SFGH, **18% blood cultures + in hospitalized pts.** Predictors of + culture: pneumonia, UTI, abscess, central line or neutropenia. Without 1 predictor, only 1.5% were +. **Sensitivity of AFB bc related to CD4 count:** <100 19% +, 101–200 7% +, >200 0% +. 17% of febrile pts in Malawi had pos. AFB blood cultures (Int J Tuberc Lung Dis 6:1067, 2002). **Fungal bc of no value:** Serum CRAG + in 3%; all <200 CD4. **Chest x-ray** of value when respiratory sx present 85–95% sensitive but specificity only 16–30%. **Urine culture** of value with dysuria. In pts with abn LFTs, liver bx revealed cause of fever in 13/24 pts (CID 20:606, 1995). **Diagnostic value of bone marrow aspirate & biopsy appears to vary from study to study, geographical location, & likely availability of other dx tests. Bone marrow bx** pos. in 52/123 FUO pts in Spain but could have probably been dx through other means (ArIM 157:1577, 1997). In Brazil, specific dx in 33/99 with AFB in 12, histo 5, & lymphoma 6 (Pathol Res Pract 200:591, 2004). In London yield of BM exam was 30% in pts on ARV RX and 23% without ARV RX. ↑ yield with fever & cytopenias (Int J STD AIDS 16:686, 2005). In 72 pts with AIDS & FUO in U.S., BM exam of low diagnostic yield even with abnormal hematological parameters (J AIDS 37:1599, 2004). In endemic areas when **LDH >600 units/L**, 32% had pos. bone marrow stain for histoplasmosis vs 8% with LDH <600 (South Med J 93:692, 2000). In pts with high prolonged fever & ↑ bilirubin, bone marrow aspiration, biopsy & culture more sensitive & rapid for dx mycobacteria & histo than blood cultures (Am J Hematol 67:100, 2001). When fever assoc. with hepatosplenomegaly & pancytopenia: think leishmania in endemic areas; bone marrow smear pos. for amastigotes (Hum Pathol 31:75, 2000). Think lymphoma with prolonged fever, cytopenias & hemophagocytic syndrome (AIDS Pt Care STDs 17:495, 2003). **High resolution sonography** revealed multiple microabscesses in 32 pts with FUO in Spain: 14 TBc, 7 leishmania, 5 MAC, 2 salmonella, 2 lymphoma, 1 rhodococcus (Eur J Clin Microbiol Inf Dis 18:374, 1999). When fever remains unexplained, think MAC, lymphoma, Bartonella, PCP or fungus.
M. avium is the most common cause of FUO in the U.S. when CD4 count <50. It appears to be rare in East Central Africa (JID 162:208, 1990; J AIDS 8:195, 1995) but point prevalence 10% in South Africa (CID 33:2069, 2002). Infection due to Mycobacterium avium-intracellulare complex [M. avium 52%, M. intracellulare 21%, M. xenopi 7%, M. fortuitum 2% (CID 20:73, 1995)] [M. genavense, an unrelated organism which clinically behaves like MAC].	M. avium usually presents as disseminated infection with symptoms of fever, weight loss, night sweats, **diarrhea, anemia & neutropenia,** but may be asymptomatic even with positive blood cultures. Highest concentration of organisms (6.7 $\log_{10}$/gm) in mesenteric nodes (JID 173:942, 1996). Lab: Colonization of respiratory secretions & GI tract is common & may precede disseminated disease. When symptomatic, blood cultures are usually positive for MAC (BACTEC system is very sensitive). Dual infection with M. tbc recognized. Prevalence of MAC but not MTB has declined in ARV RX era in Brazil (Braz J Infect Dis 9:459, 2005) but isolated from 6% of deaths from AIDS in France (Scand J Infect Dis 37:482, 2005)

TABLE 11A (16)

CLINICAL SYNDROME, ETIOLOGY, EPIDEMIOLOGY	CLINICAL PRESENTATION, DIAGNOSTIC TESTS, COURSE
Gastrointestinal Tract	
Mouth[1] (*Bull World Health Organ* 83;700, 2005; *Top HIV Med* 13;143, 2006; *Adv Dent Res* 19:63 & 57, 2006) Oral manifestations very common in HIV-infected persons worldwide. 90% of 101 HIV+ Cambodians had oral lesions: oral candidiasis 52%, hairy leukoplakia 36%, necrotizing ulcerative gingivitis 28% (*J Oral Pathol Med* 31:1, 2002). In Kenya, all of 61 pts had periodontal disease, 80% candidiasis, 28% angular chelosis, 13% KS (*East Afr Med* 78:398, 2001). Oral manifestations ↓ with ARV RX (*Oral Dis* 10:145, 2004; *BMC Oral Health* 6:12, 2006) but reappearance of oral lesions may indicate failure of ARV See www.iasusa.org (Retnick slides for pictures of lesions).	
Oral lesions without soreness (or mild soreness)	
Acute retroviral syndrome (see *Acute HIV*, page 23)	Oral ulcerations (aphthous ulcers), anathemas and oral candidiasis. Lab: Thrombocytopenia 74%. HIV antibody test initially + in 7/30 (23%).
Candidiasis Response to ARV RX with ↑ CD4 assoc. with ↓ oropharyngeal candidiasis (31% at baseline to 1% after 48wks ARV RX)] (*AIDS* 14:979, 2000). The presence of Oral Candidiasis predicted immune failure in patients on ARV RX (*AIDS patient Care STDS* 19;70, 2005).	Cigarette smoking a risk factor for OC; OR 2.5 in 631 adults (*Community Dental Oral Epidemol* 33;35, 2005)
Pseudomembranous form (thrush) (most common form) (82% had CD4 <200)	Small 1–2mm to large white plaques on any mucosal surface. Can be wiped off, leaving erythematous to bleeding base. Lab: Dx established by KOH prep of scraping & culture. Oral candidiasis was predictor for TB in Thailand (*J Oral Pathol Med* 31:163, 2002).
Erythematous form (58% had CD4 <200)	Smooth red patches on soft or hard palate, dorsal tongue &/or buccal mucosa. Lab: Dx established as above.
Angular cheilitis (60% had CD4 <200)	Erythematous cracks & fissures at corner of mouth. Lab: Dx established as above.
Hyperkeratotic form (candidal leukoplakia)	White lesions on tongue, palate &/or buccal mucosa that cannot be wiped off. Clinically resembles hairy leukoplakia (see *below*). Lab Biopsy of lesion will show fungi.
Kaposi's sarcoma (100% had CD4 <200) Oral shedding of HHV-8 (KS-assoc. herpesvirus) found in 22% of 196 HIV+ MSM (*J AIDS* 35:233, 2004), & 32% of 174 HIV+ CSWs in Kenya (*JID* 190:484, 2004) without KS. ↑ HHV-8 VL also found in oral secretions in HIV-pos. & -neg. pts with KS (*AIDS Res Hum Retrovir* 20:704, 2004).	Red to purple macules, papules or nodules, occasionally the same color as adjoining tissue, on tongue, palate or buccal mucosa. Usually asymptomatic but may become painful with ulceration & inflammation [*Oral AIDS* 8 (Suppl.2):88, 2002]. Sublingual lesion in HIV+ children in Zimbabwe may be Ranula; biopsy! (*Oral Dis* 10:229, 2004). Lab Biopsy necessary for dx since bacillary angiomatosis also reported (*J Oral Pathol Med* 29:91, 2000).

[1] J.S. Greenspan, D. Greenspan, J.R. Winker, Chapter 11, *ibid*.

TABLE 11A (17)

CLINICAL SYNDROME, ETIOLOGY, EPIDEMIOLOGY	CLINICAL PRESENTATION, DIAGNOSTIC TESTS, COURSE
Gastrointestinal Tract/Mouth (continued)	
Hairy leukoplakia (HLP) (66% had CD4 <200) Epstein-Barr virus can be detected by immunochemistry, in situ hybridization or EBV-DNA by PCR in nearly 100% of lesions (*J Oral Pathol Med* 29:118, 2000; *Am J. Clin Pathol* 114:395, 2000). EBV produces both replicative & non-productive infection in tongue epithelial cells from pts with hairy leukoplakia (HLP) (*JID* 190:387, 2004), transcription of specific EBV genes appear to be assoc. with expression of HLP (*JID* 190:396, 2004), & active infection assoc. with ↓ oral epithelial Langerhans cell count, thereby evading local mucosal immune response (*JID* 189:1656, 2004).	**Lesions usually asymptomatic. White thickening of oral mucosa &/or lateral tongue margins with vertical folds or corrugations.** Lesions range from few mm to covering entire dorsal surface of the tongue. ↑ frequency in smokers (*J AIDS* 21:236, 1999). **Lab: Biopsy; epithelial hyperplasia with thickened parakeratin layer with hair-like projections & vacuolated prickle cells.** Rx: Usually not treated, but can be rx with high-dose acyclovir (see *Table 13, page 168, & Table 12, page 152*). Lesions respond but recur. 10/10 pts responded to one application of topical podophyllin resin within 4-5days; remissions of 2-28wks (*J AIDS* 4:543, 1991).
Warts [human papillomavirus (HPV)] Oral warts may ↑ in size & frequency in response to ARV RX [*Oral Dis* 8 (Suppl.2):91, 2002]. (*AIDS Pt Care STD* 18:443, 2004; *Am J Med Sci* 328:57, 2004)	Usually asymptomatic. Present as single or multiple papilliform warts with multiple white spike-like projections, or as pink cauliflower masses, or as flat lesions resembling focal epithelial hyperplasia. Lab: Biopsy. Types 7, 13 & 32, but usually not 6, 11, 16 & 18 which are associated with anogenital warts. Rx with topical cidofovir gel 1% successful in 1 recalcitrant case (*Cutis* 73:191, 2004).
Secondary syphilis (often multiple) (*Med Oral* 9:33, 2004)	Dx by VDRL &/or biopsy of lesion (see *Clinics* 61:161, 2006).
Lymphoma	Poorly demarcated swelling on alveolar ridges &/or discrete oral masses. Lab: Biopsy. May be EBV+ (*Oral Oncol* 38:96, 2002).
Carcinoma, squamous cell: ↑ risk suggested by 3 epidemiological studies especially of lips & tongue (*Adv Dent Res* 19:57, 2006).	Squamous cell carcinoma of tongue reported in HIV disease. Lab: Biopsy
Cytomegalovirus (CMV) oral ulcers	A rare manifestation of CMV (*AnIM* 119:924, 1993). Usually with disseminated infection. Lab: Biopsy & immunohistochemistry
Histoplasmosis, Geotrichosis, Cryptococcosis, Penicillium marneffei, Leishmaniasis. Oral histo was a clue to presence of HIV infection in Brazil (*Oral Surg, Oral Med* 93:654, 2002) & found in 3% of 733 HIV+ pts in Argentina (*J Oral Pathol Med* 33:445, 2004). In endemic areas, think oral leishmaniasis (*Oral Dis* 8:59, 2002); reported as a cause of gingival ulcers (*AIDS* 22:160,2008).	Rare in occurrence. Lesions painless, clean ulcerations on palate, gingiva & oropharynx. Lab: Biopsy; organism identified on culture & stains.
Sore mouth without discrete lesions	
HIV-associated gingivitis & periodontitis: Common with advanced HIV. Pts at all stages of HIV infection have ↑↑ numbers of PMNs & mast cells throughout the gingiva & ↑ macrophages below the gingival epithelium (*AIDS* 16:235, 2002). Chronic periodontitis assoc. with ↑ cells with ↑ expression of HIV receptors/co-receptors/α defensins perhaps ↑ susceptibility of HIV infection via oral route (*J Dent Res* 83:371, 2004). Was associated with ↑ aggregations of spirochetes (87%), yeast (65.6%), & "herpes-like viruses" (56%) in 1 study (*J Periodontal Res* 38:147, 2003). Response to Rx improved with ARV RX (*Eur J Med Res* 11:232, 2006).	Marked halitosis, spontaneous bleeding & deep-seated gingival pain are usual. Gingiva show fiery red margins with necrosis & ulceration of interdental papillae. May rapidly progress to loss of gingival soft tissue & destruction of supporting bone leading to loss of teeth & necrotizing stomatitis. Is similar to noma (gangrenous stomatitis). Dx: Based on clinical features. Cultures not helpful. Entamoeba gingivalis has been isolated, ? significance (*CID* 27:471, 1998). Rx: Start with curettage/debridement, followed by topical povidone-iodine (Betadine) irrigation, then chlorhexidine gluconate (Peridex) mouthwash + oral antibiotics effective against anaerobes (metronidazole, clindamycin, AM/CL).

TABLE 11A (18)

CLINICAL SYNDROME, ETIOLOGY, EPIDEMIOLOGY	CLINICAL PRESENTATION, DIAGNOSTIC TESTS, COURSE
Gastrointestinal Tract/Mouth (*continued*)	
Oral lesions, painful	
Recurrent aphthous ulcers (RAU) More common in HIV disease, last longer & produce more painful symptoms than in immunocompetent persons (*Am J Clin Dermatol 4*:669, 2003)	Recurrent crops of superficial painful ulcers (1 mm to 1 cm) on non-keratinized oral or oropharyngeal mucosa. Lab: Biopsy; shows only non-specific inflammation. Rx: Topical steroids in 50% Orabase may ↓ pain & swelling. Thalidomide (200 mg po q24h x14d), 13/14 pts responded (*CID 20*:250, 1995). In ACTG 251, 14/23 healed with thalidomide rx vs 1/22 on placebo but ¼ had significant side-effects (*CID 28*:892, 1999).
Herpes simplex virus (HSV)—*See rx, page 156* HSV-1 most common cause, rarely HSV-2; both can be shed in oral secretions (*Sex Trans Inf 80*:272, 2004) Drug-associated lesions	Recurrent crops of small painful vesicles that ulcerate, usually on palate or gingiva. Usually heal but tend to recur. Herpetic geometric glossitis [extremely tender longitudinal fissures occur, heal with acyclovir IV (*NEJM 329*:859, 1993)]. Lab: Smears from lesions reveal multinucleate giant cells, + for HSV on immunofluorescent staining. Painful mouth lesions occur in 10–15% of patients on zalcitabine (ddI).
Xerostomia (dry mouth)	
Sjögren's-like syndrome—may be drug-associated	Clinical: Dry mouth occurs in 2% of patients on didanosine (ddl). *See Salivary gland enlargement, below.* Rx: Saliva substitutes (Orex®, Xero-Lube®, Moi-Stir®, Salivart®) (electrolytes in carboxymethylcellulose base) & nasal spray may help.
Salivary gland enlargement	
Benign parotid lymphoepithelial lesions (diffuse infiltrative CD8 lymphocytosis syndrome or DILS; *may have systemic features* (*ArthrRheum 55*:466, 2006) CD4 counts 200–500/mm³ ↑prevalence in Africans with HIV infection reported (*Arch Path Lab Med 124*:1773, 2000) Other possibilities: CMV (17%), candida, PCP, adenovirus, lymphoma, Kaposi's sarcoma, tuberculosis; 10 cases reported (*J Oral Pathol Med 34*: 407,2005), MAC, sarcoid	Presents as painless (80%) bilateral parotid swelling due to infiltration with CD8 + T lymphocytes. Submandibular glands not involved. 80% have generalized lymphadenopathy, bilateral cervical. Resembles Sjögren's syndrome with sicca symptoms (dry mouth & eyes). Associated findings may include lymphocytic interstitial pneumonia (60%), aseptic meningitis. Most black pts were HLA-DR5. In contrast to Sjögren's, none had anti Ro/SS-A or anti La/55-B antibodies, rheumatoid factor usually negative. Dx based on fine needle aspiration. More common in children. All initially responded to radiation but 11/12 relapsed after 5 months. Uni- or bilateral painful parotid swelling (*CID 22*:369, 1996). KS present as painless mass in parotid or submandibular region (*Cancer 88*:15, 2000).
Esophagus[1]: Esophageal motility disorders common (16/18, 88%) with or without symptoms of dysplasia or odynophagia (*Dig Dis Sci 48*:962, 2003)	
Dysphagia (difficulty swallowing with a sensation of food sticking)	
Candidiasis Frequency 50–70%; decline in ARV RX era (*Am J Gastro 100*:1455, 2005) Annual incidence of fluconazole-refractory mucosal candidiasis 4.2% (*CID 30*:749, 2000) (*See Table 12 page 137*). The most common cause of dysphagia in HIV+ patients (42–79% of pts).	In HIV+ pt with new onset dysphagia/odynophagia, especially if oral thrush present, fluconazole 100 mg po q24h x2 weeks, followed by 200 mg po q24h x2 weeks in non-responders. If still no response, then endoscope: 40% will have CMV ulcers, 27% idiopathic (aphthous) ulcers—*See below (Dig Dis Sci 45*: 1301, 2000; *ArIM 154*:2705, 1994). X-ray: Barium swallow; typically evidence of plaques & ulceration ("moth-eaten" appearance). Findings supportive but not diagnostic. Endoscopy: Large yellow-white plaques usually seen throughout the esophagus. Biopsy/brushing: Will show tissue-invasive pseudomycelia. Secondary prophylaxis: Recurrence rates (20–80%) in 45–90days. Fluconazole: dosage not defined; 100 mg po biweekly, 10% recurrence over median of 9mos (*32nd ICAAC Abst 1116*:297, 1992).150 mg po weekly, 42% recurrence over 6mos (*Med J Aust 158*:312, 1993).
Drug-associated	Dysphagia occurs in 2–3% of patients on zalcitabine (ddC).

---

[1] Adapted from J.P. Cello, Chapter 13, *ibid.*

TABLE 11A (19)

CLINICAL SYNDROME, ETIOLOGY, EPIDEMIOLOGY	CLINICAL PRESENTATION, DIAGNOSTIC TESTS, COURSE
Gastrointestinal Tract/Esophagus *(continued)*	
Odynophagia (pain on swallowing) or esophagospasm (retrosternal episodic pain without swallowing)	
Cytomegalovirus (CMV) esophagitis Frequency 5–15% Common 8–13% HIV+ pts.	Symptoms are odynophagia, usually without dysphagia, weight loss. Endoscopy: Large solitary (>10 cm² in surface area), shallow, superficial ulcers especially in distal esophagus (*AnIM* 113:589, 1990). Histology necessary to establish diagnosis. If no inclusions, rx as aphthous ulcer. Present in 24/74 pts who had failed antifungal rx for odynophagia (*AJM* 101:599, 1996). Rx: Therapeutic trial with ganciclovir in symptomatic pt may be warranted. 27/35 pts responded, relapse rate high. 5/8 non-GCV responders responded to foscarnet (*AJM* 98:169, 1995). Stricture may occur after healing.
Idiopathic (aphthous) esophageal ulceration (IEU) Frequency 10–30% In one series, 50%pts with esophageal ulcers due to IEU.	Pts present with odynophagia. Differential diagnosis: CMV, HSV, drug-induced ulcers. Found in 25/74 pts who failed antifungal rx for odynophagia (*AJM* 101:599, 1996). Endoscopy: Large discrete ulcers. Rx: Prednisone 40 mg po q24h, taper by 10 mg/wk, total course 4wks. 11/12 pts responded clinically (*AJM* 93:131, 1992). Thalidomide (200mg po q24h x14d), 5/5 pts healed or improved, 1 relapsed (*CID* 20:250, 1995). In a randomized double-blind controlled trial of 200 mg/day x4wks, 8/11 had complete healing vs 3/13 placebo (p <0.03). Side effects: 4 somnolence, 2 rash, 2 peripheral neuropathy (*JID* 180:61, 1999).
Herpes simplex virus (HSV) esophagitis Frequency 5–10%	Clinical: Acute onset, intense pain, widespread involvement. May be associated with oral herpes (*AIDS Clin Care* 7:2, 1995). Median CD4 15/mm³ (*CID* 22:926, 1996). Endoscopy: Shallow erosive ulcers (like reflux esophagitis) Rx: Acyclovir
Esophageal ulcers associated with acute HIV infection	Clinical: Acute retroviral syndrome (fever, myalgia, macular or papular rash) *(page 74)* + odynophagia or dysphagia. Lesions heal spontaneously. Pts are not predisposed to recurrent esophageal ulceration. Endoscopy: One or more discrete ulcers. On biopsy: retroviral virions. Rx: Viscous lidocaine may ↓ symptoms.
Lymphoma, Kaposi's sarcoma, squamous cell carcinoma, histoplasmosis	Clinical: Occur occasionally in esophagus in HIV (*South Med J* 97:383, 2004).
Stomach: nausea, vomiting, early satiety, hematemesis, melena;	
Gastritis 2° to Helicobacter pylori *Dig Dis* 49:1836, 2004	Gastritis more severe in 102 HIV+ pts with H. pylori than 107 HIV-neg. (p <0.0001). CD4 counts higher in H. pylori pts with HIV than those without H. pylori (p <0.0001).
Kaposi's sarcoma (KS) Occurs in 40% of patients with cutaneous or nodal KS.	Usually asymptomatic, occasional hematemesis. Endoscopy: Submucosal reddish nodules with intact overlying mucosa. Biopsy necessary to confirm dx but many lesions (¾) cannot be biopsied because of submucosal location & limited depth of endoscopic biopsies. Assoc. with phlegmonous gastritis from Gp A strep in 1 case (*Ar Pathol Lab Med* 128:801, 2004).
Lymphoma *J Clin Oncol* 22:4227, 2004	May produce obstructed gastric outlet syndrome or hemorrhage (hematemesis, melena). In HIV lymphomas often multifocal with disease throughout abdomen. **X-ray: Larger masses often show "target lesions" with central umbilicated ulcerations.** Endoscopy: Mass lesions, biopsy.
Cytomegalovirus (CMV) gastritis	Endoscopy: See CMV esophagitis above, lesions are similar
Drug-induced abdominal pain	Consider antiretroviral drugs as the cause: zidovudine (500 mg/day, dyspepsia 6%), didanosine (250mg q12h, abdominal pain 7%), zalcitabine (0.75 mg q8h, abdominal pain 3%), foscarnet (60 mg/kg IV q8h, abdominal pain ~5%); drugs for opportunistic infection: TMP/SMX, ketoconazole, fluconazole, neomacrolides (abdominal pain 2–3%); other drugs, especially NSAIDs.

TABLE 11A (20)

CLINICAL SYNDROME, ETIOLOGY, EPIDEMIOLOGY	CLINICAL PRESENTATION, DIAGNOSTIC TESTS, COURSE
Gastrointestinal Tract/Stomach *(continued)*	
Leishmaniasis (stomach, duodenum)	Dysphagia, odynophagia, epigastric & abdominal pain, diarrhea, GI bleeding reported in AIDS pts with CD4 <100/mm³ in endemic areas (*CID 19:48, 1994*).
Gastric ulcers caused by Strongyloides stercoralis reported in HIV+ pts (*Dig Liver Dis 36:760, 2004*)	
Gastric ulcers/nodules caused by bacillary angiomatosis producing hematemesis reported (*Int J Surg Path 11:241, 2003*)	
Abdominal pain, acute onset (*J Emer Med 23:111, 2002*)	
Pancreatitis (See page 113) • Drug-associated most common (46%), e.g., didanosine, pentamidine; lamivudine (3TC) in children, ddI & d4T, and others. • Infection common (90%) in 109 postmortem on AIDS pts in Brazil: mycobacterium 22%, toxoplasmosis 13%, CMV 9%, Pneumocystis jiroveci (carinii) 9%, & HIV p24 antigen in macrophages 2%—all had normal serum amylase premortem (*AIDS 14:1879, 2000*)	APACHE II criteria best predicted outcome in severe cases—accuracy 75% (Glasgow 69%, Ranson 48%), similar to pancreatitis in non-HIV infected populations (*Am J Gastro 98:1278, 2003*).
Bowel perforation/peritonitis Most common cause is CMV in advanced HIV infection	AIDS pts with perforation usually febrile, with rigid abdomen, rebound tenderness. Perforations most common in large bowel. Also lymphoma, typhlitis, KS, tuberculosis, salmonellosis (*Emerg Med Clin NA 7:575, 1989*). Immune reconstitution from ARV RX assoc with perforation of ileocecal TB (*Dis Col Rect 15:977, 2002*).
Small bowel disease: cramping paraumbilical abdominal pain, weight loss, large volume diarrhea	
Diarrhea (See *Curr Opin Gastroenterol 22:18, 2006*) Diarrhea occurs in 30–96.6% (after 3yrs) of U.S. & Euro. HIV+ pts & approx. 90% in developing countries (*ArIM 159:1473, 1999*). Frequency of chronic diarrhea ↑ with ↓ CD4 (*J AIDS 20:154, 1999*). If diarrhea persists for >5 days, evaluation should include microscopic exam of stool (wet mount for Isospora & E. histolytica, modified acid-fast stain for cryptosporidia & cyclospora, modified trichrome f or microsporidia), cultures for routine pathogens & C. difficile	toxin. If above negative, consider endoscopy of colon & small bowel for treatable causes such as CMV, MAC, KS, lymphoma (*Rev Gastroenterol Disord 2:176, 2002*). The frequency of chronic diarrhea is ↓ in pts receiving ARV RX (*Am J Gastro 94:3553, 1999*); however, these antiretroviral drugs themselves have become a common cause of diarrhea (*CID 28:701, 1999; Epidemiol 128:73, 2002; CID 39:717, 2004*) & reduce the quality of life (*Qual Life Res 13:243, 2004*). In Brazil, diarrhea & wasting were associated with ↓ serum levels of d4T & ZDV. Most common causes of diarrhea were cryptosporidium & Isospora belli (*Braz J Inf Dis 7:16, 2003*). Glutamine & alanyl-glutamine ↓ diarrhea & ↑ ARV drug levels (*CID 38:1764, 2004*). But saquinavir (hardgel) absorption (AUC serum level) actually ↑ in pts with diarrhea &/or wasting (*AAC 48:538, 2004*).

Acute infectious diarrhea[1] *(for specific treatment, see Table 12)* (Major site of infection may be small bowel or colon) (*Gastro Clin N.A. 26:259, 1997*) Mean annual incidence of bacterial diarrhea; 7.2 cases per 1000 person-yrs in 9 major US cities from 1992-2002 (*CID 41:1621, 2005*)

---

[1] Adapted from R.W. Goodgame, *AnIM 124:429, 1996*; J.G. Bartlett, et al., *CID 15:726, 1992*; J.P. Cello, *Medical Mgmt of AIDS*, 6th Ed., 1999.

TABLE 11A (21)

Gastrointestinal Tract/Stomach/ Acute infectious diarrhea[1] (continued)

Agent	Prevalence/CD4 Stage	Clinical Features	Diagnostic Clues/Comments
Campylobacter jejuni, C. coli, C. upsaliensis (*Emerg Inf Dis* 8:237, 2002)	4–15% (isolated from 7/43 pts with diarrhea, *CID* 24:1107, 1997) & was most common bacterial pathogen (20%) isolated from HIV+ pts in South African study (*J Health Popul Nutr* 20: 230, 2002). Any CD4	Watery or bloody diarrhea, fever, ± fecal WBC	Stool culture, most labs cannot detect C. cinaedi, C. fennelli, ↑ sensitivity using membrane filter technique on non-selective blood agar.
Clostridium difficile	Most common cause of bacterial diarrhea among persons infected with HIV: 4.1 cases/1000 person years (*CID* 41:1621, 2005) Any CD4	Watery diarrhea, fecal WBC, fever, leucocytosis, cramps, hypoalbuminemia; disease spectrum: nuisance diarrhea, colitis, megacolon. Endoscopy usually shows pseudomembranous colitis but may be normal. C. difficile toxin usually positive. Both toxin A&B should be tested. CT scan shows colitis with thickened mucosa. May present with leukemoid reaction (*South Med J* 97:388, 2004).	Antibiotic exposure: most common—cephalosporins, clindamycin, ampicillin; rare—TMP/SMX, ZDV, albendazole, rifampin
Enteric viruses: Noro, roto, adeno, corona, astro, picobirna, & calicivirus (*Molecular Med Today* 6:483, 2000)	4–15% Any CD4	Acute watery diarrhea but 1/3 become chronic. Adenovirus isolated in 16% of pts with diarrhea & associated with ↑ mortality in 1 study (*J Med Virol* 58:280, 1999).	Stool electron microscopy: detection of viral particles has limited value because viruses produce a self-limiting infection & are untreatable (*J AIDS & HR* 13:33, 1996)
Enteroadherent E. coli Enteroaggregative E. coli & enteroinvasive E. coli also found more commonly in HIV pts with diarrhea than those without in Senegal (p=.000001) (*JID* 189: 75,2004)	10–20%. Common cause of diarrhea in Central African Republic & in19% of pts in Senegal (*J Clin Micro* 40:3086, 2002; *Int J Inf Dis* 5:192, 2001). Any CD4, mean 26	Watery diarrhea, weight loss, ↓ D-xylose absorption, acute but may be chronic, usually in right colon, most pts on TMP/SMX prophylaxis	Adherence to Hep-2 cells (research labs only). Cytotoxic phenotypes assoc. with diarrhea in AIDS pts (*Trans R Soc Med Hyg* 97:523, 2003).
Idiopathic	25–40%. Variable CD4. Non-infectious causes; rule out drugs, diet, inflammatory bowel disease, anxiety, food poisoning	No clues but in 13 HIV+ Puerto Rican pts with noninfectious chronic diarrhea Rx with mesalamine (2.4 gm/day x 6d) vs. placebo impressive response in all parameters examined in Rx group (*Dig Dis Sci* 51:161, 2006)	Negative studies include culture, ova & parasites, C. difficile toxin assay. Lactobacillus no better than placebo in controlling diarrhea in placebo-controlled crossover study (*HIV Clin Trials* 5:183, 2004).
Salmonella S. enteritidis S. typhimurium	5–15% 100x ↑ when compared to general population, any CD4 count, more common with lower CD4	Watery diarrhea, fever, ± fecal WBC	Blood culture, stool culture (sensitivity approx. 90%)
Shigella	2%, ↑ in HIV+, MSM, direct oral-anal contact & foreign travel (*CID* 44:327, 2007). Any CD4	Watery or bloody diarrhea, fever, fecal WBC	Stool culture

[1] Adapted from R.W. Goodgame, *AnIM* 124:429, 1996; J.G. Bartlett, et al., *CID* 15:726, 1992; J.P. Cello, *Medical Mgmt of AIDS*, 6th Ed., 1999.

TABLE 11A (22)

Gastrointestinal Tract/Stomach/ Acute infectious diarrhea[1] (continued)

Agent	Prevalence/CD4 Stage	Clinical Features	Diagnostic Clues/Comments
\multicolumn{4}{l}{Certain parasites may also cause acute diarrhea, including Isospora belli & Entamoeba histolytica/dispar (Int J STD AIDS 14:487, 2003) (see below & next page)}
\multicolumn{4}{l}{Chronic infectious diarrhea.10% of pts with CD4 <200—unchanged with ARV RX but with change in etiology: ↓ OI (53 to 13%) & ↑ non-infectious causes (30 to 70%) (Am J. Gastro 95:3142, 2000; Curr HIV Res 4:87, 2006). A 2-wk course of albendazole given to 153 HIV+ pts with chronic diarrhea in Zambia resulted in 60% complete or partial response & cleared parasites in 46% of those pos. (cryptosporidium 7%, isospora 37%, & microsporidium 16%) (Aliment Pharm Ther 16:592, 2002). TMP/SMX ↓ mortality & diarrhea episodes in 509 HIV+ individuals in Uganda (Lancet 364:1428, 2004).}
Cryptosporidia See NEJM 346:1723, 2002 & CID 36: 903, 2003). Appear to be spread sexually between men who have sex with men (Sex Trans Inf 79:412, 2003). Most frequent cause of diarrhea in HIV+ pts in Peru (JID 191:4, 2005 & 191:11, 2005).	13–20% (E Afr Med J 80:398, 2003) CD4 <150 40% of pts with chronic diarrhea in Cambodia had cryptosporidium but also found in 40% of HIV+ pts without diarrhea (CID 43:925, 2006).	Enteritis; watery diarrhea, noninflammatory diarrhea (fecal WBC neg.), afebrile, malabsorption, wasting, large stool volume with abdominal pain, remitting symptoms for months, years	Water-borne, low infectious dose, in healthy adults only 132 oocysts (NEJM 332:855, 1995). AFB smear of stool to show **oocyst 4–6 μm.** In pts with CD4 >180/mm^3, C. parvum cleared spontaneously in 7–28days; with CD4 <180, 87% persisted. Rx with ARV RX was associated with clearance of organism from stools except when cholangitis (5th Conf Retrovir & Ols 1998, Abst 480). Nitazoxanide effective in Zambian children who were HIV-neg. but not in HIV+ (Ln 360:1375, 2002). Rx: See Table 12
Cyclospora cayetanensis	US <1%, Haiti 11% CD4 <100	Enteritis, watery diarrhea, up to 18x q24h for 10mos. (World J Gastro 10:1844, 2004).	Stool AFB smear, oocyte 8–10 μm, resembles cryptosporidia (CID 23:429, 1996; NEJM 328:1308, 1993; AnIM 121: 654, 1994)
Cytomegalovirus (CMV)	13–20% (E Afr Med J 80:393, 2003) CD4 <100	Fever, fecal WBC, ± blood, enteritis, colitis, perforation with toxic megacolon, solitary rectal ulcer, small bowel mass. Most common cause of lower GI bleeding (AIDS Pt. Care 13:343, 1999). Bleeding may be massive & assoc. with focal ischemia (AIDS Pt Care STD 18:497, 2004).	Sigmoidoscopy with rectal biopsy (best initial invasive test), 10–30% of CMV colitis will affect only right side, further steps include colonoscopy with small bowel biopsy, CT segmental lesions or pancolitis. Failure of ganciclovir rx may be due to drug resistance mutations (J Gastro 138:643, 2003). Rx: See Table 12
Entamoeba histolytica Seroprevalance was 11.2% in asymptomatic HIV+ MSM in Taiwan vs. 0.17% controls (Am J Trop Med Hyg 74:1066, 2006).	1–3%. Infection in HIV+ women in Tanzania assoc. with ↓ birth weight in neonate (Curr Inf Dis Rep 4:124, 2002). Any CD4 count	Colitis, bloody stool, cramps, pos. fecal WBC, most are asymptomatic carriers (AIDS 13:2431, 1999). Course may be protracted (J Clin Gastro 33:64, 2001)	Travel history (Latin America, SE Asia). Stool ova & parasites. Was overdiagnosed by microscopy when compared to DNA amplification: 91/232 pos. with only 21/91 confirmed (Trans R Soc Trop Med Hyg 97:309, 2003).
Giardia	1–5%. ↑ isolation from HIV+ than HIV-neg. pts in Bahia, Brazil (Braz J Inf Dis 5:339, 2001). Any CD4 count	Enteritis, watery diarrhea, flatulence, bloating, malabsorption	History of drinking mountain stream water. Stool ova & parasites.
Idiopathic	More common with lower CD4 (<200)	Watery diarrhea, malabsorption, no fecal WBC	Biopsy shows villous atrophy, crypt hyperplasia, no identifiable cause despite endoscopy with biopsy & electron microscopy for microsporidia.

[1] Adapted from R.W. Goodgame, AnIM 124:429, 1996; J.G. Bartlett, et al., CID 15:726, 1992; J.P. Cello, Medical Mgmt of AIDS, 6th Ed., 1999.

TABLE 11A (23)

Gastrointestinal Tract/Stomach/ Acute infectious diarrhea[1] (continued)

Isospora belli	U.S. 1.5%, developing countries 10–12%. Caused diarrhea in 17% of 94 Indian HIV+ pts (Nat/ Med J India 15:72, 2002), 14/107 in Malawi (E Afr Med J 80:398, 2003) CD4 <100	Enteritis, watery diarrhea, wasting, noninflammatory diarrhea (no fecal WBC), no fever	AFB stool smear, **oocytes 20–30 μm**
Microsporidia Septata intestinalis Enterocytozoon bieneusi hellum	20% CD4 <50 HIV pts more susceptible to clinical disease (JID 180:2003, 1999). Isolated from 25% HIV+ Thai children & 17.4% of Ugandan children (SE Asian J Trop Med Pub Health 33:241, 2002; Am J Trop Med Hyg 67:299, 2002).	Enteritis; watery diarrhea, noninflammatory diarrhea (fecal WBC neg.), fever is uncommon, remitting disease over years, malabsorption, wasting common. Pts improve with response to ARV RX. May disseminate to kidneys, brain, lungs, etc. Microsporidia detected in urine & may respond to albendazole (8/12 pts) (HIV Med 1:155, 2000). Rx with fumagillin[NFDA-f] 60 mg po q24h x2wks cleared stool in 6/6 vs 0/6 placebo, ↑ absorption of D-xylose & ↓ diarrhea; 3/6 had side-effects (NEJM 346:1963, 2002)	Food/water-borne infection **spores 1–2 μm**, fluorescence with calcofluor (excellent screening test), confirmation with Giemsa stain. Special trichrome stain also diagnostic. Complications: disseminated disease, biliary disease.
Mycobacterium avium (cause & effect for diarrhea not always clear)	10% CD4 <50	Enteritis, watery diarrhea, no fecal WBC, common fever & wasting (Curr Opin Gastroenterol 22:18, 2006), diffuse abdominal pain in late stage	Stool culture unreliable, colonization may occur without diarrhea. Diagnosis: positive blood cultures, biopsy may show changes like Whipple's disease, hepatosplenomegaly, adenopathy, thickened small bowel
Small bowel bacterial overgrowth		Watery diarrhea, malabsorption, wasting, often associated with hypochloridia.	Hydrogen breath test, culture of small bowel aspirate

CLINICAL SYNDROME, ETIOLOGY, EPIDEMIOLOGY	CLINICAL PRESENTATION, DIAGNOSTIC TESTS, COURSE
Diarrhea due to alternative mechanisms (↑ to 70% with ARV RX)	Considerations: HIV disease per se, autonomic denervation, Crohn's disease, pancreatic insufficiency (HIV Med 1:33, 2005), overgrowth of normal microbial bowel flora, & antiretroviral drugs (may now be most common cause). Rx of latter: d/c or some success reported with oat bran, psyllium, loperamide, and others (CID 30:908, 2000).
Typhlitis (acute cecitis, inflammation of cecum)	Clinically resembles acute appendicitis, but involves the cecum, which is ulcerated, edematous, necrotic. Associated with Clostridium septicum & Pseudomonas aeruginosa (AnIM 116:998, 1992). Can be a manifestation of C. difficile. Consider especially in severely neutropenic patients.
Colorectal disease: left lower quadrant &/or suprapubic cramping, rectal urgency (tenesmus), frequent small volume stools, occasional proctalgia & dyschezia (painful defecation)	
Drug-associated diarrhea (CID 28:701, 1999)	See adverse effects, Table 6B & Table 13. **Diarrhea is a common complication of rx with antimicrobial agents (including antiretroviral agents)**. May be a direct effect of drug on GI motility (macrolides), overgrowth of GI flora (clinda), C. difficile
Infectious agents (as above)	Adenovirus has been found on biopsy & easily overlooked, may be assoc. with symptoms (Arch Path Lab Med 125:1042, 2001)
Idiopathic (aphthous) proctitis	Endoscopy—large, discrete ulcers. Biopsy to exclude other causes. Thalidomide (200 mg po q24h x21d), improvement in 2/2 pts (CID 20:250, 1995). See Table 12, page 158.

[1] Adapted from R.W. Goodgame, AnIM 124:429, 1996; J.G. Bartlett, et al., CID 15:726, 1992; J.P. Cello, Medical Mgmt of AIDS, 6th Ed., 1999.

TABLE 11A (24)

CLINICAL SYNDROME, ETIOLOGY, EPIDEMIOLOGY	CLINICAL PRESENTATION, DIAGNOSTIC TESTS, COURSE
Gastrointestinal Tract/Colorectal disease *(continued)*	
Cytomegalovirus (CMV)	Endoscopy—focal ischemic colitis with submucosal hemorrhages & discrete shallow ulcers in distal colonic mucosa. Ganciclovir is effective in most patients. Rx: See Table 12
Herpes simplex virus (HSV) Types 1 & 2	Painful recurrent small to persistent progressive large necrotizing ulcers in perirectal area. Emergence of acyclovir-resistant strains on rx is common. Lab: Smears from lesions reveal multinucleate giant cells, + for HSV on immunofluorescent staining.
Histoplasmosis (52 cases reported) *(Diag Microbiol Infect Dis 55:193, 2006)*.	Diarrhea, fever, abdominal pain & wt loss. Most commonly involving colon or cecum. Bx of lesions + 89%, blood or other site culture + 72%. Median CD4 34
Mycobacterium tuberculosis	Tuberculosis in ileocecal area & colon may be seen in HIV patients without evidence of pulmonary TBc on chest x-ray. 14% of diarrhea caused by TBc in India *(CID 23:482, 1996)*. Immune reconstitution from ARV RX assoc. with perforation of ileocecal TB *(Dis Col Rect 15:977, 2002)*.
Other considerations: Idiopathic inflammatory bowel disease (ulcerative colitis), Kaposi's sarcoma, lymphoma, epidermoid carcinoma & other neoplasms	Kaposi's sarcoma may be confined to the rectum & present as hemorrhagic rectocolitis *(Clin Imaging 28:33, 2004)*.
Proctitis Neisseria gonorrhoeae Herpes simplex virus Syphilis, primary or secondary Lymphogranuloma venereum (LGV) Chlamydia trachomatis (non-LGV immunotypes) Human papillomaviruses Cytomegalovirus Enteric pathogens, e.g., Shigella, Entamoeba histolytica, Campylobacter	Lab: Numerous PMNs on smear of exudate. Specific diagnosis depends on laboratory studies. Empiric rx for GC & chlamydia recommended but should also consider herpes & lues *(CID 38:300, 2004)*.
Genital Tract/Sexually Transmitted Diseases *[MMWR 55(RR-11): 1-94, 2006]*	
Arthritis, Septic: N. gonorrhoeae	Part of disseminated gonorrhoea with several possible presentations: petechiae, asymmetric arthralgia, tenosynovitis, occasionally perihepatitis. **Diagnosis**: Nucleic acid amplification test (NAAT) of sample from cervix, male urethra or urine for both N. gonorrhoeae & C. trachomatis. NAAT not approved for rectal or pharyngeal test. Test for C. trachomatis, syphilis and HIV.
Cervicitis/Urethritis: N. gonorrhoeae and/or C. trachomatis High frequency of dual infection. Ref: *CID 44(Suppl 3): S77, S84 & S102, 2007*.	**Males**: Painful urination and purulent urethral discharge; gram stain sensitive (>95%) and specific (>99%). **Females**: May not have cervical discharge. Gram stain less reliable. **For both males and females**: NAAT on urine, urethral swab and/or cervical swab for both N. gonorrhoea and C. trachomatis.
Genital ulcers (For H. simplex, see genital vesicles) **Chancroid**: H. ducreyi: Discrete outbreaks; cofactor for HIV transmission; 10% coinfected with syphilis or HSV	**Painful** genital ulcer + tender suppurative lymphadenopathy. Do darkfield to rule out syphilis. Even with special culture media, culture sensitivity is <80%. Retest for syphilis 3 months after treatment.
Granuloma inguinale: [Klebsiella (Formerly Calymmatobacterium) granulomatis] Rare in US	**Painless** progressive ulcerative lesions without regional lymphadenopathy. Ulcers bleed easily. Hard to culture; rely on visualization of Donovan bodies on biopsy.

TABLE 11A (25)

CLINICAL SYNDROME, ETIOLOGY, EPIDEMIOLOGY	CLINICAL PRESENTATION, DIAGNOSTIC TESTS, COURSE
Genital Tract/Sexually Transmitted Diseases/Genital ulcers *(continued)*	
Lymphogranuloma venereum: C. trachomatis C. trachomatis serovars L1, L2 or L3. *Ref: CID 44 (Suppl 3): S147, 2007.*	Unilateral inguinal/femoral lymphadenopathy. Self-limited papule/ulcer at site of inoculation. Rectal exposure leads to proctitis (rectal discharge, pain, constipation, fever and/or tenesmus). Can result in fistulas or stricture. **Diagnosis**: Culture or PCR or lymph node aspirate.
Syphilis: Treponema pallidum *Ref: CID 44(Suppl 3): S130, 2007*	**Presentation**: Early/primary syphilis: painless ulcer (chancre) Secondary syphilis: rash, mucocutaneous lesions, and lymphadenopathy Latent: no clinical manifestations Late/tertiary manifestations: cardiac, ophthalmic, auditory, paresis, tabes dorsalis or organ gummas Meningovascular syphilis **Diagnostic Tests**: Darkfield or direct fluorescent antibody Positive VDRL, RPR or FTA-ABS (Fluorescent treponema antibody absorbed) VDRL, RPR or FTA-ABS: positive darkfield VDRL, RPR or FTA-ABS CSF VDRL specific but not sensitive. Elevated CSF WBC consistent. Some suggest CSF FTA-ABS (less specific than CSF VDRL but highly sensitive).
Idiopathic genital ulcers: "Aphthous-like"	Painful shallow ulcers. May have concomitant oral ulcers.
Genital vesicles: Mostly human herpes virus 2 (HSV-2); others HSV-1	Viral culture ideal but not sensitive; if positive, can type isolate. Cytology (e.g., Tzanck prep) insensitive; PCR for HSV DNA sensitive and specific. FDA approved type-specific glycoprotein G antibody tests available. Some experts suggest type sensitive specific antibody testing on all HIV positive patients.
Neurologic syndromes: T. pallidum Serologic tests positive	Cranial neuropathy: Bell's palsy, deafness, optic neuritis Meningovascular syphilis: ischemic event (stroke) Paresis: presenile dementia Tabes dorsalis: inability to perceive vibration, deep touch and position stimuli
Pelvic Inflammatory Disease (PID): Acute: N. gonorrhea and C. trachomatis – esp. 1st episode Acute or recurrent: vaginal flora (anaerobes, enteric gm-neg bacilli, Streptococcus agalactiae *Ref: CID 44(Suppl 3): S11, 2007*	Any combination of **endometritis**, **salpingitis**, **tubo-ovarian abscess** and **pelvic peritonitis**. Early diagnosis and treatment important to avoid scarring of upper genital tract with sequelae (infertility, dyspareunia). **Diagnosis**: Cervical motion tenderness or uterine tenderness or adnexal tenderness. Majority have mucopurulent cervical discharge. Urine nucleic acid amplification test for N. gonorrhoea and C. trachomatis.
Perihepatitis (Fitzhugh-Curtis syndrome): Either N. gonorrhea and C. trachomatis	Right upper quadrant pain. Do NAAT for N. gonorrhoea and C. trachomatis.
Proctitis, proctocolitis: **Proctitis**: N. gonorrhoea, C. trachomatis, to include LGV, T. pallidum & HSV **Proctocolitis**: Campylobacter, shigella, E. histolytica & rarely LGV **AIDS pts**: add CMV, MAI, cryptosporidium, microsporidia and isospora	Proctitis: Anorectal pain, tenesmus and/or rectal discharge. Proctocolitis: Proctitis plus diarrhea and abdominal cramps. Try to make a specific diagnosis: Urine NAAT for N. gonorrhoea & C. trachomatis, stool C&S, stool ova & parasites, antigen detection for cryptosporidia, whole blood CMV-PCR.
Rashes (selected) Petechiae-distal-with arthritis: N. gonorrhoea Pruritic nodules (Scabies) Variform skin lesions to include palms and soles + mucous membranes	Blood cultures. Urine NAAT Open burrow, scrap, microscopic exam T. pallidum: RPR

TABLE 11A (26)

CLINICAL SYNDROME, ETIOLOGY, EPIDEMIOLOGY	CLINICAL PRESENTATION, DIAGNOSTIC TESTS, COURSE
Genital Tract/Sexually Transmitted Diseases *(continued)*	
Vaginal discharge:	
Bacterial vaginosis: overgrowth of anaerobes, mycoplasmas and Gardnerella vaginalis. Associated with multiple sex partners, douching & lack of vaginal lactobacilli.	Malodorous vaginal discharge. **Diagnosis:** "Clue" cells on microscopic exam, vaginal fluid pH > 4.5 & fishy odor before and after adding 10% KOH to vaginal discharge. Gram stain: curved gm-neg rods consistent with Mobiluncus sp. Routine treatment of sex partners **not** recommended.
Trichomoniasis: T. vaginalis	Diffuse yellow-green, malodorous vaginal discharge. **Diagnosis:** Microscopic exam of wet mount of vaginal secretion has 60-70% sensitivity. FDA approved tests for women: 1) OSOM Trich. Rapid and 2) Affirm—a nucleic acid probe for T. vaginalis, G. vaginalis & C. albicans. Both >83% sensitivity and >97% specific. **Sex partners should be treated.**
Vulvovaginal candidiasis: C. albicans and rarely other species	Pruritus, vaginal discharge, vaginal soreness, dyspareunia and/or external dysuria. **Diagnosis:** Microscopic exam of wet prep and/or gm-stain of vaginal secretion: shows yeast or pseudohyphae Normal vaginal pH (<4.5). If wet mount negative, can culture for yeast.
Venereal (genital) warts: human papillomavirus—multiple types, but type 6 & 11 most common	Diagnosis is usually by appearance: flat, papular or pedunculated growth on genital mucosa
Heart (Note: Many reports of cardiovascular disease preceded availability of ARV RX. Hence, current relevance is unclear.)	
Pericarditis: Many possible etiologies: typical/atypical mycobacteria, fungi, S. aureus, nocardia, listeria, rhodococus, neoplasms: lymphoma & Kaposi's sarcoma. Ref: *Am Heart J* 137:516, 1999; *Angiology* 54:469, 2003.	Most frequent cardiovascular disease (CVD) in patients with AIDS (10-40%); most small and asymptomatic. Fever, "pleuritic" chest pain, friction rub; less commonly signs and symptoms of tamponade. Often need culture to make definitive diagnosis. In roughly 25%, no etiology established. Overall, M. tuberculosis most common.
Myocardial disease: Etiology: variety of opportunistic pathogens in 10-15%. Speculate remainder due to cardiotropic viruses, e.g., coxsackie, CMV, EBV and perhaps HIV (*NEJM* 339:1093, 1998).	Ref: Prog Cardiovasc Dis 43:151, 2000. Ranges from myocarditis at autopsy to clinical myocardopathy. Separate from atherosclerosis in successfully treated ARV RX patients. Only 10% have symptomatic heart failure. Diagnosis can be complicated by concurrent use of cocaine, alcohol and/or methamphetamine. Drugs used to treat HIV and OIs may be directly toxic to myocardium: e.g., pentamidine and zidovudine (AZT).
Atherosclerotic coronary artery disease:	Suggested that long-term successful ARV RX therapy may accelerate atherosclerotic disease. See *Table 6C, page 43*
Pulmonary hypertension (AIDS patients): Multifactorial etiology: multiple lung infections, esp. PCP, toxic effects of illicit drugs (cocaine), recurrent thromboembolism, veno-oclusive disease and idiopathic (*CID* 39:1549, 2004).	Fatigue, dyspnea, right heart failure. Cardiac ECHO: RVH, RVD, tricuspid insufficiency and pulmonary hypertension. Poor prognosis; may benefit from ARV RX. Suggested therapies: bosentan (*AJRCCM 170*:122, 2004) & inhaled prostacyclin, iloprost (*Eur Resp J* 23:321, 2004).
Valvular disease:	
Infective endocarditis: Almost always IV drug user. High frequency of S. aureus **Cardiac neoplasms:** Kaposi's sarcoma & AIDS; Non-Hodgkin's lymphoma	Can present with bacteremia, heart failure or embolic phenomena. Kaposi's sarcoma: Can involve myocardium and/or pericardium. Non-Hodgkin's lymphoma: Can be diffusely infiltrative, cause nodules/masses and/or heart block.

TABLE 11A (27)

CLINICAL SYNDROME, ETIOLOGY, EPIDEMIOLOGY	CLINICAL PRESENTATION, DIAGNOSTIC TESTS, COURSE
Heart (continued)	
Hematologic abnormalities: (possibly due to altered stem cell differentiation, *Curr HIV Res* 2:275, 2004)	
Anemia (etiologies by category):	
Infection:	
Disseminated mycobacteria & fungi	Infiltrate bone marrow. Inhibit progenitor cells. Diagnosis by culture and biopsy.
Parvo B19 virus (*NEJM* 350:586, 2004)	Infects RBC precursors with lysis. Bone marrow shows giant pronormoblasts. **Diagnosis:** serology and blood PCR
Malignancy: Non-Hodgkin's lymphoma, rarely Kaposi's	Due to marrow infiltration. Diagnosis by marrow biopsy.
B12 & Folate:	Due to poor dietary intake and reduced intestinal absorption.
Iron: anemia of chronic disease:	Chronic disease: Decreased serum iron, decreased iron binding capacity but normal or increased serum ferritin. True iron deficiency: Decreased serum iron, increased iron binding capacity and decreased ferritin. Look for G-I pathology.
Hemolysis: With AIDS, positive direct Coomb's common (18%) but hemolysis rare. Can be drug-induced.	Ref: Transfusion 46:1237, 2006.
Drug-induced bone marrow suppression: Zidovudine & less often ganciclovir, valganciclovir, ampho B and TMP/SMX	Zidovudine most common: majority of pts develop macrocytosis & roughly 25% develop anemia.
Neutropenia (etiologies by category): Defined as absolute neutrophil count (ANC) less than 1500/µL. Infection risk increases with ANC < 1000/µL.	
Antineutrophil antibodies	In nearly 1/3 of HIV pts. But presence **does not** correlate with ANC.
Ineffective granulopoiesis	Marrow dysfunction due to infiltration by, or influence of, systemic infection or malignancy.
Drugs contribute in 80% of patients (*AIDS* 11:995, 1997).	Drugs commonly involved:
	Zidovudine TMP/SMX Pentamidine
	Ganciclovir 5-flucytosine Ribavirin
	Valganciclovir Ampho B
	Pyrimethamine
Eosinophilia (etiologies in alphabetical order):	
Drug reaction Malignancy: e.g., Hodgkins disease	
Ecto-parasite: e.g., Norwegian scabies Parasites: e.g., round worm like strongyloides	
Fungal infection: e.g., Coccidioidomycosis Skin disease: e.g., HIV-associated eosinophilic folliculitis	
Thrombocytopenia:	
Primary HIV-associated thrombocytopenia (PHAT): Three etiologic factors:	
Reduction in platelet life span	Mechanism: Antiplatelet antibodies in serum & on platelet surface.
Doubling of splenic uptake	Coated platelets removed by RES macrophages.
Decrease in platelet production	HIV can infect megakaryocytes; associated with increased apoptosis.
Secondary thrombocytopenia: Differential diagnosis includes malignancy, OIs, co-morbid disease (e.g., hepatic cirrhosis) and drug toxicity.	*Common drug causes of decreased platelets:*
	Acyclovir Valganciclovir Pyrizinamide
	Ganciclovir TMP/SMX Ketoconazole
	Rifampin Pyrimethamine
	Rifabutin Pentamidine
Thrombosis: CID 39:1214, 2004. Increased frequency of various thrombi	Associated factors: CD4 count < 200/µL, antiphospholipid antibodies, acquired deficiency of proteins C&S, elevated levels of factor VIII and homocysteine.
Thrombotic thrombocytopenic purpura—hemolytic uremic syndrome:	Less common in the era of ARV RX. Look for E. coli 0157:H7 in stool.

TABLE 11A (28)

CLINICAL SYNDROME, ETIOLOGY, EPIDEMIOLOGY	CLINICAL PRESENTATION, DIAGNOSTIC TESTS, COURSE
Hepatic Disease (↑ transaminase levels in 2–3.8% asymptomatic HIV+ pts)	
Drug-associated hepatic dysfunction [CID 38(Suppl.2):S43, 2004] (Avoid acetaminophen) Multiple drugs used in HIV patients are associated with abnormalities in LFTs: TMP/SMX (½ pts), acyclovir, nevirapine, didanosine (ddI), ZDV, ddC, all PIs, esp. high-dose ritonavir (Semin Liver Dis 23:183, 2003) hydroxyurea, ganciclovir, foscarnet, ketoconazole, fluconazole, INH, rifampin (see Table 12). Most require dose reduction or discontinuation if abnormalities exceed about 5x normal values.	**Clinical:** 10% of 8851 pts treated by ACTG between 1989-1999 developed ↑ 5X ALT or ↑ 2.5X bilirubin within year following initiation of ART. Predictors of hepatotoxicity were: baseline ↑ aminotransferases, concomitant hepatotoxic medications, thrombocytopenia, renal insufficiency & Hep C coinfection (OR 2.7) (J Acq Imm Def Synd 43:320, 2006). Hepatic necrosis & death has been reported with nevirapine. **Nevirapine hepatotoxicity may be severe, esp. in pts with ↑ CD4 counts.** ↑ ALT also noted at 6wks in neonates who received nevirapine at birth (AIDS 16:851, 2002). **Co-infection with Hep B & C, ↑ baseline ALT elevation & previous hx of parenchymal liver disease ↑ likelihood of drug toxicity.**
Peliosis hepatis (bacillary angiomatosis) (see J. Koehler in MEDICAL MANAGEMENT OF AIDS, 6th Edition, 1999). Manifestation of Bartonella henselae in AIDS patients.	**Clinical:** Fever, abdominal pain, weight loss, hepato- & splenomegaly. About ½ pts will have skin lesions: painful, erythematous plaques or nodules. ½ have lymphadenopathy. 2/3 pts give history of cat bite or scratch (JAMA 269:770, 1993). **Lab:** Alkaline phosphatase ↑ >hepatocellular tests. Etiologic agent: Bartonella henselae (usual), B. quintana (uncommon). Can be isolated from blood, 5–15 days of incubation and then lysis-centrifugation on blood agar under CO_2 (J Clin Micro 30:275, 1992). Rx: Table 12, page 122.
Viral hepatitis	
Hepatitis A (HAV) Hep A in HIV-infected persons is clinically indistinguishable from Hep A in HIV-uninfected persons but viremia lasts longer and alkaline phosphatase is higher. (CID 34:380, 2002).	Risk factors include homosexual activity, injection drug use. Hepatitis A vaccine indicated for non-homosexual men.

Hepatitis B (HBV): CID 44:996, 2007

Diagnostic Issues: Tests & interpretation are same in HIV-infected and non-infected patients

Isolated positive test for Anti HBc: (JID 195:1437, 2007)
- More common in HIV pts, especially if Hep B / Hep C coinfection
- Unclear as to whether occult Hep B viremia is occurring.
- Unclear whether to give Hep B vaccine.

Pathogenesis & HIV:
- After recovery from acute disease, can detect Hep B nucleic acid by PCR. Hep B controlled by cellular & humoral immunity.
- Flares of Hep B can occur with immunosuppression.
- HBV DNA levels and reactivation rates higher in HIV pts than pts with only HBV; HIV pts more likely to develop chronic infection.

HIV/HBV co-infection & progression of liver disease/HIV:
- Co-infected patients have increased risk of cirrhosis.
- No accelerated progression of HIV in co-infected pts.
- Immune reconstitution inflammatory syndrome (IRIS)

Serologic markers and HBV DNA in response to HBV infection*

	HBsAg	HBeAg	IgM Anti-HBc	IgG Anti-HBc	Anti-HBs	Anti-HBe	HBV DNA	Interpretation
Acute Hep B:								
	+	+	+				+++	Early infection
			+	+		+	+	"Core" window
				+	+	+	±	Recovery
Chronic Hep B:								
	+	+		+			+++	Active replication
	+	±		+		+	±	Low/non-replicative
	+			+		+	+	Chronic HBV flare
	+			+		+	++	Pre-core/core promoter mutants

* Blank space means negative test. Hepatitis D not included "Occult Hep B" (JAIDS 44:309, 2007)

IRIS described in co-infected pts treated with ARV RX. Can be life threatening if limited residual hepatic function.

TABLE 11A (29)

CLINICAL SYNDROME, ETIOLOGY, EPIDEMIOLOGY	CLINICAL PRESENTATION, DIAGNOSTIC TESTS, COURSE
Hepatic Disease/Viral hepatitis/Hepatitis B (HBV) *(continued)*	
Hepatitis D: CID 44:988, 2007	
• Defective virus that requires HBV to exist.	Suggested that HIV/HBV co-infected patients should have baseline anti-HDV serology at baseline and/or with flares of hepatitis.
HIV/HBV co-infection & ARV RX associated liver toxicity: Applies to HIV/HCV co-infection as well. *CID 38(Suppl2):S90, 2004.*	1) Cirrhosis and decreased cytochrome p450 activity leads to toxic drug levels; 2) IRIS; 3) Lamivudine withdrawal can lead to flare of hepatitis; 4) resistance to Hep B drugs.
Hepatitis C/HIV co-infection: • Hep C induced liver injury complicates treatment of HIV; concomitant HIV accelerates progression of HIV-induced liver injury. *(Ln 356:1800, 2000; JAIDS 41:63, 2006).* • Liver ultrasound and serum alpha fetoprotein every 6-12 months to check for hepatocellular carcinoma. • Determine Hep C quantitation and genotype. • HCV infection increases hepatic toxicity of ARV RX: see *Hep B above & CID 38(Suppl2):S90, 2004.*	• Screen pts for past exposure to Hep A & Hep B. If no evidence of past infection, give Hep A & Hep B vaccine. • Look for occult Hep B—order antibody to HB core (IgG Anti-Hbc). Co-infection with HB and HC increases risk of hepatocellular carcinoma *(AnIM 146:649, 2007).* • Assess degree of hepatic fibrosis by liver biopsy or consider non-invasive marker of fibrosis: e.g., panels of common laboratory tests or liver stiffness by elastography (Fibro scan).
Hepatitis D (delta agent) Antibodies to delta agent in 25% of HIV+, HBV– individuals	Prolonged antigenemia. ↑ liver injury *(CID 18:339, 1994).*
Hepatitis E (HEV)	HEV antibodies by EIA found in 33/162 (20%) homosexual men (Italy), 60/198 (30%) (Spain) *(Ln 344:1433, 1994; ibid, 345:127, 1995).* In the U.S., HEV prevalence is <1%.
Hepatitis G *(see Semin Liver Dis 23:137, 2003)* Transmitted by parenteral or sexual route *(CID 34:1033, 2002).* ↑ IVDUs (75%), following blood transfusions & in hemophiliacs (38%), hemodialysis pts (17%), homosexuals (55%) *(J Med Virol 58:373, 1999).*	Clinical: No significant consistent correlation between active infection with Hep G as determined by HGV RNA in serum & either hepatocellular necrosis (↑ ALT), fulminant hepatitis or hepatocellular carcinoma has been found *(Blood 94:1460, 1999; Am J Neph 19:535, 1999).* The virus appears to infect lymphocytes & not hepatocytes *(J Gastro 34:680, 1999).* Serum HGV RNA reduced by interferon alfa but not ZDV *(JID 180:1334, 1999).* Infections (past or current) with **HGV were associated with ↑ CD4 counts & better AIDS-free survival rates** in one study of 131 hemophilia pts with HIV *(AnIM 132:959, 2000),* & slower progression & ↓ mortality in others *(NEJM 345:707 & 715, 2001; AnIM 139:26, 2003; CID 38:405, 2004).*
Hepatitis, viral, other	There are isolated reports of hepatitis associated with other viruses: EBV *(PIDJ 7:383, 1988),* HSV *(JID 157: 597, 1988);* VZV *(Scan J Inf Dis 38:929, 2006),* adenovirus *(RID 12:303, 1990).*
Influenza-like Symptoms: Acute & self-limited illness (lasting <10 days) consisting of fever, myalgias, malaise with either sore throat + cervical adenopathy, rhinitis, or conjunctivitis	Viruses were detected in 15 (50%) & Mycoplasma pneumoniae in 9 (30%) of 30 HIV+ pts during such episodes but in only 12 (40%) was isolation in close temporal relationship. These include CMV in 6, M. pneumoniae in 3, herpes simplex without cold sores in 3, & enterovirus in 1. Pts with ↑ CD4 counts were more likely to have "flu-like" symptoms than those with advanced disease (↓ CD4 counts). No cases of influenza were identified even though an epidemic of influenza A was present in the geographical area of study *(AIDS 12:751, 1998).*
Lipomatosis/Lipodystrophy *(See Table 6C & Table 11B)*	

TABLE 11A (30)

CLINICAL SYNDROME, ETIOLOGY, EPIDEMIOLOGY	CLINICAL PRESENTATION, DIAGNOSTIC TESTS, COURSE
Lung Most common causes are Pneumocystis jiroveci (carinii) pneumonia, bacterial pneumonia, tuberculosis (Ln 348:307, 1996) (See Sanford Guide to Antimicrobial Therapy for non-HIV pulmonary infections). Viral pneumonia dx increasingly common in older adults but not unique in HIV infected patients (CID 42:518, 2006) see Curr Opin Infect Dis 18:165, 2005, review of HIV pneumonia. See AIDS 20:1095, 2006. Decreased incidence in ARV RX era (0.8/100 pt yrs). Risk factors: ↑ age, IVDU, smoking, non-adherence to ARV RX (HIV Med 7:261, 2006).	
Bronchitis, bronchiectasis, bronchiolitis obliterans (BOOP) In addition to mycoplasma & respiratory viruses, H. influenzae, S. pneumo, & P. aeruginosa were cultured from sputum in 1 study; relationship to etiology not proven (ArIM 154:2087, 1994).	Mean CD4 600/μl. In pts with chronic productive cough or recurrent pneumonia in same site, consider bronchiectasis. Dx based on CT scan, not evident on CXR in 84% (Quart J Med 85:875, 1992; J Comp Asst Tomo 17:260, 1993). Whether prevalence is ↑ has not been defined but suspected (ArIM 154:2086, 1994). Acute bronchitis most common dx in HIV clinic pts in Kenya (Int J STD AIDS 15:120, 2004). BOOP rare in HIV+ but described (J Inf 49:159, 2004).
Emphysema-like bullous disease	On high-resolution CT scan, 42% pts had bullous lesions (Radiol 173:23, 1989). Pulmonary function tests: ↑ residual volume, ↑ functional residual capacity, ↓ diffusing capacity but no airflow obstruction (AnIM 116:124, 1992). 40 pts with HIV infection & emphysema were found to have ↑ disease in upper lobes with ↑ concentrations of glutathione, suggesting a response to excessive oxidant stress vs non-HIV infected individuals (Chest 126:1439, 2004).
Pneumonia (infiltrate on CXR) (Good review of lab evaluation of OIs of lung: AnIM 124:585, 1996; Clinics in Chest Dis 4:713, 1996)	
Any CD4 level	
Pulmonary tuberculosis (mycobacterium tuberculosis[1]) **Common:** **ANY PT SUSPECTED OF TB SHOULD BE ISOLATED** [private room, negative pressure, health care workers (HCW) & visitors entering should wear high efficiency disposable masks] [See Table 23]. In the Western world the number of new cases of HIV-associated TBc & MDR TBc has declined (1998–2001), likely due to the implementation of rigorous infection control measures & Directly Observed Therapy (DOT) (CID 29:1138, 1999; AnIM 130: 971, 1999).	Clinical presentation varies with stage of HIV infection: • **Early HIV infection** (CD4 >400/mm³): Reactivation. Typical presentation **with upper lobe cavitary disease most common.** Extrapulmonary disease uncommon. PPD (5 TU) is + (≥5 mm induration) in 80%. Always consider in pts with chronic cough (CID 40:1818, 2006). • **Later HIV infection** (CD4 <400/mm³): Either reactivation or progressive primary disease (30–50%). Clinical: Fever, cough (may be absent), shortness of breath, weight loss, night sweats. ½ to ⅔ involve extrapulmonary sites, especially lymph nodes & bone marrow (granulomas in 50% of bone marrow biopsies). A papulopustular rash reported (CID 27:205, 1998). Mycobacterial blood cultures + in ¼ to ½ of patients. (BACTEC system is sensitive & rapid.) Caution: patients reported with blood + for both M. tbc & MAC. Cultures of urine, joint fluid, CSF, liver, GI mucosa & ascites may also be +. Mass lesions of brain (tuberculoma) may mimic CNS toxoplasmosis. PPD (5 TU) positive (≥5mm induration in <25% with clinical AIDS). Malnutrition ↑ severity of pulmonary TB in Malawi (Int J Tuberc Lung Dis 8:211, 2004). Sepsis syndrome from disseminated TB also reported (Int J STD AIDS 17:562, 2006).

[1] H.F. Chambers, Chapter 23, Medical Mgmt of AIDS, 6th Ed, 1999.

TABLE 11A (31)

CLINICAL SYNDROME, ETIOLOGY, EPIDEMIOLOGY	CLINICAL PRESENTATION, DIAGNOSTIC TESTS, COURSE
Lung/ Any CD4 level/ Pulmonary tuberculosis (continued)	
In the 3rd World TBc & HIV are closely linked: 50% of pts who have TBc in parts of sub-Saharan Africa are also infected with HIV (*Int J Tuberc Lung Dis* 5:405, 2001) & likewise TBc was found in 50% of autopsies done in AIDS pts (*JAIDS* 24:23, 2000). Point prevalence of active TBc in 100 hospitalized pts with HIV in South Africa was 54% (*CID* 33:2068, 2002) & the leading cause of death in Botswana (*Int J Tuberc Lung Dis* 6:55, 2002), 48% had TBc in Malaysia (*Jpn J Inf Dis* 56:187, 2003), 47% in New Delhi, India (*Inf* 31:336, 2003), 26% in Cambodia (*Inf J STD AIDS* 14:411, 2003), & 14% in Guatemala (*Inf J STD AIDS* 14:810, 2003). The proportion of new cases of TB attributed to HIV was 72% in men in northern Thailand (*J AIDS* 31:80, 2002). Incidence of TB & mortality similar with HIV-1 & HIV-2 (*AIDS* 18:1933, 2004). There appears to be an ↑ in notified TB incidence following ARV RX (3 mos) in resource poor countries (*AIDS* 20:1275, 2006).	**X-ray: Mediastinal-hilar adenopathy most common with progression to diffuse, somewhat coarse interstitial densities or localized infiltrates,** especially in mid or lower lung fields. Pleural effusion in 10–20%. Disseminated (reticulonodular infiltrates, not classic "miliary" since "millets" are granulomata, usually not seen in HIV with low CD4) the most common with CD4 <200/mm3. Hilar/peritracheal adenopathy uncommon with PCP or bacterial pneumonia, common in TB. Cavity formation ↑ with multidrug-resistant disease (*J Comput Asst Tomo* 28:366, 2004). In 1 study in Ethiopia, 10% of sputum-pos. cases had normal chest x-ray (*Infection* 32:333, 2004) Sputum: Smears + for AFB in 40–50% pts with pulmonary TB, BAL + in 50–60%, culture + in 80–90%. The "string test" used to retrieve enteropathogens (giardia or salmonella) was used to obtain swallowed sputum; 14 pts pos. by string test vs 8 from induced sputum (p 0.03) (*Lancet* 365:150, 2005).
Tuberculosis often occurs before pt has AIDS-defining illness, but ARV RX sig. ↓ risk (*AIDS* 14:1985, 2000). Most cases due to reactivation but primary tuberculosis being recognized with increasing frequency. 10% of HIV+ individuals are tuberculin +. In U.S., ~4% AIDS pts have had TB, in Italy 11% (*J Infect* 28:261, 1994). **Rate of development of TB is 8%/year in PPD+ patients, reduced to 0.51% following INH prophylaxis for 12mos.** (*AIDS* 13:2069, 1999). Average CD4 count is 375/mm3. TBc has been shown to accelerate the course of HIV (*AIDS* 14:1219, 2000), ↑ HIV viral load (*JID* 190:1627, 2004) & induces expression of CXCR4 on alveolar macrophages while suppressing CCR5 by ↑ CC chemokine expression, thus encouraging switch from macrophage-trophic to lymphocytotrophic HIV phenotype which is assoc. with acceleration in HIV disease progression (*J Immunol* 172:6251, 2004). In 2006-7, a highly drug-resistant form of TB emerged in S. Africa; about 330 cases of these XDR verified with 85% mortality in HIV+ pts. By March 2007, 28 countries had reported XDR strain isolation including 47 cases in the U.S. This presents a particularly difficult problem for HCW in Africa (*CID* 44:324, 2007).	• Rx with ARV RX resulted in immune reconstitution inflammatory syndrome (IRIS) characterized by worsening of chest x-ray after 1–5wks in 45% of 31 pts receiving antituberculous rx; 23% were severe. 4/7 of the latter converted PPD to + (*Am J Roentgenol* 174:43, 2000). Severe respiratory failure reported. Bx demonstrates necrotizing granulomas with AFB. Corticosteroids produce rapid clinical improvement (*Int J Tuberc Lung Dis* 3:944, 1999). Some recommend starting ARV RX early for pts with very advanced disease (CD4 <100/mm³) & delaying ARV RX until continuation phase (>2mos.) for those who are clinically stable (CD4 >100/mm³) (*AIDS* 16:75, 2002). However, AIDS events are common during 1st 2mos of anti-TB rx in those with CD4 <100, suggesting early rx with ARV RX could be beneficial (*CID* 190:1670, 2004). IRIS assoc. with ↑ CD4, ↑ ratio of CD4 to CD8 1 month after ARV RX & with dissemination of TB (*CID* 39:1709, 2004). Rx: *Table 12, pages 123–126.*
Community-acquired pneumonias (*AIDS* 16:85, 2002). Attributable mortality 9.3%; shock, CD4 <100, pleural effusion, cavity & multiple lobe involvement ↑ mortality (*AJRCCM* 162:2063, 2000).	
Pneumococcal pneumonia is common in HIV+ patients (*CID* 38:1623, 2004) (86% S. pneumo serotypes isolated included in pneumococcal vaccine, Table 20). In several studies pneumococcal immunization reduced risk of pneumonia by 50–70% even when vaccine given to pts with <100 CD4 cells (*AriM* 160:2633, 2000; *Vaccine* 22:2006, 2004). Annual incidence of invasive disease due to S. pneumoniae is 1100 per 100,000 men with AIDS, age 25–44yrs (*JAMA* 265:3275, 1991). In another U.S. study incidence 1127 per 100,000 HIV infected pts pre- vaccine and 919 per 100,000 in vaccine era; a reduction in invasive disease of 19% (p=0.002)(*Ann Intern Med* 144:1, 2006). in Uganda, surprisingly ↑ of all-cause pneumonia in African-Americans & CD4 <200. In Uganda, surprisingly ↑ of all-cause pneumonia in vaccine group, but a survival advantage in vaccine group (*AIDS* 18:1210, 2004). Others have also found insignificant protective effect of pneumococcal vaccine in HIV+ persons in Spain (*J Med Virol* 72:517, 2004; *Lancet ID* 4:445, 2004).	**Etiologies:** Streptococcus pneumoniae [35–70%; 25% in Cameroon & 31% in Uganda (*CID* 36:652, 2003)]. **Clinical:** Typical presentation with fever, chills, productive cough, pleuritic chest pain & dyspnea can be seen at all stages of HIV infection. **Most (up to 95%) of HIV+ patients with pneumococcal pneumonia will have positive blood cultures** (*Chest* 117:1017, 2000). Leucocytosis may not occur, but look for left shift bands. Although value of sputum cultures controversial, they were of value in establishing dx in 1 study in Africa (*Eur J Clin Micro Inf Dis* 21:362, 2002). Use of induced sputum with gram stain & quantitative cultures useful for Dx in one study in Brazil: sensitivity 60%, specificity 40%, positive predictive value 80%, negative predictive value 20%, accuracy 56% using BAC as gold standard (*Braz J Inf Dis* 10:89, 2006). X-ray: Usually consolidation (homogeneous densities) with either segmental or lobar distribution (41/50 had lobar). Also similar in HIV+ & HIV-neg. in Kenya study (*AIDS* 16:2095, 2002; *COPD* 10:183, 2004).

TABLE 11A (32)

CLINICAL SYNDROME, ETIOLOGY, EPIDEMIOLOGY	CLINICAL PRESENTATION, DIAGNOSTIC TESTS, COURSE
Lung/ Any CD4 level/ Pulmonary tuberculosis/ Community-acquired pneumonia/ Pneumococcal pneumonia *(continued)*	
Prevalence of multidrug-resistant Strep. pneumoniae among HIV+ individuals is increased (24 vs 6.4%) & more likely to be invasive (40x ↑) vs non-HIV infected children in South Africa (*PID* 19:1141, 2000). Mortality rate of pneumococcal disease particularly high in resource-restricted areas: in 217 pts in Malawi, mortality of those with meningitis was 65%, pneumococcemic pneumonia 26%, & pneumococcemia without localizing signs 26% (*AIDS* 16:1409, 2002).	Course: Response to appropriate antibiotics is usually prompt (48–96hrs to become afebrile, radiographic resolution is much slower, as it is in non-HIV+ patients). If patient fails to respond as above, consider concomitant PCP or TBc. CD4 ↓ during acute S. pneumo infection (*Clin Microbiol Inf* 10:587, 2004). Macrolide failures now being reported for infections due to macrolide resistant strains (*J Chemother* 19:536, 2007). Rx: Table 12.
Haemophilus influenzae pneumonia/bacteremia: occurs with ↑ frequency. Incidence of invasive disease is 80/100,000. In one series, most pts (57%) had bilateral pneumonia, in another only 30% had pneumonia. 1/3 to ½ reported were b-lactamase negative. Response to appropriate antibiotics is prompt. Mortality is 11.5% (*CID* 30:461, 2000)	**Etiologies:** Haemophilus influenzae (common, 3–40%)
Pseudomonas aeruginosa: Pneumonia 8.7%/year. Clinical: median CD4 9/μl. ½ to ¾ community-acquired but ½ pts had been hospitalized in prior 30 days Common cause of nosocomial pneumonia (*Inf* 38:9, 2006). CXR: 60–80% segmental, 40% bilateral infiltrates, 10–50% cavities. Only 9% bacteremic respond to rx but relapse recurs in ~/3. Mortality 33%. (*CID* 18:886, 1994; ibid. 19:417, 1994; *J AIDS* 7: 823, 1994; *JID* 171:930, 1995). Risk ↑ with advanced HIV, central venous & urinary caths, ↓ WBCs, prior antibiotics & steroids (*Chest* 117:1017, 2000).	**Etiologies:** Pseudomonas aeruginosa (3–10%) most common pathogen in one series (30%) (*Chest* 117:1017, 2000) but has ↓ in era of ARV RX (*Postgrad Med J* 79:691, 2003).
Legionella sp.: 77% community-acquired. Risk in AIDS 42x ↑ (*ArIM* 154:2417, 1994). Nosocomial Legionella pneumophila pneumonia uncommon but reported in several small series (*CID* 27:97, 1998). 83% developed respiratory failure with 22% mortality in 18 Spanish pts (*Med Clin* 123:582, 2004).	
Other bacterial: Bacterial pneumonia ↑ in HIV (5.5 cases/100 person years vs 0.9/100 OR 0.22 person years), mortality 4x ↑; TMP/SMX prophylaxis ↓ pneumonia by 67% (*NEJM* 333:845, 1995; *JID* 181:158, 2000). Cigarette smoking ↑ risk of bacterial pneumonia (RR 1.57), oral candidiasis (RR 1.37) & AIDS dementia complex (RR 1.80) (*J AIDS & Human Retro* 13:374, 1996). HIV RNA copies: ↑ from a median of 60,000 copies/ml plasma to 245,000 copies/ml in 13 pts with bacterial pneumonia. Titers dropped to baseline after recovery (*J AIDS & HR* 13:23, 1996). Bacterial pneumo also ↑ risk of progression to death (*CID* 43:90, 2006).	
• Staphylococcus aureus (7%) (uncommon except with IDU, right-sided endocarditis) but common cause of nosocomial pneumonia (*Inf* 38:9, 2006) MRSA on the rise. • Moraxella catarrhalis (<1%) (*J Chemo Ther* 12:406, 2000) • E. coli (6–7%) • Serratia marcescens (<1%) (*Eur J Clin Microbiol Inf Dis* 19:428, 2000) • Other Gram-negative (7–9%) • **Aerobic Gram-negative bacilli** [TMP/SMX resistance ↑ markedly from 1988 to 1995 in HIV+ pts (*JID* 180:1809, 1999)]	HIV infection/disease not reported to alter the prevalence or course of nosocomial, usually ventilator-acquired, Gram-negative bacillary pneumonia. M. avium may be acquired from hot water systems (*Ln* 343:1137, 1994) but does not cause pneumonia.

TABLE 11A (33)

CLINICAL SYNDROME, ETIOLOGY, EPIDEMIOLOGY	CLINICAL PRESENTATION, DIAGNOSTIC TESTS, COURSE
Lung/Pneumonia *(continued)*	
• **Influenza virus, A or B** (common in outbreaks). Vaccine effective: incidence 6.1% in vaccinated vs 21.2% unvaccinated (p=0.001). Ab response ↑ when CD4 >200 on ARV RX. Recommended! *(JAIDS 39:167, 2005)*.	No evidence that influenza in general is more severe in HIV-infected patients. 1 study demonstrated ↑ morbidity & mortality from influenza in women <65yrs of age with certain chronic medical conditions including HIV; annual excess mortality 2/10,000 *(JAMA 281:901, 1999)*.
• **Mycoplasma pneumonia** (uncommon but may cause "flu-like" illness)	Mycoplasma infection may be less severe in HIV-infected pts & prolonged secretion of organism & relapsing infection reported as in other immunosuppressed pts. Presence of cough, myalgias and cervical adenopathy correlated with + culture. ↑ with ↓ CD4 & anemia. ELISA & culture useful for Dx in HIV+ pts. *(Int J Infect Dis Aug 14, 2006)*. Macrolide resistance now being reported in M. pneumoniae *(AAC 52:348, 2008)*.
• **Chlamydia pneumoniae**	Reported to cause 2.5% of pulmonary infections in 1 Italian study, 2/159 in Atlanta *(AIDS 16:85, 2002)*. May be cause of severe diffuse interstitial pneumonia *(Eur J Clin Microbiol Inf Dis 16:720, 1997)*.
• **Ehrlichiosis** (Ehrlichia chaffeensis)	In a case report, pt presented with fever, tachypnea, neutropenia with 17% bands, thrombocytopenia, ↑ hepatic enzymes. Chest x-ray: diffuse bilateral infiltrates. ↓ PaO_2. Patient deteriorated. Diagnosis suspected on last day, optimal antibiotic rx not given *(NEJM 329:1164, 1993)*.
• **Measles**	In U.S., 9/11 pts had pneumonitis; 3 had no rash & 8 had atypical exanthems; mortality 3/11 *(JAMA 267:1237, 1992)*. Immunization of HIV+ children recommended, although immune responses may be ↓. Ribavirin aerosol has been used but efficacy not proven *(ibid.)*.
• **Adenovirus**	Adenovirus diarrhea important *(see page 93)*. Frequently cultured from HIV+ pts but association with respiratory illnesses not clear *(AIDS 12:751, 1998)*.
• **Bordetella bronchiseptica**	9 cases reported by 1999; respiratory illness ranged from mild URI to pneumonia. All had prior AIDS-defining illness & 3/9 had close contact with pets (2 dogs, 1 cat) *(CID 28:1095, 1999)*.
• **Human herpesvirus 6** (HHV-6)	HHV-6 infected cells detected in tissues obtained at necropsy in 9/9 pts. In one pt, probably primary cause of fatal pneumonitis. Relevance is that HHV-6 infections may be treatable with ganciclovir & foscarnet *(Ln 343: 577, 1994)*.
• **Varicella**	7/12 pts with advanced HIV hospitalized for chickenpox developed pneumonia with typical diffuse reticulonodular infiltrates; 3 died (43%) despite acyclovir rx *(Int J Inf Dis 6:6, 2002)*.

CD4 <200/mm³

Pneumocystis jiroveci (carinii¹) (PCP pneumonia) *(see reviews: NEJM 350:24, 2004; Proc Am Thorsc Soc 3:655, 2006)*: Still common cause of pneumonia in U.S., 30% of 160 pts *(AIDS 16:85, 2002)* & death in those not receiving ARV RX *(CID 36:1030, 2003)*. Less common in Africa except children: 51/105 admitted for severe pneumonia in S. Africa *(CID 34:1251, 2002; Int J Infect Dis Feb2, 2006)*. Cause of 26% of Zambian children deaths *(Ln 360:985, 2002)*; 48% of HIV-infec infants <1yr in Botswana *(PIDJ 22:43, 2003)*. PCP also found in adults: 30% of HIV-infec adults with neg. AFB smears were pos. by nested PCR for PCP in Ethiopia *(AIDS 17:435, 2003)* & 9/27 (33%) BAL specimens pos. in Tunisians *(Tunis Med 80:29, 2002)*. In 1 report from China, 8/9 pts with pulmonary symptoms had PCP *(Respirol 5:419, 2000)* It appears PCP is ↑ in dev. world as it ↓ in industrialized nations *(CID 36:70, 2003; CID 36:652, 2003)*. Single study demonstrated 33 % ↓in mortality in 534 Zambian children receiving Cotrimoxazole prophylaxis; role of PCP prevention not known *(Cochrane Database Syst Rev Jan25; CD003508, 2006)*

---

¹ J.D. Stansell, L. Huang, H. Masur, Chapter 20, *ibid.*

TABLE 11A (34)

CLINICAL SYNDROME, ETIOLOGY, EPIDEMIOLOGY	CLINICAL PRESENTATION, DIAGNOSTIC TESTS, COURSE

Lung/Pneumonia/CD4 <200/mm³/Etiology of community-acquired pneumonia *(continued)*

AIDS 16:85, 2002:
Predicting etiology of community-acquired pneumonia:

Dx	Bact Pn (94)		PCP (101)		TBC (37)	
(OR=Odds Ratio)	%	OR	%	OR	%	OR
Fever >7 days	11%	1.0	34%	4.3†	54%	9.9†
Cough >7 days	20%	1.0	50%	3.9†	51%	4.2†
Yellow-green sputum	54%	2.8†	30%	1.0	30%	1.0
DOE	43%	1.5	81%	9.0†	32%	1.0
Weight loss	23%	1.0	44%	2.2†	68%	6.8†
Night sweats	23%	1.0	46%	2.7†	54%	3.9†
Tachycardia	57%	2.8†	39%	1.3	32%	1.0
Abn auscultation	77%	3.5†	62%	1.8	49%	1.0
LDH >400	29%	1.0	62%	4.0†	43%	1.9
pO₂ <75	36%	1.8	66%	6.0†	24%	1.0
Interstitial infiltrate	17%	1.3	69%	14.5†	14%	1.0
Lobar infiltrate	54%	59†	22%	1.0	32%	24.8†

OR: 95% CI does not include 1.0 when indicated by †

With ARV RX, incidence of PCP was dramatically ↓ *(Chest 118:704, 2000).* Use of ARV RX (either before or during hospitalization) ↓ mortality from PCP from 63% to 25% (p=0.03) in 58 ICU pts at San Francisco General Hospital *(AIDS 17:73, 2003).* ARV RX did not influence PCP mortality in another study in NYC *(J IntensiveCare Med 20:327, 2005).* Still accounts for 24% of hospitalization in Miami *(Int J Infect Dis 10;47, 2006).* Most cases (67%) now occur in pts with previously undiagnosed HIV (Scand J Infect Dis 37; 482, 2005) or in those supposedly taking PCP prophylaxis. Pts receiving TMP/SMX prophylaxis less likely to fail than other regimens. Still common initial presentation for HIV, especially in elderly!
(CID 30:S5, 2000)

Geographical clustering of cases reported *(Am J Resp CCU 162:1617, 2000)* but evidence for person-to-person transmission weak *(AIDS 16:1821, 2002).* Recently acquired infection more common cause of disease than previously thought *(JAMA 286:2950, 2001).*

Clinical: Dry cough, fever, progressive dyspnea of 1–4wks duration
Laboratory: CD4: 1st episode mean CD4 79/mm³, med. 36/mm³; 2nd episode mean 34/mm³, med. 10/mm³. Arterial blood gas—↓ pO₂¹ (<70 mmHg in 80% patients); pulmonary function tests—restrictive type defect with ↓ vital capacity ↓ & ↓ total lung capacity. Diffusion abnormalities common; single breath diffusing capacity for CO <80% of predicted (90% sensitivity but only 25% specificity). ↓ PaO₂ with exercise may be of particular value.

Chest x-ray¹: 5–10% have normal chest x-ray (in these pts, CO diffusing capacity, ↓ PaO₂ with exercise may be of particular value.

Most common: **diffuse bilateral symmetrical fine heterogeneous reticular infiltrates**

Less common: Unilateral/focal distribution of same quality infiltrates or focal alveolar consolidation (especially upper lobe in patients on aerosolized pentamidine prophylaxis) or an interstitial pattern with fine nodular infiltrates or miliary lesions or focal nodules without cavitation, thick-walled cysts or pneumatoceles or pneumothorax (may predispose to mycetoma: *Chest 122:886, 2002).*

Rare: pleural effusion &/or intrathoracic adenopathy.

After 4 days TMP/SMX treatment, there is commonly an ↑ infiltrate resembling pulmonary edema. This complication is significantly ↓ when corticosteroid rx used with TMP/SMX in pts with low pO₂ (see *Table 12, page 146).*

Sputum, induced: detection of P. jiroveci (carinii)—**sensitivity 77%,** negative predictive value 64%; use of fluorescent antibody technique markedly improves detection over that with Giemsa stain *(Eur Resp J 20:982, 2002).* Also *effective in non-AIDS immunosuppressed pts (CID 37:1380, 2003).*

Bronchoalveolar lavage (BAL): do not delay initiation of rx if BAL not immed available. Treatment for several days does not ↓ diagnostic sensitivity. Detection of P. jiroveci (carinii)—sensitivity 85–89%. Addition of real time PCR ↑ sensitivity to 100% & specificity to 84.9% *(J Med Microbiol 53:603, 2004).* Many now use empiric rx without bronchoscopy for typical clinical presentation *(CID 37:1549, 2003).* Transbronchial biopsy: detection of P. jiroveci—sensitivity 88–97%. Rarely found on transbronchial biopsy if not found on BAL. PCR on respiratory secretions may ↑ sensitivity but false + still a problem *(CID 30:141, 2000).*

Response: With effective rx, improvement is expected in 7–10 days. Mutations in dihydropteroate synthase gene (essential for folate biosynthesis) found in 20% of PCP isolates: In one study assoc. with ↓ survival (hazard ratio for death 3.1) *(Ln 354:1347, 1999)* but **no** correlation with either response to TMP/SMX rx or survival in 2 others *(Ln 358:545, 2001, AIDS 19;801, 2005).* In 2002, 80% of HIV+ pts tested had DHPS mutations, while only 7% in clinics where sulfa drug prophylaxis not common *(JID 189:1684, 2004),* 13% in South Africa *(CID 39:1047, 2004).* DHFR mutations also arise under TMP/SMX pressure *(AAC 48:4301, 2004) (also see EID 10:1721, 2004).* Pneumothorax is a common complication of PCP pneumonia & is associated with a high mortality *(CID 23:624, 1996).* Permanent ↓ in pulmonary function (↓ FEV, FVC, & FEV/FVC) & ↓ diffusion to CO reported *(Am J Resp Crit Care Med 162: 612, 2000).* PCP requiring mechanical ventilation & ICU admission still has high mortality (53%) independent of ARV RX *(Thorax 61:726, 2006 & HIV Med 7:193, 2006).* **May coexist with TBc** *(CID 32:289, 2001).*

Disease process may blossom (pO2 ↓ pulmonary infiltrates) with robust response to ARV RX (↑ CD4), **immune reconstitution.** Biopsy of lung infiltrate neg. for organisms but strongly pos. for PCP DNA *(CID 35:491, 2002; BMC Inf Dis 4:57, 2004).*

---

[1] P. Goodman, *ibid.*;

TABLE 11A (35)

CLINICAL SYNDROME, ETIOLOGY, EPIDEMIOLOGY	CLINICAL PRESENTATION, DIAGNOSTIC TESTS, COURSE
Lung/Pneumonia/CD4 <200/mm³ (continued)	
Kaposi's sarcoma (KS)[1] (common) DNA sequences of a herpesvirus, HHV-8, have been identified in >90% of AIDS-associated Kaposi's sarcoma & in classic endemic African, Mediterranean KS, suggesting a role in pathogenesis of KS (*NEJM* 332:1181, 1995; *AIDS* 17:215, 2003)	**Clinical:** Usually but not always associated with cutaneous &/or mucosal KS. Present with cough (92%), dyspnea (82%) & fever (67%); less likely than pts with concurrent OI to have temp >38.3 & RR >20 breaths/min. Symptoms prolonged (>2 mos) in 18% (*AJRCCM* 153:1385, 1996). X-ray: Findings are somewhat distinctive: **coarse, poorly defined nodular densities throughout the lungs with concomitant coarse linear densities in the perihilar regions.** Nodules increase slowly in size, rapid ↑ suggests hemorrhage. Pleural effusions common (up to 50%). Hilar adenopathy rare (<10%). **Dx:** Bronchoscopy will usually show typical violaceous endobronchial lesions. **Rx:** *Table 18.* May respond to antiretroviral rx or specific antiviral Rx (*Curr Top Microbiol Immunol* 312:289, 2007).
Lymphoma: HHV-8 also identified in body cavity lymphomas— see above	Lymphomas associated with advanced HIV infection are becoming increasingly common, are usually non-Hodgkin B cell type, with extranodal involvement the rule. Thoracic involvement is uncommon (10%) but when it occurs produces pleural effusion in 50%, hilar &/or mediastinal adenopathy in ¼ & either reticulonodular interstitial infiltrates or alveolar consolidation in 25%.
Lymphoid interstitial pneumonia (LIP) (children) (*Chest* 112:2150, 2002)	A disease of unknown etiology which may present with shortness of breath in children with HIV infection (see *Table 8E*). **X-ray: Resembles PCP with diffuse or focal, fine to medium reticular interstitial infiltrate. Findings gradually worsen over mos.** Dx: Lung biopsy is necessary for dx; shows an accumulation of lymphocytes & plasma cells in interstitial areas. Rx: Corticosteroids may be beneficial.
Pulmonary alveolar proteinosis found on lung biopsy in 2 HIV+ pts (*Pathol Res Pract* 200:699, 2004)	
Nocardiosis (Nocardia asteroides) Uncommon, 43 cases reported (*Med* 71:128, 1992). CD4 <200/mm³.	Fever, malaise, cough, weight loss. Chest x-ray: 83% abnormal, cavitation 62%, lobar consolidation 52%, pleural effusion 33%, reticulonodular infiltrates 33%. Lab: Blood cultures rarely +. May mimic TBc (*J Postgrad Med* 47:30, 2001; *S Afr J Surg* 42:17, 2004).
CD4 <100/mm³ (*For ATS statement on fungal infection in HIV+ persons, see Am J Resp Crit Care Med* 152:816, 1995)	
Cryptococcosis (Cryptococcus neoformans) (common) Most common cause of death (44%) in HIV+ South African gold miners (*CID* 34:1251, 2002). See *Meningitis* C. neoformans is a ubiquitous soil fungus which usually affects the CNS (see *Meningitis*) in patients with CD4 <100/mm³. Pneumonia more common in HIV-neg. (*J Med Microbiol* 53:935, 2004).	Site of entry is usually the lungs & pneumonia has been reported. X-ray: Variable pattern; single (*CID* 23:810, 1996) or multiple well-defined nodules with or without cavitation or diffuse reticular infiltrates &/or hilar/mediastinal adenopathy. Occasionally a reticulonodular pattern or isolated pleural effusion may occur. Other cryptococcal species may also cause pneumonia & pleural effusion (*Can Respir J* 13:275, 2006). Dx: Isolation of C. neoformans from respiratory secretions or blood cultures. Rx: *Table 12, page 139.* Serum CRAG may be positive.

---

[1] L.O. Kaplan, D.W. Northfelt, Chapter 28, *ibid.*

TABLE 11A (36)

CLINICAL SYNDROME, ETIOLOGY, EPIDEMIOLOGY	CLINICAL PRESENTATION, DIAGNOSTIC TESTS, COURSE
Lung/ CD4 <100/mm^3 *(continued)*	
Coccidioidomycosis (Coccidioides immitis) (common—endemic areas) (see *CID* 41;1174 & 1217, 2005) Risk factors include Afro-American race & ↑ level of immunosuppression (oral-esophageal candidiasis). Rx with ARV RX &/or azole rx ↓ risk (*JID 181:1428, 2000*). A common reactivation or primary infection in patients from "cocci belt" (southwest U.S.) with CD4 <150/mm^3. In HIV-negative individuals, annual incidence of symptomatic infection is 0.43%, in HIV+ individuals 25% developed symptomatic cocci over 41 months (*AJM 94:235, 1993*). 15% pts had simultaneous PCP (*Med 69:384, 1990*).	**Presentation is similar to histoplasmosis—fever, chills, night sweats & weight loss; severe shortness of breath is common.** Cutaneous lesions common: generalized ----, erythema nodosum, granulomatous dermatitis and Sweet's syndrome (*J Am Acd Dermatol 55:929, 2006*). X-ray: Diffuse bilateral reticulonodular infiltrate (65%) similar to histoplasmosis or focal pulmonary infiltrate (14%) or normal (16%) (*CID 23:563, 1996*). Dx: While complement fixation antibody tests are frequently positive (68%), dx is established by identification of large spherules of C. immitis in sputum, BAL, biopsy or on culture. Rx: *Table 12, page 138.*
Histoplasmosis (Histoplasma capsulatum) (common—endemic areas) (see *CID 24;1195, 1997*) A common reactivation infection when CD4 <200/mm^3 in pts with geographical history of having been in the "histo belts" (Ohio-Mississippi River Valley, southeastern U.S., St. Lawrence River Valley, Central America & northern South America) (*Curr Opin Infect Dis 19:443, 2006*). Annual incidence in Missouri 4.7% in HIV-infected.	Usually presents with nonspecific systemic complaints: fever, weight loss, night sweats, but lungs commonly involved with shortness of breath. Hepatosplenomegaly & rarely focal cutaneous pustules or ulcers may be presenting findings. Pts may also present with "septic shock" including DIC. CD4 count <150. X-ray: Commonly shows diffuse, bilateral poorly defined small (1–2 mm) nodular infiltrates with or without hilar/mediastinal adenopathy. Dx: Identification of H. capsulatum in WBC on peripheral blood smear or bone marrow (PAS or silver stain) & culture (about 90% are positive). If suspected & blood/bone marrow not positive, biopsy lymph node, liver, lung or lesions. About 80% will have + immunodiffusion or complement fixation test for antibodies. Measurement of H. capsulatum antigen in urine + in 95% AIDS pts with disseminated histo, test useful in following rx & relapse (*CID 19(S1):S19, 1994*). (Available at *MiraVista Diagnostics, 1-866-647-2847*). However, cross-reactivity with paracocci, blastomyces, cocci, & penicillium has been detected (*CID 24:1169, 1997*). Rx: *Table 12, page 141.*
Blastomycosis (uncommon)	Uncommon, largest series is 15 cases (*AnIM 116:847, 1992*). CD4 <200/mm^3. Pulmonary (7 cases): 4 dyspnea, 2 chest pain, CXR 3 focal, 3 diffuse reticulonodular. BAL cultures + Disseminated (8 cases): CNS involvement (5 cases), multiple organs (6 cases). Rx: *Table 12, page 142.* Reported in Brazil (*Pathol Res Pract 199:811, 2003*).
Paracoccidioidomycosis (South America)	12 cases reported from Brazil: 10 had lymphadenopathy, 7 with interstitial lung disease, 6 with papule-nodular skin lesions with central ulceration & 5 with ulcerative lesions of the mouth (*J Infect 51:248,2005*).
Mycobacterium kansasii (may also occur at higher CD4 counts)	Clinical: Fever 76%, cough 57%, weight loss 45%, dyspnea 31%, night sweats 31%, looks like typical tuberculosis. ½ X-ray: Infiltrates "atypical": alveolar, interstitial or diffuse parenchymal or pleural effusion. Upper lobe cavities. ½ have extrapulmonary dissemination. Cavitation more common at ↑ CD4 counts, hilar adenopathy with dissemination more common at ↓ CD4 counts (*Am J Resp Crit Care Med 160:10, 1999; Eur J Clin Microbial Inf Dis 18:582, 1999*). Mortality rate 53% in 1 series of 127 pts; pts on ARV RX did better (*AJRCCM 170:793, 2004*).
Mycobacterium genavense	Usually presents with fever, weight loss, diarrhea, abdominal pain, hepatosplenomegaly, anemia, pancytopenia, & occ. painful cutaneous nodules (*Ann Int Med 128:409, 1998*).
Penicillium marneffei	Primarily presents as fever, anemia, weight loss & skin lesions (70%) with lymphadenopathy but ½ have cough & organism cultured from lung in 15%. Pulmonary infiltrates (densities, abscesses & cavities) have been seen. Essentially all cases from SE Asia. Dx by isolation from skin, blood or bone marrow (*CID 23:125, 1996*). Rx *Table 12, page 142.*

TABLE 11A (37)

CLINICAL SYNDROME, ETIOLOGY, EPIDEMIOLOGY	CLINICAL PRESENTATION, DIAGNOSTIC TESTS, COURSE
Lung/ CD4 <100/mm³ (continued)	
Rhodococcus equi (uncommon) 3% of pts thought to have TBc had rhodococcus in Uganda (*J Inf* 41:227, 2000). Also reported from Thailand; confused with TB (*J Inf Chemother* 6:229, 2000).	One-half of pts with Rhodococcus equi present with slowly progressive mass lesion which cavitates (*Rev Inf Dis* 13:91, 1991). Others present with consolidation with & without cavitation, ground glass opacities, peribronchial nodules and centrilobular nodules ("tree in bud" pattern) (*J Bras Pneumol* 32:405, 2006). Has tendency to relapse, may require surgery & long-term suppressive rx. Rx: *Page 131*. ARV RX helps rx (*AIDS* 16:509, 2002).
Toxoplasma gondii (uncommon)	Rare in U.S., in France represents up to 5% of cases of suspected PCP. Febrile illness, minimal cough, ↑ dyspnea. Reported to be associated with ARDS (*CID* 19:169, 1994) and septic shock (*HIV Med* 7:415, 2006). Chest x-ray: Diffuse interstitial or diffuse coarse nodular (resembles PCP). Pleural effusion in 2/6 patients. Lab: ↑ transaminase, ↑ LDH. Sputum: BAL + for T. gondii (*CID* 23:1249, 1996). Rx: *Table 12, page 147*.
CD4 <50/mm³	
Aspergillosis (uncommon) Aspergillus sp. are commonly isolated from respiratory sites (4%), but invasive aspergillosis developed in only 15% of colonized patients, more common in pts with AIDS & associated neutropenia (*CID* 14:141, 1992; *ibid*, 19(S1):S41, 1994; *Mycoses* 41:453, 1998).	33 patients reported in one series. 64% had an episode of infectious pneumonia ≤1 year before. CD4 <50/mm³. All were febrile, cough 97%, dyspnea 80%, chest pain 20%, hemoptysis 17%, 21% CNS signs. Chest x-ray: cavities 42% (most upper lobe), bilateral interstitial infiltrates 54%, pleural effusion 15%. Despite rx, mean time to death was 8wks (*AJM* 95:177, 1993). Rx: *Table 12, page 136*.
M. avium (pulmonary findings uncommon but systemic symptoms without pos. blood cultures will occur in up to ¼ of all pts with AIDS in developed countries) (*Int J Infect Dis* 10:47, 2006).	CD4 usually ≤50/mm³, marked ↓ with ARV RX (1.4 to 0.2/100 pt yrs) (*Am J. Resp Crit Care Med* 162: 865, 2000) (see *Table 12, page 127*, & above, *Fever of unknown origin*). X-ray: When lungs involved, heterogenous interstitial infiltrates with or without hilar lymphadenopathy. Rx: *Table 12, page 127*. Following initiation of highly active antiretroviral rx, pts with MAC infection have developed unusual systemic & pulmonary syndromes: painful generalized lymphadenopathy-like scrofula, massive abdominal & thoracic adenopathy with pulmonary infiltrates, fever, leucocytosis, & cutaneous nodules (*Ln* 351:252, 1998) (*Table 11B*).
Cytomegalovirus (CMV) (uncommon) **CMV pneumonitis in HIV+ pts is rare but 90% of AIDS pts have evidence of CMV in the lungs at autopsy.** (See *Sem Resp Inf* 14:353, 1999)	Viral cultures of BAL fluid are frequently positive. CMV has been isolated from 30% of pts with PCP, & associated with ↑ mortality (*AJM* 78:429, 1985), but rx with ganciclovir does not appear to affect outcome (*NEJM* 314:801, 1986). Consider lung bx when CMV infection elsewhere, fever, cough & dyspnea, persistent interstitial/alveolar infiltrates (*Abst* 158, *3rd CRV*, 1996). Syndrome of ↑dyspnea (over 1-3mos), interstitial infiltrates, hypoxemia, hemolytic anemia, siderophages on BAL reported (*CID* 22:616, 1996). Would rx if biopsy revealed interstitial inflammation with CMV inclusions & no other pathogens. Lung cancer appears to be ↑ with ARV RX (*AIDS* 17:371, 2003).
Pulmonary nodules (1 or more on CT scan)	Common condition (87/242 HIV+ pts had pulmonary nodules). 57 had OI: bact. pulmonary nodules in 30, TB in 14. If pt had fever, cough & nodule <1 cm = bact. pulmonary nodules likely. If homeless, had weight loss, & adenopathy on CT = TB likely (*Chest* 117:1023, 2000). M. bovis reported (*CID* 39:e53, 2004).
Mass lesion ± necrosis (abscess) Histoplasmosis, coccidioidomycosis, cryptococcosis, anaerobes, S. aureus, M. kansasii, Rhodococcus equi, (Tsukamurella reported, *J Infect* 49:17, 2004), Mycobacterium tuberculosis, Pneumocystis jiroveci (carinii), lymphoma, Kaposi's sarcoma, aspergillus, MAC, Nocardia asteroides, P. aeruginosa, CMV (*AIDS Pt Care Stds* 15:353, 2001)	Cavitary lesions: PCP uncommon manifestation of common disease. Frequent: aspergillosis, M. kansasii, M. tuberculosis (in earlier HIV infection), bacterial pneumonia (P. aeruginosa, N. asteroides, R. equi). Unusual: crypto, coccidioido, histo (*CID* 22:671, 1996; *CID* 22:81, 1996) & Pseudallescheria boydii. Definitive dx essential: BAL & transbronchial bx. A sarcoid-like response to ARV RX with non-caseating granulomatosis appearing like diffuse interstitial micro-nodular lesions on chest x-ray has been reported (*Am J Resp Crit Care Med* 159:2009, 1999). Lung cancer appears to be ↑ with ARV RX (*AIDS* 17:371, 2003).

TABLE 11A (38)

CLINICAL SYNDROME, ETIOLOGY, EPIDEMIOLOGY	CLINICAL PRESENTATION, DIAGNOSTIC TESTS, COURSE
Lung/ CD4 <50/mm³ *(continued)*	
Hilar &/or mediastinal adenopathy Mycobacterium tuberculosis, Mycobacterium avium-intracellulare Fungal: Histoplasmosis, coccidioidomycosis, cryptococcosis, blastomycosis Lymphoma, Kaposi's sarcoma. (*Curr Opin Pul Med 11:208, 2005*). In 45 pts with HIV & intrathoracic lymphadenopathy, 22 had infections (17 from mycobacterial disease & 5 from "bacterial pulmonary nodules") & 17 had tumors (7 lymphomas followed by lung cancer, germ cell tumor, KS). CD4 ↑ in tumor vs. infection (314 vs 62). Cavitary lesions = infection (*AIDS Pt Care STDS 13:645, 1999*).	Following ARV RX & ↑ CD4 (immune reconstitution) pts may develop hilar adenopathy with MAC, M. Tbc, crypto & other pathogens. Clinically useful predictors of etiology in 110 HIV+ pts: • Cough + necrosis of nodes = mycobacteria (51) • ≤7 days symptoms, dyspnea, airway disease = bacterial pneumonia (26) • >7 days symptoms, no cough or pulmonary nodules = lymphoma (2) (*AIDS 31:291, 2002*) "Sarcoid" diagnosed several months following ARV RX in 9 cases in France, possibly representing immune reconstitution disease (*CID 38:418, 2004*).

Pleural effusion (*Sex Trans Infect 76:122, 2000*)
Infections (66–70%):
  Bacterial pneumonia   31–57%
  P. jiroveci (carinii) pneumonia   15%
  M. tuberculosis   8–16%
  Others (each <5%): Septic embolism, aspergillosis, C. neoformans, MAC, nocardia—PCP rarely
Non-infectious (31%): (*see Curr HIV Res 1:385, 2003*)
  KS   10–40%
  Hypoalbuminemia   19%
  Heart failure   5%
  Others: Kaposi's sarcoma (10% in 1 series), non-Hodgkin lymphoma (18% in 1 series), atelectasis, uremia, ARDS, pulmonary emboli (4%)
	Incidence in 222 pts was 27% (*AnIM 118:856, 1993*). Large effusions & bilateral associated with Kaposi's sarcoma & lymphoma (*South Med J 92:400, 1999*). Tuberculosis ↑ likely when associated with miliary nodules or mediastinal adenopathy. Pleural TB usually occurs soon after primary infection in normal host, however ↑ in reactivation disease in HIV+. Dx usually requires pleural bx for histology & culture. Usually responds to conventional antituberculosis chmo Rx (*Monaldi Arch Chest Dis 65:26, 2006*).
	
	Carcinomatous lymphangitis presented with acute respiratory failure in 2 HIV-infected individuals; both had bronchogenic carcinoma (*Intensive Care Med 30:1956, 2004*).

Pneumothorax P. jiroveci (carinii) pneumonia (more common with aerosolized pentamidine) Pulmonary eosinophilia (Loeffler's syndrome)	Occurred in 2% of a large series of patients (*AnIM 114:455, 1991*). Has high mortality rate if associated with PCP (*CID 23:624, 1996; Lancet ID 4:120, 2004*). Can be caused by drugs commonly used in HIV+ pts: sulfonamides, dapsone, penicillin (*Ln 343:860, 1994*).
Lymph Nodes **Generalized lymphadenopathy** (applies to lymphadenopathy without an obvious primary source) Etiologies: acute HIV infection, TBc, atypical mycobacteria, histoplasmosis, coccidioidomycosis, lymphoma, Kaposi's sarcoma, syphilis, Epstein-Barr virus, toxoplasma, tularemia, sarcoid, CMV, & Castelman's disease (*AIDS 10:61, 1996*)	History & physical exam direct evaluation. If nodes fluctuant, aspirate & base rx on Gram & acid-fast stains. Pts receiving ARV RX may demonstrate fever & generalized lymphadenopathy from MAC infection following robust ↑ CD4 cells; **immune reconstitution inflammatory syndrome (IRIS)** (*Ln 351:252, 1998*) (*Table 11B*). Percutaneous ultrasound-guided fine needle aspiration effective in abd. adenopathy in AIDS pts in Thailand (*J Med Assoc Thai 87:400, 2004*).
Musculoskeletal System (*see Skeletal Radiol 33:311, 2004; Infect Dis Clin North Am 19:881, 2005; AIDS Reader 14:175, 183, 2004*) **Pyomyositis** (*Am J Med 117:420, 2004; Infect Dis Clin North Am 19:881, 2005*) Staphylococcal; aerobic Gm-neg. bacilli (uncommon) (*CID 22:372, 1996*) Immune reconstitution with ARV RX produced pyomyositis & cutaneous abscesses from M. avium (*CID 38:461, 2004*).	May follow exercise, local trauma or injections. Swelling in muscular area, localized pain & fever. ESR usually ↑. Erythema often absent, can be indolent. ↑ bilateral in HIV. WBC may be normal & blood cultures usually negative (*AJM 90:595, 1991*).

TABLE 11A (39)

CLINICAL SYNDROME, ETIOLOGY, EPIDEMIOLOGY	CLINICAL PRESENTATION, DIAGNOSTIC TESTS, COURSE
Musculoskeletal System (continued)	
Osteomyelitis (Brit J Rheum 31:381, 1992) S. aureus, Strep. species, enterobacteriaceae, M. kansasii, H. capsulatum, nocardia Septic arthritis (Clin Orthop Relat Res 451:46, 2006)	Sinus tract cultures may give misleading results regarding etiology of osteomyelitis—bone biopsy necessary to establish dx. Septic arthritis has a similar course in HIV+ & non-HIV pts (Rheumatol 38:139, 1999). M. kansasii ↑ in AIDS (CID 29:1455, 1999). Think MRSA & mycobacteria.
Osteonecrosis (avascular necrosis) was found in 15/339 (14%) asymptomatic HIV+ pts (AnIM 137:17, 2002, J AIDS 25:19, 2000), osteoporosis, & osteopenia, assoc. with advanced HIV & traditional risk factors (↓ body mass, weight loss, steroid use, & smoking) but not ART (CID 36:482, 2003). Bone density ↓ in 84 HIV+ women vs HIV-neg, age-matched controls: osteopenia 54% vs 30% control (p 0.004). Bone density did not differ according to ARV RX exposure (AIDS 18:475, 2004). Above confirmed in men (J Bone Miner Res 19:402, 2003). However, in 51 pts on ARV RX ↓ in bone density correlated with ↑ central obesity & glucose intolerance (post-load hyperglycemia) (JCEM 89:1200, 2004).	Evaluate for osteonecrosis in pt with persistent groin & hip pain. Plain films not usually revealing; usually requies MRI for definitive diagnosis. In 1 study of 25 HIV+ pts, 22 had other risk factors: ↑ lipids 32%, alcoholism 28%, corticosteroid rx 12%, hypercoagulable state 12%—4/25 receiving megestrol acetate. Multiple joints involved in 72%. All associated with ARV RX but results conflicting. In the Swiss HIV Cohort Study, 27 cases of avascular necrosis found; they had more severe immunosuppression & ↑ body mass index than 260 HIV-infected controls (AIDS Res Hum Retrovir 20:909, 2004). In a review of 56,393 pts from the French Hospital Database on HIV, 104 subjects had symptomatic osteonecrosis (4.5/10,000 person yrs): Risk factors: 1) prior AIDS-defining illness (RR 3.1); 2) degree of immunosuppression (CD4<50, RR1.8, 50 to 200 RR1.6 vs. those >200) and duration of exposure to ART: <12 mo, RR 2.6, 760 mo RR5.1 (AIDS 201627, 2006). In a prospective multicenter randomized open-label study, alendronate 70mg qw + Vit. D 500 intl units q24h & calcium 1000mg q24h improved lumbar bone mineral density & minimized femoral bone mineral density decrease after 52wks vs Vit. D & calcium alone in 41 HIV+ persons on ARV RX (HIV Clin Trials 5:269, 2004). Other studies also confirm use of Bisphophonates while hormonal therapies such as raloxifane testosterone and growth hormone-releasing hormone promising but require more study (see CID 42:108, 2006).
Arthritis, polyarticular Reiter's syndrome: urethritis or cervicitis, conjunctivitis, arthritis, & mucocutaneous lesions (circinate balanitis, keratoderma blennorrhagica). For review of rheumatic diseases, see Semin Arth Rheum 30:47, 2000.Reiter's syndrome occurs in 0.5–10% of HIV+ patients, 75% are HLA B-27 positive (Rheumatol Int 9:137, 1989).	Typically, non-bacterial urethritis 7–14 days after sexual exposure. Asymmetric polyarticular arthritis involving large joints of legs, including toes, develops over several weeks. Typically resolves in 3–4mos but ~50% have recurrences. HLA B27 uncommon in Africans but reactive spondyloarthropathies still common in HIV+ persons (Curr Opin Rheum 12:281, 2000). Lab: Synovial fluid typically is translucent, 2000–100,000 cells/µl, >50% PMNs, culture negative, glucose <50mg/dl lower than blood glucose. Rx: Since often assoc. with C. trachomatis, empirical rx for chlamydia (see Table 12, pg 122) is appropriate. In non-HIV+ patients, methotrexate or folic acid antagonists have been used; they should not be used in HIV+ pts.
Psoriatic arthritis	Psoriasis noted in 1–5% HIV+ population. Frequency of arthritis ↑ in HIV+ pts with psoriasis (Rheum Dis Clin NA 17:59, 1991; J Rheum 27:1699, 2000). Rx with infliximab reported in several cases (Br J Dermatol 150:784, 2004).
"Lightning pain" syndrome	Severely painful acute attack of arthralgia or myalgia lasts a few hours to a few days. Often requires narcotics for relief. Clinical exam normal. Cause unknown, no sequelae (Med J Aust 158:114, 1993).
Rheumatoid arthritis	Virtually never occurs in pts with HIV. Several pts with rheumatoid-factor positive RA have gone into remission after infection with HIV.
Systemic Lupus Erythematosis	Also not reported in HIV patients. SLE appears to be protective against acquisition of HIV infection, perhaps through mechanism of anti-phospholipid like antibodies 2F5 and 4E10 (Science, 308: pp 1906-08, 2005)
Arthritis, oligoarticular	Usually asymmetrical, lower limbs. HLA B27 negative. Synovial fluid: low WBC with PMNs (Med J Aust 158: 114, 1993). HIV-associated arthritis occurred in 7.8% of 270 pts at various stages of HIV. Course was acute, of short duration (2 wks), without recurrences or erosive changes (J Rheumatol 26:1158, 1999). A similar aseptic inflammatory arthritis reported from Congo: 83 pts (80% polyarthritis, 20% oligo), asymmetrical & non-erosive, knees 84%, ankles 59%, great toes 23%, wrists 41%, elbows 29%, small joints of hands 25%. All responded to NSAIDs in 4–8 wks (Joint Bone Spine 71:300, 2004). Septic arthritis also usually monoarticular, MRSA & mycobacteria most common (Clin Orthop Relat Res 451:46, 2006).

TABLE 11A (40)

CLINICAL SYNDROME, ETIOLOGY, EPIDEMIOLOGY	CLINICAL PRESENTATION, DIAGNOSTIC TESTS, COURSE
Musculoskeletal System (continued)	
Myopathy (progressive proximal muscle weakness) HIV-1 associated myopathy (see Curr Neurol Neurosci Rep 4:62, 2004)	Proximal muscle weakness, ↑ creatinine kinase levels. Muscle biopsy: ½ had inflammatory infiltrates. ½ pts rx with & responded to prednisone (AnIM 113:492, 1990; Neurol 53:241, 1999).
Drug-associated: zidovudine (ZDV), ddI & ddC (AIDS 12:2425, 1998), may be assoc. with d4T, lactic acidosis & mitochondrial toxicity (AIDS 18:1403, 2004)	Proximal muscle weakness & atrophy (legs >arms, "saggy butt" syndrome) occurred in 5/86 pts (6%) rx with ZDV >6mos (mean 45wks). Creatinine kinase ↑ (average 777 units/L). Typically associated with high-dose zidovudine use in the past (200 mg every 4 hrs while awake, circa 1988). Muscle biopsy: "Ragged red fibers" on histology, abnormal mitochondria on EM. Improves with discontinuation of ZDV, recurs with rechallenge. ddC also causes a selective loss of mitochondrial DNA in vitro (Ln 337:508, 1991). Now reported with most NRTIs (Ln 354:1084, 1999). Rhabdomyolysis rarely associated with TMP-SMX (Am J Med Sci 331:339, 2006).
Polymyositis—also reported from IRIS (Clin Exp Rheumatol 22:651, 2004; Sex Trans Inf 80:315, 2004)	A dermatomyositis-like disease has been described in AIDS (Rheum Dis Clin NA 17:117, 1991; ArIM 159:1012, 1999).
Pancreatitis (see above Endocrine System/Pancreas) **Hyperamylasemia with or without abdominal pain:** 52/86 asymptomatic HIV+ pts had at least 1 ↑ amylase or lipase in serum; risk factors were Hep B or C or IV TMP/SMX. No associated clinical pancreatitis (Am J Gastro 94:1248, 1999). 44 cases: usual major causes—alcohol 39%, gallstones 2%; drugs: pentamidine 27%, ddI 9%, TMP/SMX 5%, 3TC esp. in children; opportunistic infections: CMV 5%, MAC 2%, other 9% (AJM 98:243, 1995). 334/920 HIV+ Italian pts had at least 1 pancreatic lab abnormality (36.3%) in an observational case-controlled study. The 128 who had highest & most prolonged abnormalities were related to ddI, d4T, 3TC, pentamidine, TMP/SMX, anti-TBc rx, ETOH, OIs, liver or biliary disease, PI-based ARV RX & ↑ triglycerides. No difference in risk factors seen between symptomatic (32 pts) & asymptomatic (96). After withdrawal of inciting agent, gabexate &/or octreotide administration appeared to be of benefit (Eur J Med Res 9:537, 2004).	Pancreatitis due to ddI can be fatal (0.35%). In pts with history of pancreatitis, 8/27 pts on ddI developed pancreatitis. All NRTIs implicated & likely due to mitochondrial toxicity (J AIDS 37:S30, 2004). Pancreatitis 2° to NRTI may be ↑ in older pts (Expert Rev Anti-Infect Ther 2:733, 2004). Tenofovir + ddI assoc. with pancreatitis in 6 cases (2.7%) (An Pharmacother 38:1660, 2004) & reduction in ddI dose recommended (Lancet 364:65, 2004). Pts rx for both Hep C & HIV receiving ribavirin & ddI ± d4T at ↑ risk for mitochondrial toxicity including pancreatitis (CID 38:e79, 2004). Also reported in 1° HIV infection (South Med J 97:393, 2004). In a recent review of 8,451 subjects enrolled in ACTG trials, overall pancreatitis rates were 0.61 per 100 person-years. Highest rates seen in pts on indinavir/DDI/d4T (J AIDS 39:159, 2005). IV pentamidine is associated with pancreatic islet cell damage (hypoglycemia with later diabetes mellitus).
Peritoneal Disease Ascites, sudden onset	Symptoms & signs of underlying process.
Transudative ascitic fluid (<3 gm protein/100 ml) Concomitant hepatic cirrhosis (alcoholic), congestive heart failure, inferior vena cava obstruction, Budd-Chiari syndrome, hypoalbuminemia, vasculitis, hep B or C	
Exudative ascitic fluid (>3gm protein/100ml) (>**500 cells/mm suggests infection, neoplasm**) Tuberculosis, lymphoma, cytomegalovirus, nocardia (S Afr J Surg 42:17, 2004), strongyloides (Acta Cytol 48:211, 2004)	Collect large volume (500–1000 ml), centrifuge; may reveal AFB on smear Biopsy: Etiology most often found on biopsy. Elevated adenosine deaminase (10X ↑ vs cirrhosis or malignancy) found in TBc peritonitis (Eur J Gastro 11:337, 1999).

113

TABLE 11A (41)

CLINICAL SYNDROME, ETIOLOGY, EPIDEMIOLOGY	CLINICAL PRESENTATION, DIAGNOSTIC TESTS, COURSE
Renal (see *Am J Neph 24:511, 2004* for dialysis issues; for kidney transplantation, *Scand J Inf Dis 36:680, 2004*). For nice review of HIV-associated renal disease, see *CID 42:1488, 2006*.	
Proteinuria & azotemia [screen for proteinuria semi-annually (*AnIM 164:333, 2004*)] 14% black & 6% white pts in U.S. dying from AIDS have renal disease & 10% overall have renal failure (*Curr Inf Dis Rep 4:449, 2002*). Proteinuria & ↑ serum creatinine were risk factors for progression to AIDS & death (RR 2.5) in >400 HIV+ ♀ (*J AIDS 32:203, 2003; CID 39:1199, 2004*).	
HIV-associated nephropathy (glomerulosclerosis) (HIVAN) (*AnIM 139:214, 2003; Adv Chronic Kidney Dis 13:307, 2006*—excellent reviews). Prevalence 12% in HIV+ African-Americans in Galveston, TX (*Am J Neph 19:655, 1999; Am J Kidney Dis 35:884, 2000*). 85% pts are black. In 3,926 HIV+ pts, incidence HIVAN 8/1000 person yrs but 26.4/1000 person yrs in those with AIDS. ARV RX ↓ risk of HIVAN by 60% & no pt developed HIVAN if ARV RX started before AIDS developed (*AIDS 18:541, 2004*). Etiology likely due to direct infection of HIV shown to infect podocytes causing proliferation & de-differentiation. HIV accessory gene ref itself causes injury to mature podocytes through Src kinase-dependent activation of the signal transducer & activator of other signaling pathways (*Curr Opin Nephrol Hypertens 15:450, 2006*). HIV also shown to infect renal tubular epithelial cells with production of the various proinflammatory mediators (*J AIDS 42:1, 2006*).	Usually occurs in advanced HIV with ↑ viral load (*CID 43:377, 2006*). Massive proteinuria of sudden onset, hypoalbuminemia, renal insufficiency rapidly progressing to endstage renal disease. Peripheral edema & hypertension minimal or absent. Biopsy recommended to differentiate from other causes of GN. Renal bx: Focal glomerulosclerosis with mesangial deposits of C3 & IgM, tubular ectasia & tubulo-interstitial disease. Significance of antiglomerular basement membrane antibody uncertain (*Am J Kidney Dis 48:e55, 2006*). Bx may be of value in HIV+ pt with varying degrees of proteinuria: 6 of 25 pts from S. Africa with classic findings of HIVAN had only microalbuminuria and in 6 of 7 with persistent microalbuminuria (*Kidney Int 69:2243, 2006*). Course: Death in 3–6mos. even with dialysis. 60mg prednisone for 1mo. followed by 2mos. taper ↓ serum creatinine, ↓ proteinuria, & preserved renal function at 6mos: in 7/13 pts vs. 0/8 control (*Kidney Int 58:1253, 2000*). Angiotensin-converting enzyme (ACE) inhibitor have also had some limited success (*Pharmaco Therapy 25:1761, 2005*). ARV RX rx improves outcome of HIV-assoc. nephropathy but not other renal diseases found in HIV+ pts (*AnIM 139:214, 2003; AIDS Reader 14:443, 2004; Kidney Int 66:145, 2004; Clin Nephrol 64:124, 2005*).
HIV-associated IgA nephropathy Rarer than HIV glomerulosclerosis. Majority of pts are white.	Microscopic hematuria, minimal proteinuria. ↑ serum IgA. Progression of disease is slow. Thought to be immune complex disease (*NEJM 327:702, 1992*).
Nephrotoxic drugs: pentamidine, foscarnet, aminoglycosides, amphotericin B; tenofovir	Causes renal tubular damage (*Scand J Inf Dis 36:389, 527, 2004, CID 42: 283, 2006*) with Fanconi's syndrome (*J Gen Intern Med 21:C3, 2006*).
Hemorrhagic cystitis	Hem. cystitis caused by adenovirus reported (*Am J Hematol 63: 32, 2000*).
Urolithiasis: Renal colic occurred in 27/1155 pts rx with PIs (*CID 39:248, 2004*)	24 HIV+ pts with nephrolithiasis: 14 on indinavir but only 4 (28%) had indinavir-containing stones. Others contained Ca oxalate, ammonia acid urate & uric acid. Abnormalities included hypocitraturia (5), hypomagnesuria (4), hypercalcuria (3), supersaturation of Ca oxylate (3), & hyperuricosuria (2) (*J Urol 169:475, 2003*). Occasional reports of kidney stones with atazanavir.
Immune reconstitution syndrome (IRIS)	Inflammatory response following 8 wks of ARV RX in pt with miliary TB with AFB urinary shedding, developed acute renal failure (*CID 38:e32, 2004*).
"Sepsis"/Bacteremia (M. tuberculosis, non-typhi salmonella & S. pneumo were most common causes in Nairobi, Kenya (*CID 33:248, 2001*)	
Disseminated pneumococcal disease	30–85% of pts with pneumococcal pneumonia have bacteremia. Rate of S. pneumoniae bacteremia is 100-fold ↑ in HIV+ pts. It often occurs in early stage HIV disease. 86% of serotypes are included in current vaccine (*Am J Epidem 138:909, 1993*). Outcome of rx has been good, although rare relapsing infections reported (*CID 14: 1050, 1992*). In addition, S. pneumoniae may cause soft tissue infections (*JID 163:897, 1991*) (See page 104).
Disseminated histoplasmosis may mimic sepsis syndrome	*CID 24:1195, 1997*
	See page 105
Haemophilus influenzae bacteremia	Nasopharyngeal carriage rates for Staph. aureus in HIV+ 44% vs 23% in hospital personnel; rates of Staph aureus bacteremia ↑ (*Europ J Clin Micro-ID 11:985, 1992*). Nosocomial bacteremia still common in ARV RX era (2.45/1000 pt days) (*CID 34:677, 2002*).
Causes include those seen in the non-HIV+ patient, especially the febrile neutropenic patient: enterobacteriaceae, Pseudomonas sp., Staph. aureus, Staph. epidermidis	

TABLE 11A (42)

CLINICAL SYNDROME, ETIOLOGY, EPIDEMIOLOGY	CLINICAL PRESENTATION, DIAGNOSTIC TESTS, COURSE
"Sepsis"/Bacteremia/Disseminated histoplasmosis may mimic sepsis syndrome *(continued)*	
Recurrent bacteremia	
Non-typhi salmonella, especially S. typhimurium (outside of U.S., Salmonella typhi)	In U.S., 20-fold ↑ in risk in HIV+ individuals (*Rev Inf Dis 9:925, 1987*). With CD4 >200/mm³ clinical presentation & response to rx similar to HIV-negative individuals. With CD4 <200/mm³, diarrhea is a less prominent symptom. 1–16% relapse within several months (*AJM 151:381, 1991*).
Mycobacterium avium-intracellulare (MAC)	See page 110
Bartonella henselae, quintana	See pages 101 & 116
Rhodococcus equi	**See page 110**
Sinuses, paranasal (*Rhinol 39:136, 2001*)	
Sinusitis: microbial flora similar to HIV-negative (S. pneumoniae, H. influenzae, M. catarrhalis) plus other Gram-positives (Staph. epidermidis, P. acnes), aerobic Gram-negatives (Pseudomonas aeruginosa), fungi [aspergillus, rhizopus (mucor), Alternaria alternata, H. capsulatum] (*CID 24:1178, 1997*). Rarely parasites (microsporidium, cryptosporidium, CMV, & mycobacteria (*CID 25:267, 1997*). Sinusitis occurs in 1/3 to 2/3 of adults with AIDS (*Ear, Nose, Throat J 69:460, 1990*).	Sinusitis may be part of acquired atopy in AIDS (*JID 167:283, 1993*). 2/3 pts are symptomatic (fever, nasal congestion, discharge). X-ray: 79% had air fluid level, usually more than one sinus. Despite rx, 60% pts had recurrent or persistent infection (*AJM 93:163, 1992*). Antral puncture required for accurate cultures & indicated if rx against common pathogens fails (*CID 16:404, 1993*). Think fungal if facial pain or headache out of proportion to clinical or x-ray finding, if CD4 <50 & ANC <1000, indolent course & subtle x-ray findings of invasion. Most common fungus Aspergillus fumigatus (*Otolaryng Clin NA 33:335, 2000*).
Skin/Hair[1] (*See Dermatol Clin 24:473, 2006 for excellent review*)	
HIV-associated pruritus (*see Am J Clin Dermat 4:177, 2003*) Etiology: Skin infections or infestations; papulosquamous disorders; photodermatitis; xerosis; drug reactions; rarely lymphoproliferative disorders	One of the most common symptoms in pts with HIV. Workup with careful exam of skin, nails, hair & mucous membranes to establish primary dermatological diagnosis; biopsy skin if necessary. ARV RX may improve idiopathic HIV pts but some may flare with immune reconstitution.
Eosinophilic folliculitis (*see J Am Acad Dermatol 55:215, 2006*)(resembles Ofuji's disease); marked pruritus, discrete, erythematous urticarial, follicular painless papules on trunk, head, neck, proximal extremities. 90% above nipple line. ↑ eos. ↑ IgE. CD4 <250 in 10/13 pts (*Mayo Clin Proc 67:1089, 1992*). Itraconazole 200mg po q24h improves ~75% pts (fluconazole of no benefit) (*Arch Derm 131:358, 1995*). Iso-tretinoin 0.75–1 mg/kg/day may also benefit (*Arch Derm 131:1089, 1995*). Metronidazole 250mg po q8h for 3–4wks works in some (*Arch Derm 131:1089, 1995*). May represent auto-immune reaction to sebum. Difficult to differentiate from infective folliculitis; bx is useful (*Br J Dermatol 141:3, 1999*). In large study of 878 HIV-infec women, ARV RX ↓ folliculitis (*CID 38:579, 2004*).	
Macular or papular lesions	
Acute retroviral syndrome	Lesions 5–10mm diam symmetrical, esp. on face or trunk (may involve palms & soles), erythematous, non-pruritic. Stevens-Johnson syndrome (*CID 19:798, 1994*), *see page 74*. Constitutional "mono-like symptoms:" fever, (87%), skin rash (68%). Mean duration of symptoms/signs 21 days (*CID 17:59, 1993*).
Insect bites (scabies—axilla, groin, fingerweb; fleas—lower legs; mosquitoes—arms & legs) Most common cause of pruritic papular eruption in Africa: 86/102 pts from the Academic Alliance Clinic, Mulago Hospital & Reachout Clinic, Uganda had biopsy findings characteristic of arthropod bites. These lesions assoc. with ↑ peripheral eosinophile counts & ↓ CD4 counts (*JAMA 292:2614, 2004*).	Erythematous, urticarial papules. Intensely pruritic lesions are scabies until proven otherwise. Heaped up, scaly eruption is Norwegien Scabies; highly infectious! (See "crusted lesions" below) Rx with topical therapy, **Permethrin** 5% total body (Chin to toes) overnight; alternative **Ivermectin** 200 mcg/kg po 1X; may need to be repeated 14 days later.
Drugs: Common cause of rash (esp. TMP/SMX & nevirapine) HIV+ pts have ↑ frequency of skin reactions to most drugs.	When Pls were initiated in 1,251 NRTI-experienced pts with <50 CD4 cells, 66 (5.3%) developed rash; risk factors: ♀ sex & ineffective ART (*HIV Med 5:1, 2004*). On the other hand, overall ARV RX assoc. with ↓ of dermatological manifestations (*CID 38:579, 2004*).

---

[1] T.C. Berger, Chapter 11, *ibid*.; *Mayo Clin Proc 67:1089, 1992*. Also ref.: *Ln 348:659, 1996.*

TABLE 11A (43)

CLINICAL SYNDROME, ETIOLOGY, EPIDEMIOLOGY	CLINICAL PRESENTATION, DIAGNOSTIC TESTS, COURSE
Skin/Hair/Macular or papular lesions (continued)	
Molluscum contagiosum More common in young women (CID 38:579, 2004)	Occurs in 8–15% AIDS pts. 2–5mm pearly flesh-colored papules, often with central umbilication on face, anogenital region. Disseminated cryptococcosis, P. marneffei; granuloma annulare (J Am Acad Dermatol 49:S184, 2003) may mimic.
Syphilis, secondary	See above, Genital Tract.
Candidiasis (47% of AIDS pts had mucocutaneous candidal infections in 1 series)	Children: diaper-rash type rash involving trunk & extremities. Adults: red, hemorrhagic macular or papular lesions.
Cryptococcosis	Common. Widespread skin-colored, dome-shaped translucent papules 1–4mm in diameter. Resemble Molluscum contagiosum.
Histoplasmosis	Slightly pink 2–6mm cutaneous papules to larger reddish plaques & multiple shallow crusted ulcerations, usually in febrile patient. (J Drug Dermatol 2:189, 2003).
Mycobacterial infections: M. tuberculosis, M. avium-intracellulare, M. kansasii, M. marinum, M. haemophilum, M. genavense (see page 109)	Vary from acneiform plaques, pustules or indurated verrucous plaques to ulcerative nodular lesions. See page 103. A case report of painful vesiculopustular rash secondary to hypersensitivity reaction to M. tbc antigen (tuberculide) (Ln 347:372, 1996). Lupus vulgaris from disseminating Mtbc or BCG (Int J Dermatol 44:299, 2005).
Mycobacterium leprae	Clinical presentation of borderline leprosy similar in HIV+ & HIV–, but rx for neuritis less successful in HIV+ (Lep Rev 63:134, 1992).
Penicillium marneffei (See CID 23:125, 1996; 24:1080, 1997)	Clinically present with fever, weight loss, small umbilicated macular or papular skin lesions (2/3 pts), hepato-splenomegaly, adenopathy. Almost all pts lived or traveled in Southeast Asia (J AIDS 6:466, 1993; CID 15:744, 1992).
Cutaneous Pneumocystis jiroveci (carinii)	Rare but reported with underlying PCP and advanced AIDS. More common if pt on aerosolized pentamidine. Typically verrucous translucent papules anywhere on body.
Human papillomavirus (warts, condyloma acuminatum)	Diffuse flat & filiform lesions, often in unusual sites. See GI & Genital Tract, above.
Kaposi's sarcoma (CD4: mean 87/mm^3, median 37/mm^3)	Early lesions are round or irregular pinkish-red to violaceous macules to papules, usually non-tender. Often symmetrical along skin tension lines. (See below)
Lymphoid papulosis (LyP) Rare cutaneous lymphoproliferative disorder (AIDS Pt Care STDs 18:563, 2004)	Chronic recurrent pruritic eruption of papules & nodules that undergo spontaneous regression. Usually benign with minority progressing to lymphoma. May resemble pityriasis but histologically resembles lymphoma (Anaplastic T-cell or HD).
Nodular, verrucous, &/or ulcerative lesions	
Mycobacterial infections	See above
Bacillary angiomatosis (Reference: CID 22:794, 1996)	Friable vascular papules, cellulitis, plaques & subcutaneous nodules, usually tender. Pts may be febrile. May be confused with KS. Etiology: Bartonella henselae & B. quintana. May be isolated from blood (5–15 days incubation of lysis centrifugation cultures on blood agar, 5% CO_2) & identified with Warthin Stary stain. See pages 101 & 116.
Acanthamoeba, disseminated	Rare (NEJM 331:85, 1994)
Sporotrichosis	Uncommon, but reported. May cause multiple lesions with dissemination (J Inf 51:e73, 2005).
Cryptococcosis	As above
Histoplasmosis	As above
Furunculosis can be severe	Most due to MRSA. Contagious. Spread with households, partners.

TABLE 11A (44)

CLINICAL SYNDROME, ETIOLOGY, EPIDEMIOLOGY	CLINICAL PRESENTATION, DIAGNOSTIC TESTS, COURSE
Skin/Hair/Nodular, verrucous, &/or ulcerative lesions *(continued)*	
Kaposi's sarcoma: Kaposi-associated herpesvirus (KSHV) now called HHV 8 is found in biopsy samples & blood mononuclear cells of pts with AIDS-related or classical KS (*Ln 346:799, 1995*).	Skin usually 1st site of presentation. Lesions palpable, firm, non-tender nodules. Early lesions may resemble ecchymoses. Typically violaceous, hyperpigmented, involving head, neck. Later become confluent, form large tumor masses & occur throughout the body. Up to 40% GI involvement. Oral lesions may precede skin lesions. In 107 Brazilian pts with KS, 61.6% demonstrated complete response to ARV RX, 23% partial response & 15.4% progressed. None receiving Pts progressed (*Int J Dermatol 43:643, 2004*).
Non-Hodgkins lymphoma	Skin involved in 15% of pts with non-Hodgkin lymphoma. Lesions are usually papules or nodules.
Mycobacterium avium-intracellulare (MAI/MAC)	Fever & extensive cutaneous nodules (granulomas or focal necroses) have been reported in pts infected with MAC who responded to ARV RX **with immune reconstitution** (↑ CD4 counts & ↓ viral load). Steroids may be useful rx (*5th Conf Retrovir & OI 1998, Abst. 726*) (Table 11B).
Leishmania 4% of cutaneous lesions in India (*Indian J Path Micro 45:293, 2002*)	May produce a wide spectrum of localized or disseminated cutaneous, mucosal or diffuse lesions (*An Trop Med Parasitol 97:S107, 2003*). Most lesions are small, papular with ulceration but with HIV may widely disseminate with hundreds of lesions (*Am J Trop Med Hyg 7:558, 2004, J Clin Microb 44:1178, 2006*). Common in the Middle East / Iraq.
Vesicular bullous or pustular lesions	
Herpes simplex virus	Grouped vesicles on erythematous base, rapidly evolve into ulcerations or fissures. May persist as chronic large ulcerative lesions, esp. in perianal area.
Varicella-zoster virus: Common in HIV+ pts & frequently precedes AIDS; 10–20%, frequency overall (*Int J Dermatol 39:192, 2000; J Clin Epid 54:522, 2001; Am J Med Sci 321:372, 2001*)	Grouped vesicles on erythematous base. May be verrucous. In chronic form may persist as hyperkeratotic lesions. Dermatomal distribution. May be multidermatomal.
Cytomegalovirus	Rare. Small reddish-purple macules that ulcerate. May present with non-healing perianal ulceration.
Staphylococcal impetigo	Erythematous crusted papules, may be pruritic on face, trunk, groin.
"Typical scabies"	Extremely pruritic, papular & vesicular lesions characterized by linear or serpentine burrows most commonly on hands, wrists, elbows, ankles. Average number of mites is 11. As above.
Stevens-Johnson syndrome	Most often drug-related: TMP/SMX, fluconazole, ddI, anti-TBc drugs. 1 case reported with acute HIV infection (*CID 19:798, 1994*).
Porphyria cutanea tarda	Association with HIV described but the co-occurrence may reflect coexistence of risk factors, esp. alcohol use, Hep C, rather than causal association (*CID 20:348, 1995*). Lesions especially over sun-exposed areas.
Papulosquamous lesions	
Seborrheic dermatitis	Occurs in 20–80% HIV+ individuals, dandruff to patches & plaques of erythema with indistinct margins & yellowish scale on "hairy" areas. Malassezia furfur may be causative agent (*CID 22:S128, 1996*).
Xerotic eczema (dry-skin syndrome). ↑ with ↓ CD4 counts (*CID 38:579, 2004*)	Occurs in 5–20% HIV+ individuals. Often severely pruritic & resistant to antihistamines.
Dermatophytosis (T. rubrum most common, then T. mentagrophytes & E. floccosum)	Occurs in 20–35% HIV+ individuals. Widespread, often severe with scaly red pruritic papules & plaques.
Tinea versicolor	Patchy areas of fine scale & hypopigmentation. CD4 often >300/mm^3. Usually resistant to topical agents.

117

TABLE 11A (45)

CLINICAL SYNDROME, ETIOLOGY, EPIDEMIOLOGY	CLINICAL PRESENTATION, DIAGNOSTIC TESTS, COURSE
Skin/Hair/Papulosquamous lesions (continued)	
Psoriasis	Presents as (1) discrete plaques or (2) a diffuse dermatitis often associated with palmoplantar keratodermia. Distribution may be atypical: groin, axilla & scalp rather than elbows & knees. Common nail changes & psoriatic arthritis. (JRD 17:914, 1996).
Crusted (Norwegian) scabies Occurs in 1.3–5% HIV+ individuals. A marker for HIV or HTLV-1 infection in Brazil & India (AIDS 16:1292, 2002; Indian Pedi 39:875, 2002). Found in 13/109 CSWs in Nigeria—all had HIV infection (Afr J Med Sci 31:243, 2002).	**Highly contagious** to close contacts (health care workers). Usually occurs in patients with severe immunodeficiency. Characterized by erythema, hyperkeratosis & crusting. Pruritus is typically present but hyperkeratotic, crusted form may be absent. Burrows usually not seen. Gross nail thickening & subungual debris common. Alopecia, hyperpigmentation, pyoderma & eosinophilia may occur. Dx is based on demonstration of heavy mite burden (1000s) on scraping vs a few in typical scabies. Combination rx with topical benzyl benzoate & ivermectin po x1 effective in severe crusted scabies in one series of 39 pts (Br J Dermatol 142:969, 2000). Ivermectin may also be of value topically (Fundam Clin Pharmacol 17:217, 2003).
Folliculitis	
Staphylococcal folliculitis	An uncommon presentation is violaceous plaques (up to 10cm) in groin, axilla & scalp.
Eosinophilic folliculitis	See above, Skin, eosinophilic folliculitis.
Skin discoloration (reddish-brown, occ. black or bluish)	Seen in 75–100% of pts on clofazimine, but also think Addison's disease, toxoplasmosis, etc. (J Derm 31:756, 2004).
Pressure ulcers (PUs) Incidence 2.3/100 hospital admissions: ↑ with female sex, length of hospital stay (1.06/100 pt days), advanced HIV. Mortality 50% with PU vs 7.2% without PU with attributed mortality of 42.8.	Aggressive preventive strategies should be implemented.
Hair disease: Diffuse thinning, premature graying, elongated eyelashes. In African-Americans peculiar straightening of previously curly hair has been observed in advanced HIV (JRD 17:914, 1996)	
Nail disease	
Onychomycosis	
Longitudinal pigmented nail bands	Seen in almost ½ pts on higher-dose ZDV, more common in dark-skinned patients, occurs within 4–8wks of starting rx.
Splenomegaly	23% of 70 consecutive HIV+ pts were found to have splenomegaly on physical exam & 66% by ultrasound. Pts with liver disease were more likely to have ↑ (RR=1.84, P<0.001). ↑ spleen was not predictive of any clinical event during a 1-yr follow-up or with developing AIDS in a 6-yr follow-up (CID 30: 943, 2000). **Massive splenomegaly: think leishmaniasis!**
Systemic, wasting syndromes "Slim" disease (enteropathic AIDS), rule out: Cryptosporidium & other causes of chronic diarrhea Mycobacterium avium-intracellulare complex (MAC) Mycobacterium tuberculosis Histoplasma capsulatum Kaposi's sarcoma Non-Hodgkin lymphoma	Weight loss is common (29% in one series). Causes: opportunistic infections (47%), psychosocial factors (17%), drug-associated (7%), unexplained (29%) (Int J STD 4:234, 1993). In Africa, most common symptom of AIDS is slim disease: weight loss (often >30% body weight), chronic fever, intermittent watery diarrhea without blood or mucus [25% to 50% have parasites (cryptosporidium, Strongyloides stercoralis, I. belli Ethiop Med J 43:93, 2005)]. Many die without an apparent OI. Treatment unsuccessful. Nutritional deficiencies were found in 86% of 125 HIV-infected IVDUs & could account for unexplained weight loss (J AIDS & Human Retro 16:272, 1997). Rapid weight loss (>4 kg in <4 mos.) accompanied by anorexia is usually a sign of secondary infection, slower weight loss (>4 kg in >4 mos.) is often due to GI disease with diarrhea, less marked weight loss may be due to ↓ caloric intake (NEJM 333:123, 1995). Usually reversed with ARV RX response! Assoc. with ↓ survival in South Africa (S Afr Med J 91:583, 2001). **Watch for 'refeeding syndrome'.**

TABLE 11B: IMMUNE RECONSTITUTION & NOVEL SYNDROMES ASSOCIATED WITH ARV RX

As noted in Table 6A, the use of Highly Active Antiretroviral Therapy (ARV RX) has led to a marked improvement in the control of HIV infections & significant reduction in mortality from AIDS wherever it has been employed *(AnIM 135:19, 2001; CID 44:599, 2007)*. In addition, ARV RX has led to reconstitution of the immune deficiencies in the majority of patients receiving this therapy. As a result of this, the incidence of opportunistic infections & AIDS-defining illnesses has also declined *(JAMA 296:292, 2006)*. This has been noted most dramatically in multi-center studies of treatment of AIDS-associated opportunistic infections, as the rate of accrual of patients in these studies has declined markedly in the past several years. The incidence of certain other infections including invasive S. pneumoniae has also declined in the US since the advent of ARV RX *(JID 191:2038, 2005)*. Interestingly, in developed countries, non-HIV related causes of death (especially cardiovascular disease, non-HIV-related cancer and substance abuse) caused 25% of all deaths in patients receiving ARV RX between 1999 and 2004 *(Ann Int Med 145:397, 2006)*. HIV-infected patients with the metabolic syndrome are at increased risk for ASCVD *(CID 44:1368, 2007)*. In addition to the direct antiretroviral effects of ARV RX, a number of novel clinical syndromes have been seen as well. Among the syndromes associated with ARV RX are adverse effects due to protease inhibitors & other components of ARV RX, new syndromes associated with immune reconstitution, & the clinical effects of ARV RX on opportunistic disorders.

1. **Adverse effects due to drugs used in ARV RX**
   Many of the most important adverse events directly related to the agents used in ARV RX (such as renal lithiasis due to indinavir, gastrointestinal events related to ritonavir & other protease inhibitors) are detailed in Table 6B. In addition, a number of unusual syndromes (not necessarily related to a specific agent, but to classes of agents used in ARV RX) have been described in the past several years. Included among these syndromes (some of which may cause serious morbidity or even death) are lactic acidosis, abnormalities in glucose metabolism, disorders of lipid metabolism, lipodystrophy syndromes such as lipoatrophy & lipohypertrophy, osteopenia & possibly aseptic necrosis of the hip. These complications are covered in detail in Table 6C.

2. **New syndromes associated with immune reconstitution**
   Patients receiving ARV RX have reduced plasma HIV-1 viral load & increased CD4 T-lymphocyte counts. Despite this, there are reports of development of AIDS-defining events, particularly in the first several months after initiation of therapy *(JAMA 282:2220, 1999)*. It is unclear at this point as to whether this is related to a delay in restoration of immune function or the fact that ARV RX may actually promote clinical development &/or expression of such infections as well as AIDS-related malignant disease. More commonly, however, one sees a variety of inflammatory reactions associated with immune reconstitution *(Med 81:213, 2002; JAC 51:1, 2003)*. This syndrome is often termed the **immune reconstitution inflammatory syndrome (IRIS)** & occurs in up to 25% of patients with an underlying opportunistic infection after initiation of ARV RX *(JAC 57:167, 2006)*. The most frequent manifestations are dermatological, particularly involving genital herpes and warts *(CID 42:418, 2006)* or in patients with mycobacterial disease *(Lancet ID 5:361, 2005)*. In patients with disseminated MAC disease, elevations in CD4 cells & associated immune reconstitution may be coupled with the development of painful generalized lymphadenopathy resembling scrofula. Massive mesenteric adenopathy with severe abdominal pain & thoracic adenopathy associated with pulmonary infiltrates & endobronchial proliferative lesions have also been described *(JID 179:329, 1999; JID 180:76, 1999; AIDS 13:177, 1999)*. These patients are often systemically ill with fever, leukocytosis & malaise sufficient to require hospital admission *(Ln 351:252, 1998)*. We have seen one patient with disseminated MAC disease who developed a symptomatic brain abscess due to MAC after initiating ARV RX. The resultant brisk granulomatous response & macrophage activation may lead to increased levels of 1,25 hydroxy vitamin D & hypercalcemia. One of the authors has observed 5 cases of hypercalcemia in this setting. IRIS is also a well-known complication of the initiation of antiretroviral therapy in patients infected with M. tuberculosis *(JID 196:S63, 2007)*.

   "Paradoxical reactions" (hectic fevers, lymphadenopathy, worsening chest film) have also been described in patients with HIV & tuberculosis receiving concomitant therapy for both diseases *(AJRCCM 158:157, 1998)*. The development of symptomatic cytomegalovirus retinitis shortly after initiation of ARV RX is likely a manifestation of the same phenomenon. Flares in hepatitis in patients chronically infected with hepatitis B & C viruses are likely also the result of improvement in immune status *(Ln 349:996, 1997)*. Note that this syndrome must be distinguished from the mild hepatotoxicity associated with drugs used to treat ARV RX. The symptoms of the immune reconstitution syndromes usually subside spontaneously with continued therapy for the underlying disease or with the use of nonsteroidal anti-inflammatory agents. Occasionally reactions may be severe enough to be life-threatening & may require corticosteroid therapy *(CID 38:1159, 2004)*. A summary of the clinical manifestations of specific opportunistic infections in HIV-1 infected patients receiving & not receiving ARV RX is given below *(adapted from AnIM 133:447, 2000)*:

3. **Selected effects of ARV RX on opportunistic infections or other complications of HIV infection**
   (also see Table 11A for individual OIs)

TABLE 11B (2)

Opportunistic Infection	Common Clinical Presentation	Presentation After Highly Active Antiretroviral Therapy (ARV RX)
Castleman disease	Fever, lymphadenopathy	Clinical recovery with resolution of lymphadenopathy (J Inf 40:90, 2000). However, late relapse (fatal) after initial response described in 5 patients despite immune reconstitution (CID 35:880, 2002).
Cryptococcus neoformans	Meningitis usually indolent, cerebrospinal fluid leukocytosis uncommon	Overt meningitis, marked cerebrospinal fluid leukocytosis
Cryptosporidiosis, microsporidiosis	Diarrhea	Clinical, microbiological resolution associated with significant reduction in viral load (Ln 351: 256, 1998)
Cytomegalovirus	Retinitis, vitreitis, uveitis uncommon	Atypical (non-retinitis) manifestations of CMV, including pneumonitis, pseudotumoral colitis, adenitis & symptoms of viremia (Ln 351:228, 1998). Immune recovery uveitis (JAMA 282:1633, 1999; Eur J Clin Micro Inf Dis 22:114, 2003)
Eosinophilic folliculitis	Inflammatory reaction involving new hair follicles—especially on face and trunk	Inflammatory reaction to Dermodex folliculorum mites. May respond rapidly to ivermectin (AIDS 18:701, 2004; Dermatology 205:394, 2002).
Hepatitis B (chronic)	Asymptomatic or nonspecific symptoms	Acute flare of clinical hepatitis 5–12wks after beginning ARV RX. Usually resolves without change in therapy. There is a description of resolution of e-antigen in a patient with a 5-yr history of e-antigen positive hepatitis B (Ln 349:996, 1997).
Hepatitis C (chronic)	Asymptomatic	Acute hepatitis, cirrhosis or HCV-associated disorder such as cryoglobulinemia within 1–9 months after initiation of ARV RX (JID 181:2033, 2000). HCV seropositivity may be associated with smaller CD4 recovery on ARV RX (Ln 356:1800, 2000). Both ↑ & ↓ in HCV DNA levels have been described following ARV RX & overall outcomes not yet known (CID 35: 873, 2002).
Herpes simplex (ano-genital)	Painful ulcerated lesions	Recrudescence of recurrent episodes of ano-genital lesions (CID 42:418, 2006). Note reconstitution of HSV-specific T cell immunity in HIV-infected patients receiving ARV RX (JID 195:410, 2007).
Herpes zoster	May be severe accompanied by complications	Mild presentation, uncomplicated. May see increased incidence of zoster after initiation of ARV RX, possibly due to ↑ CD8 cells (Am J Med 110:605, 2001).
HIV-1 associated nephropathy	Impaired renal function	Reversal of pathology & recovery of function (Ln 352:783, 1998)
HIV-associated non-Hodgkin's lymphoma	Typical Stage I-IV lymphoma	Improved clinical outcome & survival (CID 37:1556, 2003)
Kaposi's sarcoma	Skin lesions, disseminated disease, oral lesions	Regression of lesions coincident with significant reduction in viral load (AIDS 11:161, 1997; Ln 357:1411, 2001; J AIDS 31:384, 2002; JAC 51:1095, 2003). Laryngeal obstruction from mucosal edema is rare complication of ARV RX (CID 34: 231, 2002).
Lymphoepithelial parotid cysts	Parotid cysts	Resolution on antiretroviral therapy (AnIM 128:455,1998)
Molluscum contagiosum	Disseminated skin lesions	Resolution of severe disease coincident with 10-fold increase in CD4 cells (CID 24:1023, 1997)
Mycobacterium avium complex	Disseminated disease, weight loss, diarrhea, mycobacteremia	Focal lymphadenitis, granulomatous masses, endobronchial proliferative lesions, abdominal lymphadenopathy & pain (see above for more details), clearance of bacteremia without antimycobacterial therapy (CID 26:758, 1998), development of cavitation in pulmonary nodules (CID 27:1542, 1998). Immune reconstitution lymphadenitis may occur despite azithromycin prophylaxis (CID 34:371, 2002; CID 42:418, 2006). Intraabdominal disease results in greater morbidity than peripheral lymphadenitis (CID 41:1483, 2005).
Oral candidiasis	White plaques on oral & pharyngeal mucosa (thrush)	Clinical resolution of oral candidiasis without antifungal therapy. This is independent of immune reconstitution & may be a direct effect of PIs (JID 185:188, 2002).
Oral warts	Relatively rare oral lesions	Marked ↑ in oral warts which are progressive & recur after removal (Ln 357:1411, 2001; CID 34:641, 2002)
Chronic parvovirus B-19 infection	Anemia; AIDS wasting syndrome; encephalitis	Anecdotal case reports of response in patients with each syndrome receiving ARV RX (The AIDS Reader 8:21, 1998; CID 36:1191, 2003). Case report of development of parvovirus B-19 encephalitis in 1 patient on ARV RX (CID 36:1191, 2003).

TABLE 11B (3)

Opportunistic Infection	Common Clinical Presentation	Presentation After Highly Active Antiretroviral Therapy (ARV RX)
Progressive multifocal leukoencephalopathy	Neurologic deficits, MRI demonstration of hypodensities without contrast enhancement	Neurologic deficits; neurologic deficits with enhancing lesions on MRI, frequently with peripheral enhancement *(AIDS 13:1426, 1999)*; long-term, see remission of neurologic symptoms & improvement of radiographic findings *(Ln 349:850, 1997)* & increased survival in approx. 50% of cases *(CID 36:1047, 2003; JID 180:621, 1999)*. Fatal, paradoxical worsening of PML (nonresponsive to steroids) has also been described in pts shortly after initiation of ARV RX *(CID 35:1250, 2002)*
Pulmonary tuberculosis	Pulmonary infiltrates	Fever, lymphadenopathy, worsening pulmonary infiltrates. Note: incidence of Tbc decreased with ARV RX *(CID 45:1518, 2007)*.
Sarcoidosis	Cutaneous lesions; diffuse pulmonary involvement; adenopathy	Flares of preexisting or new onset sarcoidosis described in patients on ARV RX *(Radiology 218:242, 2001; HIV Medicine Self-Directed Study Guide 275, 2005)*.
Systemic lupus erythematosus	Incidence of SLE decreased in immunosuppressed AIDS pts	Anecdotal reports of new onset of SLE & flares of preexisting SLE following ARV RX *(J Rheum 27:11, 2000)*
Tegumentary leishmaniasis	No lesions or few erythematous papules	Worsening of prior lesions or development of disseminated lesions *(JID 192:1819, 2005)*
Visceral leishmaniasis	Fever, hepatosplenomegaly	Long-term remission *(J Inf 40:94, 2000)*; development of post-kala-azar dermal leishmaniasis *(J Inf 40:199, 2000)*. Decreased incidence of VL seen in France after ARV RX in 1996 *(JID 186:1366, 2002)*.

4. **Effect on incidence of AIDS-related opportunistic infections** The immune reconstitution associated with ARV RX has clearly led to a striking decline in the incidence of AIDS-related opportunistic infections, although the spectrum of these diseases, in general, has not been altered *(CID 27:1379, 1998)*. The incidence is highest immediately after starting ARV RX & declines progressively after that *(JAMA 282: 2220, 1999)*. The decreased incidence is also manifest by a striking decline in enrollment of patients into NIH-sponsored treatment protocols for opportunistic infections. Recent studies suggest that in patients receiving ARV RX, diarrhea is more likely due to therapy itself than to any of the formerly frequent opportunistic pathogens that cause diarrhea *(CID 28:701, 1999)*. A retrospective study has also suggested a significant decrease in incidence of HIV cardiac involvement, especially pericarditis, arrhythmias & dilated cardiomyopathy in patients receiving ARV RX *(J Inf 40:282, 2000)*.

5. **Discontinuation of prophylaxis for opportunistic infections** *(Also see Table 10)* Data have now accumulated that it is possible to stop primary prophylaxis for MAI, PCP, & toxoplasmosis in patients with sustained responses (CD4 cell counts >100–200) to ARV RX *[Ln 353:1293, 1999; NEJM 340:1301, 1999; MMWR 51(RR-8):1, 2002; CMI 12:666, 2006; CID 43:79, 2006]*. It is also now possible to stop secondary prophylaxis for PCP, MAI [especially in patients who received at least 1 year of macrolide-based therapy *(JID 187:1046, 2003)*], toxoplasmosis, cryptococcosis, & CMV retinitis in patients with sustained CD4 cell responses *[JAMA 282:1633, 1999; Ln 353:1293, 1999; NEJM 342:1460, 2000; MMWR 51(RR-8):1, 2002; CID 36:645, 2003]*. Although it may be possible to stop secondary prophylaxis for other opportunistic infections including varicella zoster virus, Histoplasma capsulatum, & Coccidioides immitis, further data are necessary to ascertain that this is safe *(J Inf 41:18, 2000; NEJM 342:1416, 2000; MMWR 51(RR-8):1, 2002)*. Rare instances of recurrence of MAI infection following immune reconstitution & cessation of therapy for disseminated MAI have been described *(Eur J CMID 20:199, 2001)*. The same may be true for patients in whom secondary prophylaxis for PCP is discontinued *(CID 36:645, 2003)*. It appears that discontinuation of PCP prophylaxis is not associated with increase in community-acquired pneumonia in patients with sustained CD4 cell count increase to >200 *(CID 36:917, 2003)*.

6. **Infectivity** Although one might expect that effective suppression of viral load might decrease the chance of transmission of HIV from patients responding to ARV RX, a serious note of caution is injected by data showing that in HIV-1 infected men on ARV RX (& no detectable plasma viral RNA), the virus may persist in seminal cells & semen & may be capable of sexual transmission *(NEJM 339:1803, 1998)*. Although a recent report suggests that people on ARV RX are more likely to develop a sexually transmitted disease, an epidemiological marker for unsafe sex *(Ln 357:432, 2001)*, the increased prevalence of unsafe sex in this setting is likely related to the perception that the subjects are at low risk of transmitting HIV & not to the administration of ARV RX *(JAMA 292:224, 2004)*.

TABLE 12: TREATMENT OF SPECIFIC INFECTIONS IN HIV+/AIDS PATIENTS

CAUSATIVE AGENT/DISEASE	MODIFYING CIRCUMSTANCES	SUGGESTED REGIMENS PRIMARY	ALTERNATIVE	COMMENTS
BACTERIAL INFECTIONS				
Bartonella				
Cat-scratch disease—immunocompetent patient—lymphadenopathy Axillary/epitrochlear nodes 46%, neck 26%, inguinal 17%	Etiology: Bartonella henselae Ref: *PIDJ* 23:1161, 2004 & *AAC* 48:1921, 2004	**Azithro**: Adults (>45.5kg): 500 mg po x1, then 250 mg/day x4d Children (<45.5kg): liquid azithro po 10 mg/kg x1, then 5 mg/kg/day x4d Treatment controversial—See Comment	No rx; resolves in 2–6mos. Needle aspiration relieves pain in suppurative nodes. Avoid surgical I&D.	**Clinical**: 10% nodes suppurate. Atypical presentation in <5%, i.e., lung nodules, liver/spleen lesions, Parinaud's oculo-glandular syndrome (*CID* 28:1156, 1999), CNS manifestations in 2% (encephalitis, peripheral neuropathy, retinitis, FUO). **Dx**: Cat exposure. Positive IFA serology. Rarely biopsy. **Rx**: 1 prospective randomized blinded study, used azithro (*PIDJ* 17:447, 1998): faster ↓ node size with azithro.
Bacillary angiomatosis; Peliosis hepatis—patients with AIDS	Etiology: B. henselae, B. quintana	(**Clarithro** 500 mg q12h or **clarithro ER** 1gm q24h) or (**azithro** 250 mg q24h) or (**CIP** 500–750 mg q12h), po x8wks	(**Erythro** 500 mg q6h po or **doxy** 100 mg q12h po) x8wks. If severe, combine **doxy** with **RIF**, 300 mg po q12h	
Endocarditis (see Table 11A, page 99) Ref: *AAC* 48:1921, 2004	Etiology: B. henselae, B. quintana	[**Ceftriaxone** 2 gm IV q24h x 6 wks + **gentamicin** 1 mg/kg q8h x 14 days] + **doxycycline** 100 mg IV/po bid x 6 wks. Surgery: Over ½ pts require valve surgery; relation to cure unclear.		Diagnosis: Immunofluorescent antibody titer ≥ 1:800; blood cultures only occ. Positive, or PCR of tissue from surgery. B. Quintana transmitted by body lice among homeless. Asymptomatic colonization of RBCs described (*Ln* 360:226, 2002).
Trench fever	B. quintana	**Doxy** 100 mg po bid. Doxy alone is OK if **no** endocarditis		
For chronic suppression in AIDS patients	With CD4 count <200	**Erythro** 250–500 mg po q6h (see Comments)	**Clarithro**, **azithro**, or **CIP** in above doses	Suppression until CD4 T-lymphocyte count above 200/mm3
Campylobacter jejuni Fever in 53–83%; bloody stools 37%	CAUTION: See Comment on quinolone resistance	(**CIP** 500 mg po q12h or **azithro** 500 mg po q24h) x3d.	**Erythromycin stearate** 500 mg po q6h x5d	↑ **worldwide resistance to FQs** varies from 10% (USA) to 84% (Thailand) (*AAC* 47:2358, 2003). Erytho resistance reported (*CID* 37:131, 2003). 15% of **Guillain-Barre** may follow campylobacter (*CID* 37:307, 2003). **Reactive arthritis** occurs.
Chlamydia trachomatis (non-gonococcal or post-gonococcal urethritis, cervicitis) Refs: MMWR 55(RR-11), 2006	NOTE: Assume concomitant GC. **Evaluate & rx sexual partners.**	**Doxycycline** 100 mg po q12h x7 days OR **Azithro** 1 gm po (single dose) In pregnancy: **azithro** 1 gm po x1. **Doxy & FQ not recommended in pregnancy.**	**Erythro** 500 mg po q6h x7 days OR **Ofloxacin** 300 mg po q12h x7d OR **Levo** 500 mg po q24h x7 days	**Diagnosis**: Nucleic acid amplification test on urine, urethral swab, or cervical swab [*MMWR* 55(RR-11), 2006]. Clarithro active in vitro vs C. trachomatis, but not FDA-approved for STDs. **For recurrent or persistent disease**: either metro 2gm po x1 + (either erythro base 500 mg po q6h x7d or erythro ethylsuccinate 800 mg po q6h x7d)
Clostridium difficile toxin-mediated diarrhea (*CID* 45:222, 2007)	See *Sanford Guide to Antimicrobial Therapy* for more detail	**Metronidazole** 500 mg po q8h or 250 mg po q6h x10–14d. If severe use **vanco** (*CID* 40:1588, 1591 & 1598, 2005 & 45:302, 2007)	**Vancomycin** 125 mg po q6h x14d	Avoid anti-motility agents. **Relapse occurs in 10–20% of patients;** use vanco + RIF 300mg po q12h x7–14d for relapse or 6 weeks vanco taper. Isolate patient.
Granuloma inguinale (Calymmatobacterium granulomatis or donovanosis)	Now: Klebsiella granulomatis	**Doxycycline** 100 mg po q12h x minimum of 3–4wks or **TMP/SMX** 1 DS tablet (160 mg TMP) po q12h x21d	[(**Erythro** 500 mg po q6h x21d (can be used in pregnancy)] or **CIP** 750 mg po q12h x3wks) or **azithro** 1 gm po qwk x3wks	Rare in U.S. Should see clinical response after 1wk. Rx until all lesions healed—may require 4wks rx. Rx failure/ relapse seen with doxy & TMP/SMX. FQ & chloro reported efficacious (*CID* 25:24, 1997).
Haemophilus ducreyi (chancroid)	Painful genital ulcer(s)	**Ceftriaxone** 250mg IM (single dose) or **azithro** 1gm po single dose	**CIP** 500 mg po q12h x3d OR **Erythro** 500 mg po q6h x7d	In HIV+ pts, failures reported with single dose azithro, may require usual regimen (0.5 gm po, then 250mg po q24h x4d). Ref.: *MMWR* 55(R-11), 2006
Listeriosis Ref.: *CID* 43:1233, 2006	Bacteremia, meningitis, focal infections	**Ampicillin** 2 gm IV q4h ± **gentamicin** 2mg/kg load dose, then 1.7mg/kg q8h.	If pen allergic: **TMP/SMX** 20 mg/kg/day TMP (component) IV divided into q6–8h dosage	Some evidence suggests synergy with ampicillin + an aminoglycoside (gentamicin). Duration of rx 2–4wks. (**Cephalosporins not active vs L. monocytogenes**)

TABLE 12 (2)

CAUSATIVE AGENT/DISEASE	MODIFYING CIRCUMSTANCES	SUGGESTED REGIMENS PRIMARY	SUGGESTED REGIMENS ALTERNATIVE	COMMENTS
BACTERIAL INFECTIONS (continued)				
Lymphogranuloma venereum Ref:*MMWR 55(RR-11), 2006*	Etiology: C. trachomatis, serovars. L1–L3	**Doxycycline** 100 mg po q12h x21d	**Erythro** 500 mg po q6h x21d	Dx based on serology, biopsy contraindicated. Rectal LGV may require retreatment.
Mycobacterium tuberculosis: Treatment of latent infection (LTBI) [previously known as preventive treatment, infection without disease (pos tuberculin test)¹] **or HIV+ pt with anergy & high risk for tuberculosis** *(AnIM 119: 185, 1993).* HIV+ pts with anergy need prophylaxis only if exposed to active TB *(NEJM 337: 315, 1997)* or if they fall into a group at high risk for TBc (e.g., HIV-infected IV drug abusers) *(AIDS 13: 2069, 1999).* Therefore use of anergy testing in conjunction with PPD testing not recommended for routine screening programs for TB among HIV-infected pts in U.S. *[MMWR 46(RR-15):1, 1997; JAMA 283:2003, 2000].* Treatment of LBTI effective in HIV+ patients *(JID 196:S52, 2007).*	Organisms likely to be INH-susceptible	**INH** 5 mg/kg/day (max. 300 mg/day) po + **pyridoxine** (B6) 25–50 mg po x9mo (See Comment). For children, see Table 8F, page 66.	If compliance problem: **INH** by DOT 15 mg/kg 2x/wk x9mos *(MMWR 52:735, 2003).* **If INH not possible, options: RIF**** 600 mg po q24h OR **RFB**** 300 mg po q24h x4 mos.	For pts given ddC + INH, suggest 50 mg pyridoxine/day. Duration of preventive rx unclear; recommendations range from 2–12mos. Ugandan study suggests 6mos of INH or 3mos of INH + RIF also ↓ risk of TB *(NEJM 337:801, 1997),* 2mo regimens of RIF + PZA or RFB + PZA also shown to be effective *(AIDS 13:1549, 1999).* **However, there are recent descriptions of severe & fatal hepatitis in immunocompetent pts on RIF + PZA** *(MMWR 50:289, 2001).* Monitoring for cofactors did not seem to allow prediction of fatalities *(CID 42:346, 2006).* Therefore, regimen is no longer recommended by CDC for LTBI *(MMWR 52:735, 2003; CID 39:484, 2004).* Not all agree with CDC recommendations and recent study suggests short course therapy is safe with monitoring and more likely to be completed than longer Rx *(CID 43:271, 2006).* Resistant TBc occurred in HIV+ pts given INH + RIF by DOT presum. due to malabsorption *(NEJM 332:336, 1995; AJM 127:289, 1997; CID 25:1044, 1997),* although 1 study failed to detect direct effect on bioavailability of antimycobacterial drugs in pts with AIDS ± diarrhea *(CID 25: 104, 1997).* INH prophylaxis reported to ↓ progression of HIV *(Lancet 342:268, 1993).* Late "failures" of INH "prophylaxis" usually due to reinfection, not primary failure of regimen *(CID 34:366, 2002).*
	INH-resistant (or adverse reaction to INH), RIF-sensitive organisms likely	**RIF**** 600 mg po q24h or **RFB**** 300 mg po q24h x4 mos.		
For more details, see USPHS recommendations *[AnIM 137 No. 5 (Suppl., Part 2), 2002; CID 37:1686, 2003; NEJM 350:2060, 2004; JAMA 293:2776, 2005].*	INH- & RIF-resistant organisms likely	Efficacy of all regimens unproven. **PZA** 25–30 mg/kg/day to max. of 2 gm/day + **ETB** 15–25 mg/kg/day po x12mos.	**PZA** 25 mg/kg/day to max. of 2 gm/day + **ETB** 15–25 mg/kg/day + **CIP** 750 mg q12h or **oflox** 400 mg q12h or **levoflox** 500 mg/day, all po, x6–12 mos.	If ETB used in dose above 15 mg/kg/day, monitor pt for retrobulbar neuritis. (Visual acuity & red/green color test, ≥10% loss considered significant.) **Consultation recommended.**

¹ Tuberculin test (TST): The standard is the Mantoux test, 5 TU (intermediate) PPD in 0.1 ml diluent stabilized with Tween 80. Read at 48–72hrs, measuring the maximum diameter of induration (not erythema). A reaction of ≥5mm is defined as + in the HIV+ pt. For HIV+ pts who have received BCG ≥10 mm is cut-off for rx *(Brit Med J 304:1231, 1992).* Note that BCG immunization in HIV+ children carries significant risk of causing disseminated BCG disease *(CID 42:548, 2006).* Because up to 25% of patients with HIV are anergic, the decrease in proportion of false-negative TST results obtained by reducing cutoff for positivity from 10 to 5 mm is limited *(CID 43:634, 2006).* See also *Table 23* for details of PPD testing. Whole blood interferon-gamma release assay [QuantiFERON-TB (QFT)] approved by U.S. FDA as diagnostic test for TB *(JAMA 286:1740, 2001; CID 34:1449 & 1457, 2002).* CDC recommends TST for TB suspects & pts at ↑ risk for progression to active TB & suggests either TST or QFT for individuals not warrant testing but are deemed at low risk for LTBI *[MMWR 52(RR-2):15, 2003].* IFN-γ assay is better indicator of TBc risk than TST in BCG-vaccinated population *(JAMA 293:2756, 2005).* A more sensitive assay based on M. tbc-specific antigens (QuantiFERON-TB GOLD) was approved by the USFDA 5/2/05 and an enzyme-linked immunospot method (ELIspot) using antigens specific for MTB (do not cross-react with BCG) is under evaluation & looks promising *(Thorax 58:916, 2003; Ln 361:1168, 2003; AnIM 140:709, 2004; LnID 4:761, 2005; CID 40:246, 2005; JAMA 293:2756, 2005; MMWR 54:49, 2005).* However, none of these tests can distinguish latent from active TB and none is 100% sensitive (ELIspot slightly higher sensitivity than Quantiferon-TB Gold)*(AnIM 146:340, 2007; CID 44:74, 2007).*

** *See end of section for options regarding concomitant use of protease inhibitors & **RIF** or **RFB**.*

NOTE: All dosage recommendations are for adults (unless otherwise indicated) & assume normal renal function.

BACTERIAL INFECTIONS/Treatment, active tuberculosis (continued)

Treatment, active tuberculosis **General principles TBc therapy in pts co-infected with HIV:** • Rx of TBc in pts with HIV infec should follow same principles as for persons without HIV. • Presence of active TBc requires immediate initiation of rx. • In antiretroviral-naive pts, delay of ARV RX for 4–8wks after initiation of TBc rx permits better definition of causes of adverse reactions & paradoxical reactions. Further delay could be detrimental (JID 190: 1670, 2004). • Impact of specific initial ARV RX regimen on outcome of TBc not clear [In developing countries, 10–20% of pts who are HIV+ & have active TBc are bacteremic (AIDS 13: 2/93, 1999)] • Directly observed therapy strongly recommended for HIV/TBc co-infected. • Rifampin/rifabutin-based regimens should be given at least 3x weekly in pts with CD4 <100/mm³. • Once weekly rifapentine not recommended in HIV-infected pts. • Despite drug interactions, rifamycin should be included in pts receiving ARV RX, with dosage adjustment as necessary. • Paradoxical reaction should be treated with continuation of rx for TBc & HIV, along with use of NSAIDs. • In severe cases of paradoxical reaction, some suggest use of high-dose prednisone. (www.aidsinfo.nih.gov). However, adjunctive prednisone of no benefit in HIV+ patients with CD4 counts >200 (JID 191:856, 2005) or in patients with TBc pleurisy (JID 190:869, 2004).

	INITIAL PHASE[9]			CONTINUATION PHASE OF THERAPY (in vitro susceptibility known)[9]				Dose in mg/kg (max. daily dose)					
Rate of INH resistance known to be <4% (drug-susceptible organisms)	Regimens[1,2]	Drugs	Interval/Doses (min. duration)[2]	Regimen	Drugs	Interval/Doses (min. duration)[2,3]	Range of Total Doses (min. duration)[2]	Regimen*	INH	RIF**	PZA	ETB	SM	RFB**
			SEE COMMENTS FOR DOSAGE					Daily: Child	10–20 (300)	10–20 (600)	15–30 (2000)	15–25 (1600)	20–40 (1000)	10–20 (300)
								Adult	5 (300)	10 (600)	15–30 (2000)	15–25 (1600)	15 (1000)	5 (300)
	1	INH RIF** PZA ETB	7d/wk x56 doses (8wk) or 5d/wk x40 doses (8wk)[4]	1a	INH/RIF	7d/wk x126 doses (18wk) or 5d/wk x90 doses (18wk)[4]	182–130 (26wk)	2x/wk (DOT): Child	20–40 (900)	10–20 (600)	50–70 (4000)	50 (4000)	25–30 (1500)	10–20 (300)
				1b	INH/RIF	2x/wk x36 doses (18wk)	92–76 (26wk)[5]	Adult	15 (900)	10 (600)	50–70 (4000)	50 (4000)	25–30 (1500)	5 (300)
				1c[6]	INH/RFP	1x/wk x18 doses (18wk)	74–58 (26wk)	3x/wk (DOT): Child	20–40 (900)	10–20 (600)	50–70 (3000)	25–30 (2000)	25–30 (1500)	NA
	2	INH RIF** PZA ETB	7d/wk x14 doses (2wk), then 2x/wk x12 doses (6wk) or 5d/wk x10 doses (2wk)[4] then 2x/wk x12 doses (6wk)	2a	INH/RIF	2x/wk x36 doses (18wk)	62–58 (26wk)[5]	Adult	15 (900)	10 (600)	50–70 (3000)	25–30 (2000)	25–30 (1500)	NA
				2b[6]	INH/RFP	1x/wk x18 doses (18wk)	44–40 (26wk)	Second-line anti-TB agents can be dosed as follows to facilitate DOT:						
	3	INH RIF** PZA ETB	3x/wk x24 doses (8wk)	3a	INH/RIF	3x/wk x54 doses (18wk)	78 (26wk)	Cycloserine 500–750 mg po q24h (5x/wk) **Ethionamide 500–750 mg po q24h (5x/wk)** Kanamycin or capreomycin 15 mg/kg IM/IV q24h (3–5x/wk) CIP 750 mg po q24h (5x/wk) Ofloxacin 600–800 mg po q24h (5x/wk) Levofloxacin 750 mg po q24h (5x/wk) (CID 21:1245, 1995)						

Isolation essential! (See Table 11A, page 103.) Older observations on infectivity of susceptible & resistant M. tbc before & after rx (Am Rev Resp Dis 85:511, 1962) may not be applicable to MDR M. tbc or to the HIV+ individual. Extended isolation may be appropriate. [MMWR 54(RR-17), 2005]

General references on therapeutic options: CID 28:130, 1999; NEJM 340: 367, 1999; J Resp Dis 21:53, 2000; BMJ 325:1282, 2002; MMWR 52(RR-11):1, 2003; MMWR 53(RR-15):1, 2004; CID 40 (Suppl.1):S1, 2005; JID 196 (Suppl 1):S35, 2007; The Medical Letter 5(55):15, 2007.

Multiresistant (MDR) TBc: defined as resistant to at least 2 drugs including INH and RIF (JID 196(Suppl 1):S86, 2007).

NOTE:
1. Clinical & microbiologic response same as in HIV-neg patient although there is considerable variability among currently available studies (CID 32:623, 2001)
2. Post-treatment long-term suppression not necessary for drug-susceptible strains

(Continued on next page.)

(Continued on next page.)

* Footnotes are in the next page.

NOTE: All dosage recommendations are for adults (unless otherwise indicated) & assume normal renal function.

125

TABLE 12 (4)

** See end of Section for options regarding concomitant use of protease inhibitors & **RIF** or **RFB**

MODIFYING CIRCUMSTANCES	SUGGESTED REGIMENS	DUR. OF TREATMENT (MO.)	SPECIFIC COMMENTS		COMMENTS

BACTERIAL INFECTIONS/Treatment, active tuberculosis (continued) Review of therapy for MDR TB: *JAC 54:593, 2004; Med Lett 2:83, 2004.*

MODIFYING CIRCUMSTANCES	SUGGESTED REGIMENS	DUR. OF TREATMENT (MO.)	SPECIFIC COMMENTS		COMMENTS
(Continued from previous page.) **Extensively Drug-Resistant TB (XDR-TB):** defined as resistant to INH & RIF plus any FQ and at least one of 3 second-line drugs: capreomycin, kanamycin or amikacin *(MMWR 56:250, 2007; CID 45:338, 2007).*	4	INH RIF** ETB	7d/wk x56 doses (8wk) or 5d/wk x40 doses (8wk)[4]	4a INH/RIF[7] 7d/wk x217 doses (31wk) or 5d/wk x155 doses (31wk)[4]	(Continued from previous page.) 3. Short course (6mo) therapy, including 2x weekly DOT regimens in HIV+ pts clearly shown effective in U.S. & Africa *(AIDS 13:1899 & 1543, 1999).* However, because of **possibility of developing resistance to rifampin in pts with low CD4 cell counts who receive weekly or biweekly doses of rifabutin**, it is recommended that such pts receive daily (or at least 3x-weekly) doses of RFB for initiation & continuation phase rx of TBc *(MMWR 51:214, 2002; CID 41:83, 2005).* Low serum levels of RIF & ETB noted in HIV+ patients. Where practical, therapeutic monitoring may be useful *(CID 41:1638, 2005).*
				273–195 (39wk)	
				4b INH/RIF[7] 2x/wk x62 doses (31wk)	
				118–102 (39wk)	
INH (± SM) resistance	**RIF, PZA, ETB** (an **FQ** may strengthen the regimen for pts with extensive disease). Emergence of FQ resistance a concern *(Ln ID 3:432, 2003; AAC 49:3178, 2005).*	6	In Brit. Medical Research Council trials, 6mos regimens have yielded ≥95% success rates despite resistance to INH if 4 drugs were used in the initial phase & RIF + ETB or SM was used throughout *(ARRD 133:423, 1986).* Add'l studies suggested results were best if PZA also used throughout 6mos *(ARRD 136:1339, 1987).* FQs not employed in BMRC studies, but may strengthen regimen for pts with more extensive disease. INH should be stopped in cases of INH resistance [see *MMWR 52(RR-11):1, 2003* for add'l discussion].		NOTE: FQ resistance may be seen in pts previously treated with FQ *(CID 37:1448, 2003).* Moxifloxacin, levofloxacin have enhanced activity compared with ciprofloxacin against M. tuberculosis *(AAC 46:1022, 2002; AAC 47: 2442, 2003; JAC 53:441, 2004; AAC 48:780, 2004).* Linezolid has excellent in vitro activity, including MDR strains *(AAC 47:416, 2003).*
Resistance to INH & RIF (± SM)	**FQ, PZA, ETB, IA**, ± alternative agent[8]	18–24	In such cases, extended rx is needed to ↓ the risk of relapses. In cases with extensive disease, the use of an additional agent (alternative agents) may be prudent to ↓ the risk of failure & additional acquired drug resistance. Resectional therapy may be appropriate.		
Resistance to INH, RIF (± SM), & ETB or PZA	**FQ** (**ETB** or **PZA** if active), **IA**, & 2 alternative agents[8]	24	Use the first-line agents to which there is susceptibility. Add 2 or more alternative agents in case of extensive disease. Surgery should be considered. Survival ↑ in pts receiving active FQ & surgical intervention *(AJRCCM 169:1103, 2004).*		
Resistance to RIF	**INH, ETB, FQ**, supplemented with **PZA** for the first 2 mos. (an IA may be included for the first 2–3mos. for pts with extensive disease)	12–18	Daily & 3x/wk regimens of INH, PZA, & SM given for 9mos. were effective in a BMRC trial *(ARRD 115:727, 1977).* However, extended use of an IA may not be feasible. It is not known if ETB would be as effective as SM in these regimens. An all-oral regimen x12–18mos. should be effective. But for more extensive disease &/or to shorten duration (e.g., to 12mos.), an IA may be added in the initial 2mos. of rx.		

In order of preference. [2] When DOT is used, drugs may be given 5 days/wk & the necessary number of doses adjusted accordingly. Although there are no studies that compare 5 with 7 daily doses, extensive experience indicates this would be an effective practice. [3] Patients with cavitation on initial chest x-ray should receive a 7-month (31 wk; either 217 doses [daily] or 62 doses [2x/wk]) continuation phase. [4] 5-day a wk administration is always given by DOT. [5] Not recommended for HIV-infected pts with CD4 cell counts <100 cells/μL. [6] Options 1c & 2b should be used only in HIV-neg. pts who have neg. sputum smears at the time of completion of 2mos of rx & who do not have cavitation on initial chest x-ray. For pts started on this regimen & found to have a pos. culture from the 2-mo specimen, rx should be extended an extra 3 months. [7] Options 4a & 4b should be considered only when options1–3 cannot be given. [8] Alternative agents = ethionamide, cycloserine, p-aminosalicylic acid, clarithromycin, AM/CL, linezolid. [9] Modified from *MMWR 52(RR-11):1, 2003.* See also *IDCP 11:329, 2002.*

NOTE: All dosage recommendations are for adults (unless otherwise indicated) & assume normal renal function.

TABLE 12 (5)

BACTERIAL INFECTIONS (continued)

XDR-TB (as resistant to INH & RIF plus any FQ and at least one of 3 second-line drugs: capreomycin, kanamycin or amikacin)	See comments	18–24	Therapy requires administration of 4-6 drugs to which infecting organism is susceptible, including multiple second-line drugs (MMWR 56:250, 2007; CID 45:338, 2007). Increased mortality in HIV+ patients.

INITIAL & CONTINUATION THERAPY

INH 300 mg + **RFB** (see below for dose) + **PZA** 25 mg/kg + **ETB** 15 mg/kg q24h x2 mos.; then **INH** + **RFB** x4mos. (up to 7mos.)

Concomitant protease inhibitor (PI) therapy requires dose modification	PI Regimen	RFB Dose	PI Dose	ALT. REGIMEN
	Nelfinavir, indinavir or amprenavir	150 mg q24h or 300 mg intermittently	Nelfinavir 1250 mg q12h Indinavir—consider ↑ to 1000 mg q8h Amprenavir 1200 mg q12h	**INH + SM + PZA + ETB** x2mos.; then **INH + SM + PZA** 2–3x/wk for 7mos. May be prolonged to 12mos. in pts with delayed response. May be used with any PI regimen.
	Saquinavir	300 mg q24h or intermittently	No change	
	Ritonavir	150 mg 2x/wk	No change	
	Lopinavir/ritonavir	150 mg 2x/wk	No change	

COMMENTS

(Adapted from MMWR 49:185, 2000; AJRCCM 162:7, 2001) Rifamycins induce cytochrome CYP450 enzymes (RIF > rifapentine > RFB) & reduce serum levels of concomitantly administered PIs. Conversely, PIs (ritonavir > amprenavir > indinavir = nelfinavir > saquinavir) inhibit CYP450 & cause ↑ in serum levels of RIF & RFB. If dose of RFB is not reduced, toxicity ↑. RFB/PI combinations are therapeutically effective (CID 30:779, 2000). For detailed discussion of drug interactions in rx of TBc in HIV-infected pts, see CID 28:419, 1999. Based on new data, MMWR now recommends that RIF can be used for rx of active TB in pts on regimens containing efavirenz or ritonavir. **RIF should not be administered to pts on ritonavir + saquinavir because drug-induced hepatitis with marked transaminase elevations has been observed in healthy volunteers receiving this regimen** (www.fda.gov). RFB can also be used with efavirenz or ritonavir but dose should be ↑ to 450–600mg/day with efavirenz & ↓ to 150 2 or 3x/wk with ritonavir. (CID 41:1343, 2005) No dose modification of RFB with saquinavir (softgel) as single agent (MMWR 49: 185, 2000). RFB has no effect on nelfinavir levels at nelfinavir dose of 1250mg po q12h (Can JID 10:218, 1999).

NOTE: All dosage recommendations are for adults (unless otherwise indicated) & assume normal renal function.

TABLE 12 (6)

CAUSATIVE AGENT/DISEASE	MODIFYING CIRCUMSTANCES	SUGGESTED REGIMENS		COMMENTS
		PRIMARY	ALTERNATIVE	

BACTERIAL INFECTIONS (continued)

CAUSATIVE AGENT/DISEASE	MODIFYING CIRCUMSTANCES	PRIMARY	ALTERNATIVE	COMMENTS
Mycobacterium avium-intracellulare complex (MAC or MAI) (CID 42:1756, 2006; AJRCCM 175:367, 2007).	**Primary prophylaxis**—Pt's CD4 count <50–100/mm³ NOTE: Prophylaxis may be discontinued in pts with sustained ↑ in CD4 cells of ≥100/mm³ on ARV RX (AnIM 133:493, 2000; NEJM 342:1085, 2000)	**Azithro** 1200 mg po weekly OR **Clarithro** 500 mg po q12h	**RFB** 300 mg po q24h OR **Azithro** 1200 mg po weekly + **RIF** 300 mg po q24h	RFB reduces MAC infection rate by 55% (no survival benefit); clarithro by 68% (30% survival benefit); azithro by 59% (68% survival benefit) (CID 26:611, 1998). Azithro + RFB more effective than either alone but not as well tolerated (NEJM 335:392, 1996). Many drug-drug interactions, see Table 16B. RFB ↑ metabolism of ZDV with 32% ↓ in AUC. Clarithro ↑ blood levels of non-sedating antihistamines with attendant risk of arrhythmias. Drug-resistant MAI disease seen in 29–58% of pts in whom disease develops while taking clarithro prophylaxis & in 11% of those on azithro but has not been observed with RFB prophylaxis (J Inf 38:6, 1999). Clarithro resistance more likely to be seen in pts with extremely low CD4 counts at initiation (CID 27:807, 1998). Need to be sure no active M. tbc; RFB used for prophylaxis may promote selection of rifamycin-resistant M. tbc (NEJM 335:384 & 428, 1996).
	Treatment: Either presumptive dx or after positive culture of blood, bone marrow, or other usually sterile body fluids, e.g., liver. (CID 42:1756, 2006)	[**Clarithro** 500 mg* po q12h or **azithro** 600 mg po q24h] + **ETB** 15–25 mg/kg/day +/– **RFB** 300 mg po q24h * **Higher doses of clari (1000 mg q12h) may be associated with ↑ mortality** (CID 29:125, 1999)	**Clarithro** or **azithro** + **ETB** +/– **RFB** + one or more of: **CIP** 750 mg po q12h **Oflox** 400 mg po q12h **Amikacin** 7.5–15 mg/kg IV q24h In pts receiving protease inhibitors can use [clarithro 500 mg q12h (or azithro 600 mg q24h) – ETB 15–25 mg/kg/day] if the pt has not had previous prophylaxis with a neomacrolide (Johns Hopkins AIDS Report 9:2, 1997).	Median time to neg blood culture: clarithro + ETB 4.4wks vs azithro + ETB > 16wks. At 16wks, clearance of bacteremia seen in 37.5% of azithro- & 85.7% of clarithro-treated pts (CID 27:1278, 1998). More recent study suggests similar clearance rates for azithro (46%) vs clarithro (56%) at 24wks when combined with ETB (CID 31:1245, 2000). Azithro 250 mg q24h not effective but azithro 600 mg po q24h as effective as 1200 q24h & yields fewer adverse effects (AAC 43:2869, 1999). Addition of RFB to clarithro + ETB ↓ emergence of resistance to clari, ↓ relapse rate, & improves survival (CID 37:1234, 2003). Data on clofazimine suggests adding CLO is of no value (CID 25:621, 1997). More recent study suggests it may be as effective as RFB in 3 drug regimens containing clari & ETB (CID 29:125, 1999) although it may not be as effective as RFB at preventing clari resistance (CID 28:136, 1999). Thus, pending more data, we still do not recommend CLO for MAI in HIV+ pts. Drug toxicity: With clarithro, 23% pts had to stop drug 2° to dose-limiting adverse reaction (AnIM 121:905, 1994). Combo of clarithro, ETB & RFB led to uveitis & pseudojaundice (NEJM 330:438, 1994); result is reduction in max. dose of RFB to 300mg. Treatment failure rate is high. Reasons: drug toxicity, development of drug resistance, & inadequate serum levels. Serum levels of clarithro ↓ in pts also given RIF or RFB (JID 171:747, 1995). If pt not responding to initial regimen after 2–4wks, add 1 or more drugs. Several anecdotal reports of pts not responding to usual primary regimen who gained weight & became afebrile with dexamethasone 2–4mg/day po (AAC 38: 2215, 1994; CID 26:682, 1998).
	Chronic post-treatment suppression—secondary prophylaxis	**Always necessary.** [**Clarithro** or **azithro**] + **ETB** (lower dose to 15 mg/kg/day) (Dosage above)	**Clarithro** or **azithro** or **RFB** (dosage above)	Recurrences almost universal without chronic suppression. In pts with good response to ARV RX (robust CD4 ↑) it is possible to discontinue chronic suppression (JID 178:1446, 1998; NEJM 340:1301, 1999) (see Table 11B).

NOTE: All dosage recommendations are for adults (unless otherwise indicated) & assume normal renal function.

TABLE 12 (7)

CAUSATIVE AGENT/DISEASE	MODIFYING CIRCUMSTANCES	SUGGESTED REGIMENS		COMMENTS
		PRIMARY	ALTERNATIVE	
BACTERIAL INFECTIONS *(continued)*				
Mycobacterium celatum	Treatment; optimal regimen not defined	Easily confused with M. xenopi & MAC. May be susceptible to clarithro, FQ (*Clin Microbiol Inf 3:582, 1997*). Suggested treatment like MAI but may be resistant to RIF (*J Inf 38:157, 1999*). Most reported cases received 3 or 4 drugs—usually **clari** + **ETB** ± **CIP** ± **RFB** (*EID 9:399, 2003*).		Isolated from blood of patients with AIDS (*CID 24:140 & 144, 1997*). Usually resistant to INH, PZA, capreomycin (*JCM 33:137, 1995; CID 24:140, 1997*).
Mycobacterium chelonae, ssp. abscessus, chelonae	Treatment. Surgery is important adjunct to therapy (*CID 24:1147, 1997*).	**Clarithro** 500 mg po q12h x6mos. (*AnIM 119:482, 1993; CID 24:1147, 1997; EJCMID 19:43, 2000*). **Azithro** may also be effective. For serious, disseminated infections add **amikacin** + **IMP or cefoxitin** for first 2–6wks (*CMR 15:716, 2002; ARJCCM 175:367, 2007*).		M. abscessus susceptible in vitro to clarithro (95%), clofazimine, cefmetazole, amikacin (70%), cefoxitin (70%), IMP, azithro, cipro, doxycycline, minocycline, tigecycline (*CID42:1756, 2006*). Clarithro-resistant strains described (*JCM 39:2745, 2001*). M. chelonae susceptible in vitro to clarithro, tobramycin (100%), amikacin (80%), IMP (60%), moxifloxacin, ciprofloxacin, minocycline, doxycycline, linezolid (94%) (*AJRCCM 156:S1, 1997; AAC 46:3283, 2002; CID 42:1756, 2006*).
Mycobacterium fortuitum	Treatment	Optimal regimen not defined. **Amikacin** + **cefoxitin** + **probenecid** 2–6wks, then po TMP/SMX, or doxycycline 2–6mos (*J Inf Dis 152:50, 1985*). Surgical excision of infected areas. Nail salon-acquired skin infections in immunocompetent pts have responded to 4–6mos. of minocycline or doxycycline or CIP (*CID 38:38, 2004*).		Resistant to all standard anti-TBc drugs. Sensitive in vitro to cefoxitin, doxycycline, minocycline, imipenem, amikacin, TMP/SMX, CIP, oflox. May be resistant to RFB, azithro, variably susceptible to clarithro, linezolid (*JAC 39:567, 1997; CMR 15:716, 2007*). Usually responds to 6–12mos. of oral rx with 2 drugs to which it is susceptible (*AJRCCM 156:S1, 1997; AAC 46:3283, 2002; CMR 15:716, 2007*). For M. fortuitum pulmonary disease: treat with at least 2 agents active in vitro until sputum cultures negative for 12 mos (*ARJCCM 175:367, 2007*).
Mycobacterium genavense	Treatment	Regimens used include ≥2 drugs: **ETB**, **RIF**, **RFB**, **clofazimine**, **clarithro**. In animal model, clarithro & RFB (& to lesser extent amikacin & ETB) shown effective in reducing bacterial counts; CIP not effective (*JAC 42:483, 1998*).		Clinical: CD4 <50. Symptoms of fever, weight loss, diarrhea. Lab: growth in BACTEC vials slow (mean 42 days). Subcultures grow only on Middlebrook 7H11 agar containing 2 mcg/ml mycobactin J—growth still insufficient for in vitro sensitivity testing (*Lancet 340:76, 1992; AnIM 117:586, 1992*). Survival ↑ from 81 to 263 days in pts rx for at least 1 month with ≥2 drugs (*Arch Int Med 155:400, 1995*).
Mycobacterium gordonae	Treatment	Regimen(s) not defined, but consider **RIF** + **ETB** + **kanamycin** or **CIP** (*J Inf 38:157, 1999*) or **linezolid** (*ARJCCM 75:367, 2007*).		In vitro: sensitive to ETB, RIF, amikacin, CIP, clarithro, linezolid (*AAC 47:1736, 2003*). Resistant to INH (*CID 14:1229, 1992*). Surgical excision.
Mycobacterium haemophilum	Treatment	Regimen(s) not defined. In animal model, **clarithro** + **RFB** effective (*AAC 39:2316, 1995*). Combo of **CIP** + **RFB** + **clarithro** reported effective but clinical experience limited (*CMR 9:435, 1996*). Surgical debridement may be nec. (*CID 26:505, 1998*).		Clinical: Ulcerating skin lesions, synovitis, osteomyelitis, cervicofacial lymphadenitis in children (*CID 41:1569, 2005*). Lab: Requires supplemented media to isolate. Sensitive in vitro to: CIP, cycloserine, RFB. Over 50% resistant to: INH, RIF, ETB, PZA (*AnIM 120:118, 1994*).

NOTE: All dosage recommendations are for adults (unless otherwise indicated) & assume normal renal function.

TABLE 12 (8)

CAUSATIVE AGENT/DISEASE	MODIFYING CIRCUMSTANCES	SUGGESTED REGIMENS PRIMARY	SUGGESTED REGIMENS ALTERNATIVE	COMMENTS
BACTERIAL INFECTIONS (continued)				
Mycobacterium kansasii	Treatment	**RIF** (600 mg po q24h) + **ETB** (25 mg/kg/day × 2 mos, then 15 mg/kg/day) + **INH** (300 mg po q24h) for 15–18mos (AnIM 120:945, 1994)	If RIF-resistant, use **INH** 900 mg po q24h + **pyridoxine** 50 mg po q24h + **ETB** 25→15 mg/kg/day po + **sulfamethoxazole** 1 gm po q8h. Rx until culture negative x12–15mos. **Clari + ETB + RIF** also effective in small study (CID 37: 1178, 2003).	If organism resistant to (≥1mcg/ml) INH, discontinue (70–85% isolates resistant), **All isolates resistant to PZA**. Rifapentine, azithro, ETB effective alone or in combo in athymic mice (JAC 42:417, 2001). Highly effective either clarithro (500mg bid) or RFB (150mg/d) for RIF substitute either clarithro (500mg bid) or RFB (150mg/d) for RIF (AJRCCM 156:S1, 1997). Because of variable susceptibility to INH, some substitute clarithro 500–750mg q24h for INH. Resistance to clarithro reported (DMID 31:369, 1998), but most strains susceptible to clarithro as well as moxifloxacin (JAC 55:950, 2005) & levofloxacin (AAC 48:4562, 2004). Prog related to level of immunosuppression (CID 37:584, 2003).
Mycobacterium marinum	Treatment	(RIF + ETB) or doxycycline or minocycline or TMP/SMX or clarithro for at least 12wks (Arch Int Med 147:817, 1986; AJRCCM 156:S1, 1997; Eur J Clin Micro ID 25:609, 2006). Surgical excision.		Sensitive in vitro to clarithro, reported effective in 2 pts (1 HIV+) who failed on other regimens) (CID 18:664, 1994). Resistant to INH & PZA (AJRCCM 156:S1, 1997). Susceptible in vitro to linezolid. CIP, moxifloxacin also show moderate in vitro activity (AAC 46:1114, 2002).
Mycobacterium scrofulaceum	Treatment	Although regimens not defined, clarithro + clofazimine with or without ETB. Surgical excision.		In vitro resistant to INH, RIF, ETB, PZA, amikacin, CIP (CID 20:549, 1995).
Mycobacterium simiae	Treatment	Regimen(s) not defined. If true infection, start 4 drugs for disseminated MAI. Anecdotal reports of response in pts on ARV RX who received clarithro, ETB & CIP (J Inf 41:143, 2000).		Susceptible in vitro to RIF, strep, CLO, clarithro, CIP, oflox, amikacin, moxifloxacin, linezolid (AAC 42:2070, 1998; JAC 45:231, 2000: AAC 46:3193, 2002; AAC 50:1921, 2006). Monotherapy with RIF selects resistant mutants in mice (AAC 47:1228, 2003). RIF + Strep effective in small study (AAC 49:3182, 2005). Treatment generally disappointing—see review, Ln 354:1013, 1999. RIF + dapsone only slightly better (82% improved) than placebo (75%) in small study (IJID 6:60, 2002).
Mycobacterium ulcerans (Buruli ulcer)	Treatment	[**RIF + AMK** (7.5 mg/kg IM bid) or [**ETB + TMP/SMX** (160/800mg po tid)] for 4–6wks. Surgical excision most important. WHO recommends RIF + SM for 8 weeks but overall, value of drug therapy not clear (Ln ID 6:288, 2006; Lancet 367:1849, 2006; AAC 51:645, 2007).		
Mycobacterium xenopi	Treatment (NOTE: Recent study suggests no need to treat in most pts with HIV) (CID 37:1250, 2003)	Regimen(s) not defined (CID 24:226 & 233, 1997). INH + RIF + ETB suggested but no clinical trials available (Clin Chest Med 17:697, 1996). Nct always susceptible to these agents in vitro (CID 25:206, 1997). Macrolide + (RIF or RFB) + ETB ± SM also recommended (AJRCCM 156:S1, 1997) or RIF + INH ± ETB (Resp Med 97:439, 2003), but recent study suggests no need to treat in most pts with HIV (CID 37:1250, 2003).		In vitro: sensitive to clarithro (ACC 36:2841, 1992) & RFB (JAC 39:567, 1997) & many standard antimycobacterial drugs. Clarithro-containing regimens more effective than RIF/INH/ETB in mice (AAC 45:3229, 2001). FQs, linezolid also active.
Mycobacterium leprae (leprosy) Classification: CID 44:1096, 2007	**Therapy of HIV may "uncover"** underlying leprosy in previously infected patients. **Frequency of this phenomenon not presently known.** There are 2 sets of therapeutic recommendations here: one from USA (National Hansen's Disease Programs [NHDP], Baton Rouge, LA) and one from WHO. Both are based on expert recommendations and neither has been subjected to controlled clinical trial (M. P. Joyce & D. Scollard, Conns Current Therapy 2004; MP Joyce, Immigration Medicine, in press 2006; J Am Acad Dermatol 51:417, 2004).			

NOTE: All dosage recommendations are for adults (unless otherwise indicated) & assume normal renal function.

TABLE 12 (9)

CAUSATIVE AGENT/DISEASE	MODIFYING CIRCUMSTANCES	SUGGESTED REGIMENS		COMMENTS
		PRIMARY	ALTERNATIVE	

BACTERIAL INFECTIONS (continued)

Type of Disease		NHDP Regimen	WHO Regimen	Comments
Paucibacillary Forms: (Intermediate, Tuberculoid, Borderline tuberculoid)		(**Dapsone** 100 mg/day (unsupervised) + **RIF** 600 mg po/day) for 12 months	(**Dapsone** 100 mg/day (unsupervised)) + **RIF** 600 mg 1x/mo (supervised)) for 6 mo	Side effects overall 0.4%. In patients receiving protease inhibitors, authors suggest substituting RFB for RIF, but no clinical data exist to backup this recommendation.
Single lesion paucibacillary		Treat as paucibacillary leprosy for 12 months.	Single dose **ROM** therapy: (**RIF** 600 mg + **Oflox** 400 mg + **Mino** 100 mg) (Ln 353:655, 1999).	
Multibacillary forms: Borderline Borderline-lepromatous Lepromatous See Comment for erythema nodosum leprosum Rev.: Lancet 363:1209, 2004		(**Dapsone** 100 mg/day + **CLO** 50 mg/day + **RIF** 600 mg/day) for 24mo **Alternative regimen:** (**Dapsone** 100 mg/day + **RIF** 600 mg/day + **Minocycline** 100 mg/day) for 24 mo if CLO is refused or unavailable.	(**Dapsone** 100 mg/day + **CLO** 50 mg/day (both unsupervised) + **RIF** 600 mg + **CLO** 300 mg once monthly (supervised)). Continue regimen for 12 months.	Side-effects overall 5.1%. For erythema nodosum leprosum: prednisone 60–80mg/day or thalidomide 100-400 mg/day (BMJ 44:775, 1988; AJM 108:487, 2000). Thalidomide available in US at 1-800-4-CELGENE. Altho thalidomide effective, WHO no longer rec because of potential toxicity (JID 193:1743, 2006) however the majority of leprosy experts feel thalidomide remains drug of choice for ENL under strict supervision. CLO (Clofazimine) available from NHDP under IND protocol; contact at 1-800-642-2477. **Ethionamide** (250mg q24h) or **prothionamide** (375mg q24h) may be subbed for CLO. Oflox 400mg po q24h, bactericidal and effective clinically with 4 log ↓ in organisms in small trials (AAC 38:662, 1994; AAC 38:61, 1994). Clarithro also rapidly bactericidal (AAC 38:515, 1994; Ln 345:4, 1995). Regimens incorporating clarithro, minocycline, RIF, moxifloxacin, and/or oflox also show promise (AAC 44:2919, 2000; AAC 50:1558, 2006). High relapse rate in pts treated with q24h RIF + oflox for 4wk (AAC 41:1953, 1997). Resistance to dapsone, RIF & oflox reported (Ln 349:103, 1997). Dapsone monotherapy has been abandoned due to emergence of resistance, but older patients previously treated with dapsone monotherapy may remain on lifelong maintenance therapy. Dapsone (or acedapsone[NUS]) effective for prophylaxis in one study (J Inf 41:137, 2000).
Neisseria gonorrhoeae (gonococcus) Ref.: MMWR 55(RR-11), 2006	Gonorrhea; urethritis, conjunctivitis, proctitis; mucopurulent cervicitis; epididymoorchitis (sexually acquired); for disseminated disease, see Sanford Guide to Antimicrobial Therapy	[(**Ceftriaxone** 125 mg IM x1) or (cefpodoxime 400 mg po x1)] **PLUS—if Chlamydia infection not ruled out:** [(**Azithro** 1 gm po x1) or (**doxy** 100 mg po x2/day x7d)] **Evaluate & rx sex partner.** **Note:** Due to increasing resistance, **fluoroquinolones** no longer recommended (MMWR 56:332, 2007).		**Treat for both GC & C. trachomatis.** Other alternatives for **GC**: Spectinomycin 2gm IM x1 Other single-dose cephalosporins: ceftizoxime 500mg IM, cefotaxime 500mg IM, cefotetan 1gm IM, (cefoxitin 2gm IM + probenecid 1gm po). Azithro 1gm po x1 effective for chlamydia but need 2gm po x1 for GC; not recommended for GC due to GI side-effects & expense.
Pelvic inflammatory disease (PID), salpingitis, tuboovarian abscess. Etiology polymicrobic: gonococcus, C. trachomatis, bacteroides, enterobacteriacae, streptococci, mycoplasma. Ref.: MMWR 55(RR-11), 2006	Outpatient (limit to pts with temp <38°C, WBC <11,000/mm³, minimal evidence of peritonitis, active bowel sounds & able to tolerate oral nourishment	**Outpatient rx:** (**ceftriaxone** 250 mg IM x1 + **doxy** 100 mg po q12h ± **metro** 500 mg po q12h) OR (**cefoxitin** 2 gm IM with **probenecid** 1 gm po—both as single dose) + (**doxy** 100 mg po bid with **metro** 500 mg po bid). Treat for 14 days.	**Inpatient regimens:** [(**Cefotetan** 2 gm IV q12h or **cefoxitin** 2 gm IV q6h) + **doxy** 100 mg IV/po q12h)] (**Clinda** 900 mg IV q8h) + (**gentamicin** 2 mg/kg loading dose, then 1.5 mg/kg q8h or single daily dosing), then **doxy** 100 mg po q12h x14d	Alternative parenteral regimen: **AM/SB** 3 gm IV q6h + **doxy** 100mg IV/po q12h **FQs** not recommended due to increasing resistance (MMWR 56:332, 2007). **Remember: Evaluate & treat sex partner.**

NOTE: All dosage recommendations are for adults (unless otherwise indicated) & assume normal renal function.

TABLE 12 (10)

CAUSATIVE AGENT/DISEASE	MODIFYING CIRCUMSTANCES	SUGGESTED REGIMENS PRIMARY	SUGGESTED REGIMENS ALTERNATIVE	COMMENTS
BACTERIAL INFECTIONS (continued)				
Prostatitis—Review: *AJM* 106:327, 1999				
Acute ≤35 years of age	N. gonorrhoeae C. trachomatis	(**ceftriaxone** 250 mg IM x1, then **doxy** 100 mg po q12h x10d)		In AIDS pts, prostate may be focus of Cryptococcus neoformans. **FQs** no longer recommended for gonococcal infections
>35 years of age	Enterobacteriaceae (coliforms)	**FQ: CIP-ER** 500 mg po 1x/day or **CIP** 400 mg IV bid or **levo** 750 mg IV/po 1x/day x 3-4 wks or **TMP/SMX** 1 DS tablet 160 mg TMP) po q12h x10-14d	**TMP/SMX-DS** po bid x 3-4 wks.	Treat as acute urinary infection, 14d (not single dose regimen). Some authorities recommend 3-4 wk therapy. If uncertain, do urine NAAT for C. trachomatis & N. gonorrhoeae.
Chronic bacterial	Enterobacteriaceae (80%), enterococci (15%), P. aeruginosa	**FQ (CIP** 500 mg po q12h x4wks, OR **levo** 750 mg po q24h x4wks)—see Comment	**TMP/SMX-DS** 1 tab po q12h x1-3mos.	With rx failures, consider infected prostatic calculi. FDA-approved dose of levo is 500 mg; editors prefer higher 750 mg dose.
Chronic prostatitis/chronic pain syndrome (New NIH classification, *JAMA* 282: 236, 1999)	The most common prostatitis syndrome, etiology is unknown; molecular probe data suggest infectious etiology (*Clin Micro Rev* 11:604, 1998)	α-adrenergic blocking agents are controversial (*AnIM* 133:367, 2000)		Definition of chronic prostatitis: pt. has sx of prostatitis, cells in prostatic secretions, but routine cultures negative. Chlamydia, ureaplasma suspected Definition of chronic pain: pt. has sx of prostatitis but negative cultures & no cells in prostatic secretions. Review: *JAC* 46:157, 2000. In randomized double-blind study, CIP and alpha blocker were of no benefit (*AnIM* 141:581 & 639, 2004).
Rhodococcus equi (Corynebacterium equi)	Pulmonary infection	[**Erythro** (0.5 gm IV q6h) or **IMP** (0.5 gm IV q6h)] + **RIF** 600 mg po q24h for at least 2wks	**CIP** 750 mg po q12h ≥2wks. CIP-resistant strains SE Asia (*CID* 27:370, 1998)	¾ pts have positive blood cultures. Prolonged oral suppressive therapy (macrolide + RIF) indicated since relapses are frequent. Vancomycin active in vitro & rx success in pt who relapsed after erythro + RIF (*IDCP* 7:480, 1998). Linezolid active in vitro.
Salmonella sp., bacteremia Fever in 71-91% Bloody stool 34%	**Bacteremia, AIDS patient** For typhoid fever, see Sanford Guide to Antimicrobial Therapy	1st episode: **CIP** 400 mg IV bid until afebrile, then 500-700 mg po bid to total of 5-6 wks	Pt who relapses: Assuming in vitro susceptibility, long term suppression with **CIP** 500 mg po bid or **TMP/SMX-DS** tab po bid	Primary therapy: fluid & electrolyte replacement.
Shigellosis Fever in 58% Bloody stool 51%	Treatment Acute	**CIP** 500 mg po q12h x3d or **LEVO** 500 mg po q24h x3d	(**TMP/SMX-DS** q12h po x3d) or (**azithro** 500 mg po x1, then 250 mg/day x4d)	In immunocompromised children & adults, treat for 7-10 days.
	Recurrent in AIDS pts	**CIP** 500 mg po q12h (perhaps 750 mg po q24h) indefinitely		

NOTE: All dosage recommendations are for adults (unless otherwise indicated) & assume normal renal function.

TABLE 12 (11)

CAUSATIVE AGENT/DISEASE	MODIFYING CIRCUMSTANCES	SUGGESTED REGIMENS		COMMENTS
		PRIMARY	ALTERNATIVE	
BACTERIAL INFECTIONS (continued)				
Staphylococcus aureus: methicillin/oxacillin susceptible (MSSA) Culture furuncles if possible	Treatment: Folliculitis/ furunculosis/ subcutaneous abscess in "skin poppers"	**Dicloxacillin** 500 mg po q6h for 7–14d. If refractory/ recurrent, add **RIF** 600 mg po q24h or 300 mg po q12h **Need hot packs and I&D**	**Mupirocin** (Bactroban), apply to affected area q8h for 5d (if infection not disseminated)	**Hot packs & drainage are equal in effectiveness to antimicrobic therapy.**
	Bacteremia &/or endocarditis	PRSP [(**nafcillin** or **oxacillin** 2 gm IV q4h **x4wks**) + **gentamicin** 1 mg/kg q8h IV or IM **x3–5d**]	(**Cefazolin** 2 gm IV q8h x4–6wks) + (gentamicin 1 mg/kg IV q8h x3–5d)	In IV drug users with right-sided endocarditis, 2wks rx with nafcillin/gentamicin is usually adequate (AnIM 109:619, 1988).
	Suppression: Recurrent infections (most likely pt is a nasal carrier)	**Mupirocin** (Bactroban), apply to nasal vestibule q8h x5d	(**Dicloxacillin** 500 mg po q6h) + (**RIF** 600 mg po q24h or 300 mg po q12h) x10d	Culture nasal vestibule to determine if nasal carrier. Mupirocin effective vs both MSSA & MRSA.
Staphylococcus aureus: Methicillin resistant (MRSA) (see Sanford Guide to Antimicrobial Therapy for details)				
Possible community-acquired MRSA	Furuncles (boils) and carbuncles EMPIRIC THERAPY	If CA-MRSA: Hot packs, **incision & drainage** (with culture and sensitivities if possible) most important part of therapy		If abscess (furuncle <5 cm diameter, I&D alone may suffice; if >5 cm, benefit from antimicrobic)(PIDJ 23:123, 2004). NOTE: rarely concomitant S. pyogenes. **TMP/SMX** not active vs. S. pyogenes. Add **RIF** or Pen **V-K**
		TMP/SMX-DS 1-2 tabs po q12h ± **RIF** 300 mg po q12h x7–14d. **Don not use RIF monotherapy.**	**Doxy** or **minocycline** 100 mg po bid x 7-14d.	
Could be MSSA or MRSA; (usually MRSA)	Ventilator (hospital)-associated pneumonia. Document with quantitative cultures of lower airway.	EMPIRIC THERAPY: **Vanco** 1gm IV q12h; if vanco allergic or intolerant, **linezolid** 600 mg IV/po q12h	SPECIFIC THERAPY for: 1) MSSA: **nafcillin** or **oxacillin** 2 gm IV q4h. **Vanco** if pen allergic or vanco intolerant. 2) MRSA: vanco 1 gm IV q12h or linezolid 600 mg IV/po q12h.	Retrospective study found linezolid superior to vanco (Chest 124:1789, 2003); prospective study in progress. Check CBC at least once weekly while taking linezolid.
Could be MSSA or MRSA (usually MRSA)	Bacteremia and possible endocarditis	EMPIRIC THERAPY: **vanco** 1 gm IV q12h (see comment). Do not combine vanco with nafcillin or oxacillin.	SPECIFIC THERAPY: 1) MSSA: **nafcillin** or **oxacillin** 2 gm IV q4h. **Vanco** if pen allergic or vanco intolerant. 2) MRSA: a) **vanco** l gm IV q12h or b) if no left-sided endocarditis, **dapto** 6 mg/kg IV q24H	EMPIRIC ALTERNATIVE THERAPY PROBLEMS: 1) **Daptomycin** not approved for left-sided endocarditis. 2) **TMP/SMX** not as efficacious as vanco in bacteremic patient. 3) Do not use **clinda** until lab checks for inducible resistance.

NOTE: All dosage recommendations are for adults (unless otherwise indicated) & assume normal renal function.

TABLE 12 (12)

CAUSATIVE AGENT/DISEASE	MODIFYING CIRCUMSTANCES	SUGGESTED REGIMENS PRIMARY	SUGGESTED REGIMENS ALTERNATIVE	COMMENTS
BACTERIAL INFECTIONS/Staphylococcus aureus: Methicillin resistant (MRSA) *(continued)*				
MSSA or MRSA	Attempt to DECOLONIZE DUE TO REPEATED INFECTION or need for PROSTHETIC JOINT SURGERY	1) Culture nose and/or perineum/groin to establish S. aureus colonization or carriage. 2) Daily 2% chlorhexidine showers x 7d. 3) Mupirocin ointment 2% to anterior nares (if nares culture-positive), 3 times per day x 7d. 4) (**Doxy** 100 mg po bid or **TMP/SMX-DS** 1-2 tab po bid + **RIF** 300 mg po bid x 7d.		In randomized trial, indicated regimen reduced MRSA carriage from 74% to 32% for 3 months (*CID 44:178, 2007*). For problems & limitations see *CID 44:186, 2007*: e.g., resistance of MRSA to mupirocin as high as 24%. Could use a 0.12% chlorhexidine gel in place of mupirocin for nasal application (prevented surgical infections in the Netherlands, but not available in the U.S. *JAMA 296:2460, 2006*).
Streptococcus pneumoniae				
Pneumonia—culture & in vitro susceptibility results available	Susceptible or inter-mediate resistance to pen G in vitro	**Ceftriaxone** 1 gm IV q24h OR **Penicillin G:** 2 million units IV q4h OR **Amox** 1 gm po tid OR **Ampicillin:** 2 gm IV q6h	**Erythro** 500 mg IV q6h OR **Azithro** 500 mg IV/day OR **Clindamycin** 600 mg IV q8h	The prevalence of high-level pen G-resistant S. pneumo varies by region; average is 18%. **Resistant strains** are often cross-resistant to erythro, azithro (80%), clarithro (22%). U.S. isolates may or may not be clindamycin-susceptible. β-lactam/β-lactamase inhibitor combinations are not effective, as mechanism of resistance is target change, not β-lactamase production.
	High-level resistance to pen G in vitro	**Levo** 750 mg IV q24h or **moxi** 400 mg IV q24h	**Vancomycin** 1 gm IV q12h OR *if oral therapy:* **Telithro** 800 mg po q24h or **Gemi** 320 mg po q24h	
Meningitis—culture & in vitro susceptibility results available Ref. on steroid use: *NEJM 347:1549 & 1613, 2002* General ref: *CID 39:1267, 2004 & LnID 4:139, 2004.*	Susceptible to pen G in vitro	(**Aq. pen G** 4 million units IV q4h OR **ceftriaxone** 2 gm IV q12h OR **ampicillin** 2 gm IV q4h) + **dexamethasone**—See *Comment*	For severe penicillin allergy (IgE-mediated anaphylaxis, angioneurotic edema): **Vanco** 500-750 mg IV q6h.	**Adjunctive dexamethasone, 1st dose 15-20min. prior to, or concomitant with, 1st dose of antibiotic.** Dose: 0.4 mg/kg IV q12h x2d. (1) In children, steroids do **not** reduce CSF penetration of vanco. (2) In adults, unclear if steroids ↓ vanco CSF penetration. If steroids used, add RIF 600 mg/day IV or po. **Vanco dosage:** Due to low/erratic CSF penetration, recommended dosage in children of 15 mg/kg q6h is double usual dose; in adults a max. dose of 2-3 gm of vanco/day suggested, i.e., 500-700 mg IV q6h.
	Intermediate or high-level resistance to pen G in vitro	(**Vancomycin** 500-750 mg IV q6 (see *Comment*) + **ceftriaxone** 2 gm IV q12h) + **dexamethasone** —See *Comment*	**Meropenem** may work—2 gm IV q8h. Severe penicillin allergy: **Vanco** 500-750 mg IV q6h + **RIF** 600 mg po/IV q24h	

NOTE: All dosage recommendations are for adults (unless otherwise indicated) & assume normal renal function.

TABLE 12 (13)

CAUSATIVE AGENT/DISEASE	MODIFYING CIRCUMSTANCES	SUGGESTED REGIMENS		COMMENTS
		PRIMARY	ALTERNATIVE	
BACTERIAL INFECTIONS *(continued)*				
Syphilis (Treponema pallidum) Recommendations are for pts with normal CD4 T-lymphocyte counts. In AIDS pts, clinical course may be atypical. Higher doses/longer periods of rx may be required— *MMWR 55 (RR-11), 2006.*	Primary (chancre), secondary (rash, mucositis, lymphadenopathy), & early latent (<1 year)	**Benzathine penicillin G (Bicillin L-A)** 2.4 mUnits IM x1. Dose for children: 50,000 units/kg IM up to max. of 2.4 mUnits	**Doxycycline** 100 mg po q12h x14 d **or Tetracycline** 500 mg po q6h x14 d **or Ceftriaxone** 1 gm IM/IV q24h x8–10d For failures of initial rx, re-treat with benzathine penicillin G 2.4 mUnits IM weekly x3.	For all stages, penicillin best drug. If penicillin allergy, skin test if available or desensitize & treat with penicillin. Erythro not acceptable alternative agent.; use doxycycline if unable to desensitize. Limited data on efficacy of alternative regimens. Need baseline titered VDRL (RPR) & repeat titered serology at 3, 6, 12, 24mos. Repeat rx if (1) persistent clinical signs, (2) titer of VDRL increases 4-fold or fails to decrease 4-fold after 3–6mos. Even with recommended rx, serologic relapse frequent. Some recommend CSF exam of all HIV+ pts regardless of stage of syphilis. Definite indication for CSF exam if late latent syphilis and serum RPR ≥1:32.
Azithro resistance in California, Ireland, & elsewhere *(CID 44:S130, 2007)*	Late latent: >1 year duration & neg. CSF exam	**Benzathine penicillin G (Bicillin L-A)** 2.4 mUnits IM q wkly x3wks	**Doxycycline** 100 mg po q12h x28d **or Tetracycline** 500 mg po q6h x28d	**L.P. on all HIV-infected patients with late syphilis and serum RPR ≥ 1:32**
	Neurosyphilis or optic neuritis	**Pen G** 3–4 mUnits q4h IV x10–14d	(**Procaine pen G** 2.4 mUnits IM q24h + **probenecid** 0.5gm po q6h) both x10–14d—See *Comment*	**Ceftriaxone** 2 gm q24h (IV or IM) x14d. 23% failure rate reported (*AJM 93:481, 1992*). For penicillin allergy: either desensitize to penicillin or obtain infectious diseases consultation. **Serologic criteria for response to rx: 4-fold or greater ↓ in VDRL titer over 6–12mos.** [*CID 28(Suppl.1):S21, 1999*].

NOTE: All dosage recommendations are for adults (unless otherwise indicated) & assume normal renal function.

TABLE 12 (14)
FIGURE 3 - ACTIVITY OF SELECTED ANTIFUNGAL DRUGS AGAINST PATHOGENIC FUNGI

Microorganism	Antifungal[1-4]				
	Fluconazole[5]	Voriconazole	Posaconazole	Echinocandin	Polyenes (Amphotericin)
Candida albicans	+++	+++	+++	+++	+++
Candida dubliniensis	+++	+++	+++	+++	+++
Candida glabrata	±	+	+	+++	++
Candida tropicalis	+++	+++	+++	+++	+++
Candida parapsilosis[6]	+++	+++	+++	++ (higher MIC)	+++
Candida krusei	-	++	++	+++	++
Candida guilliermondii	+++	+++	+++	++ (higher MIC)	++
Candida lusitaniae	+	+++	++	++	+
Cryptococcus neoformans	+++	+++	+++	-	+++
Aspergillus fumigatus[7]	-	+++	+++	++	++
Aspergillus flavus[7]	-	+++	+++	++	++ (higher MIC)
Aspergillus terreus	-	++	++	++	-
Fusarium sp.	-	++	++	-	++ (lipid formulations)
Scedosporium apiospermum (*Pseudoallescheria boydii*)	-	+++	+++	±	±
Scedosporium prolificans[8]	-	±	±	-	±
Trichosporon spp.	±	++	++	-	+
Zygomycetes (e.g., *Absidia, Mucor, Rhizopus*)	-	-	+++	-	+++ (lipid formulations)
Dematiaceous molds[9] (e.g., *Alternaria, Bipolaris, Curvularia, Exophiala*)	±	+++	+++	+	+
Dimorphic Fungi[10]					
Blastomyces dermatitidis	++	++	++	-	+++
Coccidioides immitis/posadasii	+++	+++	+++	-	+++
Histoplasma capsulatum	+	+++	+++	-	+++
Sporothrix schenckii	+	++	++	-	+++

- = no activity; ± = possibly activity; + = active, 3rd line therapy (least active clinically)
++ = Active, 2nd line therapy (less active clinically); +++ = Active, 1st line therapy (usually active clinically)

1. Minimum inhibitory concentration values do not always predict clinical outcome.
2. Echinocandins, voriconazole, posaconazole and polyenes have poor urine penetration.
3. During severe immune suppression, success requires immune reconstitution.
4. Flucytosine has activity against *Candida sp.*, *Cryptococcus sp.*, and dematiaceous molds, but is primarily used in combination therapy.
5. For candidal infections patients with prior triazole therapy have higher likelihood of triazole resistance.
6. Successful treatment of infections from *Candida parapsilosis* requires removal of foreign body or intravascular device.
7. Lipid formulations of amphotericin may have greater activity against *A. fumigatus* and *A. flavus* (+++).
8. *Scedosporium prolificans* is poorly susceptible to single agents and may require combination therapy (e.g., addition of terbinafine).
9. Infections from zygomycetes, some *Aspergillus* spp., and dematiaceous molds often require surgical debridement.
10. For infections (other than cocci meningitis) caused by dimorphic fungi; itraconazole is first-line therapy and active clinically (+++).

NOTE: All dosage recommendations are for adults (unless otherwise indicated) & assume normal renal function.

TABLE 12 (15)

TYPE OF INFECTION/ORGANISM/ SITE OF INFECTION	SUGGESTED REGIMENS		COMMENTS
	PRIMARY	ALTERNATIVE	

FUNGAL INFECTIONS

Aspergillosis

Invasive, pulmonary (IPA) or extrapulmonary: (See *Am J Respir Crit Care Med* 173:707, 2006) Post-chemotherapy in neutropenic pts (PMN <500 per mm³) but may also present with neutrophil recovery.
In one study from India 5/60 patients with AIDS-related mycoses had evidence of invasive aspergillosis, one of whom had IPA (*Journal of Medical Microbiology* 56:1101, 2007).
Typical x-ray/CT lung lesions (halo sign, cavitation, or macronodlues (*CID 44:373, 2007*). Initiation of antifungal Rx based on halo signs on CT associated with better response to Rx & improved.
An immunologic test that detects circulating galactomannan is available for dx of invasive aspergillosis. Galactomannan detection in the blood relatively insensitive; one study suggests improved sensitivity when performed on BAL fluid. (*Am J Respir Crit Care Med* 177:27, 2008).

Primary therapy (See *CID 46:327, 2008*):

Voriconazole 6 mg/kg IV q12h on day 1; then either (4 mg/kg/day IV q12h) or (200 mg po q12h for body weight ≥40kg, but 100 mg po q12h for body weight <40 kg)

Alternative therapies:

Liposomal ampho B (L-AmB) 3-5 kg/kg/day IV

Or

Ampho B lipid complex (ABLC) 5 mg/kg/d IV

Or

Caspofungin 70 mg/day then 50 mg/day thereafter

Or

Micafungin ^NFDA-I 100-150 mg/day

Or

Posaconazole ^NFDA-I 200 mg qid, then 400 mg bid after stabilization of disease

Or

Itraconazole tablets 600 mg/day for 3 days, then 400 mg/day.

Voriconazole more effective than ampho B. Vori, both a substrate and an inhibitor of CYP2C19, CYP2C9, and CYP3A4, has potential for deleterious drug interactions (e.g., with protease inhibitors) and careful review of concomitant medications is mandatory.
Ampho B: not recommended except as a lipid formulation, either L-AMB or ABLC. 10 mg/kg and 3 mg/kg doses of L-AMB are equally efficacious with greater toxicity of higher dose (*CID 2007; 44:1289–97*). One comparative trial found much greater toxicity with ABLC than with L-AMB: 34.6% vs 9.4% adverse events and 21.2% vs 2.8% nephrotoxicity (*Cancer. 2008 Jan 25; Epub ahead of print*). Vori preferred as primary therapy.
Caspo: ~50% response rate in IPA. Licensed for salvage therapy. Efavirenz, nelfinavir, nevirapine, phenytoin, rifampin, dexamethasone, and carbamazepine, may reduce caspofungin concentrations.
Micafungin: Favorable responses to micafungin as a single agent in 6/12 patients in primary therapy group and 9/22 in the salvage therapy group of an open-label, non-comparative trial (*J Infect* 53: 337, 2006). Outcomes no better with combination therapy. No significant drug interactions identified for micafungin.
Posaconazole: In a prospective controlled trial of IPA immunocompromised pts refractory or intolerant to other agents, 42% of 107 pts receiving posa vs 26% controls (p.006) were successful (*CID 44:2, 2007*). Posa inhibits CYP3A with potential for drug-drug interactions. Do not use for treatment of azole-non-responders as there is a potential for cross-resistance.
Itraconazole: Licensed for treatment of invasive aspergillosis in patients refractory to or intolerant of standard antifungal therapy. Itraconazole formulated as capsules, oral solution in hydroxypropyl-beta-cyclodextrin (HPCD), and parenteral solution with HPCD as a solubilizer; oral solution and parenteral formulation not licensed for treatment of invasive aspergillosis. 2.5 mg/kg oral solution provides dose equivalent to 400 mg capsules. Parenteral HPCD formulation dosage is 200 mg every 12h IV for 2 days, followed by 200 mg daily thereafter. Oral absorption of capsules enhanced by low gastric pH, erratic in fasting state and with hypochlorhydria; measurements of plasma concentrations recommended during oral therapy of invasive aspergillosis. Itraconazole is a substrate of CYP3A4 and non-competitive inhibitor of CYP3A4 with potential for significant drug-drug interactions. Do not use for azole-non-responders.
Combo therapy: Uncertain role and not routinely recommended for primary therapy; consider for treatment of refractory disease, although benefit unproven. A typical combo regimen would be an echinocandin in combination with either an azole or a lipid formulation of ampho B.

TABLE 12 (16)

TYPE OF INFECTION/ORGANISM/ SITE OF INFECTION	SUGGESTED REGIMENS		COMMENTS
	PRIMARY	ALTERNATIVE	

FUNGAL INFECTIONS (continued)

TYPE OF INFECTION/ORGANISM/ SITE OF INFECTION	PRIMARY	ALTERNATIVE	COMMENTS
Blastomycosis	**Ampho B** 0.7–1 mg/kg IV until evidence of response, then **itraconazole** 200 mg po q24h if pt not critically ill or does not have CNS involvement	Limited data with lipid preparations of ampho B & fluconazole in HIV+ pts.	Ampho B cumulative dose >1 gm results in cure without relapse in 70–91% of pts. In HIV– pt, itraconazole is drug of choice. In HIV+ pts, because of potential for drug-drug interactions, fluconazole 400-800 mg/day may be used instead of itraconazole.

Candidiasis: Oral, esophageal & vaginal candidiasis is a major manifestation of advanced HIV & represents one of the most common AIDS-defining diagnoses. Candida is also a common cause of nosocomial bloodstream infection. A decrease in C. albicans & increase in non-albicans species show ↓ susceptibility among candida species to antifungal agents (esp. fluconazole). These changes have predominantly affected immunocompromised pts in environments where antifungal prophylaxis (esp. fluconazole) is widely used. In vitro susceptibility testing for antifungal drugs to date has not undergone rigorous in vivo validation studies, & clinical outcomes are often more dependent on host factors. Yet it seems prudent to use susceptibility profiles to help select empiric antifungal therapy. See Figure 3.

TYPE OF INFECTION/ORGANISM/ SITE OF INFECTION	PRIMARY	ALTERNATIVE	COMMENTS
Bloodstream: clinically stable with or without venous catheter & C. glabrata or C. krusei unlikely (no flu with in 30 days) (CID 42:249,2006). • **All positive blood cultures require therapy!** • **Remove & replace venous catheter** ("not over a wire") (J Clin Micro 43:1829, 2005), esp. in non-neutropenic: mortality 21% vs 4% if catheter not removed. Treat for 2wk after last pos. blood culture & resolution of signs & symptoms of infection.	**Fluconazole** ≥6 mg/kg per day or 400 mg q24h IV or po times 7 days then po for 14 days after last + blood culture	Echinocandin (see **caspo, anidula, mica** below)	Fluconazole still preferred here because of impressive efficacy in randomized studies, favorable safety profile and very low cost (CID 42:249, 2006, JAC 57:384,2006). In centers with relatively higher rates of non-albicans candida species, an echinocandin may be preferred empirical therapy. A double-blind randomized trial comparing anidulafungin to fluconazole for invasive candidiasis showed an 88% response rate in patients (n=135) treated with anidulafungin vs a 76% response rate (n=130) treated with fluconazole (p=0.02) (NEJM 356:2472, 2007). Fluconazole not recommended for treatment of documented C. glabrata or C. krusei: use an echinocandin or voriconazole or posaconazole (note: echinocandins have better in vitro activity than either vori or posa against C. glabrata).
Bloodstream: unstable • Failing to respond to flu or deteriorating (Critical to remove intravenous catheter) • Hemodynamic instability (sepsis) • C. glabrata or C. krusei likely (immunosuppressed/flu prophylaxis) • Neutropenia (controversial) Observational studies suggest flu& ampho B are similarly effective in neutropenic pts **Mortality rates inc with delay in initiation of therapy:** 15% day 0, 24% day 1, 37% day 2 & 41% >day 4-p<.0009 (CID 43:25, 2006).	**Caspofungin** 70 mg IV on day 1 followed by 50 mg IV q24h (reduce to 35 mg IV q24h with moderate hepatic insufficiency). **OR** **Micafungin**^{NFDA-I} 100 mg IV q24h **OR** **Anidulafungin** 200 mg IV times 1, then 100 mg q24h (no dosage adjustments for renal or hepatic insufficiency)	**Ampho B** 0.7 mg/kg IV q24h, (>0.7mg/kg/d IV for C. glabrata, 1 mg/kg/d for C. krusei) **OR** **Lipid-based Amphotericin** 3-5 mg/k/d **OR** **Voriconazole:** 6 mg per kg IV q12h times 2 doses, then maintenance doses of 3 mg per kg IV q12h or 200 mg po q12h, after at least 3 days of IV therapy	**Echinocandins** have efficacy similar to and perhaps better than ampho B, but are less toxic: response rates of ~70% for candins vs ~60% for ampho B. One comparative study suggests that anidulafungin may be superior to fluconazole (see above) (NEJM 356:2472, 2007). MICs of candins are higher for C. parapsilosis than for other candidal species and clinical response rates may be less. Micafungin and anidulafungin have no known important drug-drug interactions. Cross-resistance can occur between **voriconazole** and flu, especially with C. glabrata (J Clin Micro 44:529, 2006); vori still active vs C. krusei (J Clin Micro 44:1740, 2006). Vori not preferred for initial Rx in those with extensive azole exposure.

NOTE: All dosage recommendations are for adults (unless otherwise indicated) & assume normal renal function.

TABLE 12 (17)

TYPE OF INFECTION/ORGANISM/ SITE OF INFECTION	SUGGESTED REGIMENS		COMMENTS
	PRIMARY	ALTERNATIVE	
FUNGAL INFECTIONS/Candidiasis/Bloodstream: unstable (continued)			
Stomatitis, esophagitis An AIDS-defining illness: correlates with HIV RNA levels in plasma & with CD4 counts. ARV RX has resulted in dramatic ↓ in prevalence of oropharyngeal & esophageal candidiasis & ↓ in refractory disease.	**Oropharyngeal (OP)**, initial episodes (7–14d rx): • **Fluconazole** 100 mg po q24h; or • **Itraconazole** oral solution 200 mg po q24h; or • **Clotrimazole** troches 10 mg po 5x/day; or • **Nystatin** suspension 4–6 ml q6h or 1–2 flavored pastilles 4–5x/day	**Fluconazole-refractory oropharyngeal:** • **Itra** oral solution ≥200 mg po q24h; or • **Posaconazole** 200 mg qd x 1 followed by 100 mg qd x 13d; or • **Ampho B** suspension 100 mg/ml^{NUS}, 1ml po q6h; or • **Ampho B** 0.3 mg/kg IV q24h	Fluconazole-refractory disease remains uncommon & is seen in pts with low CD4 counts (<50/ mm³). MICs > 4 mcg/ml predictive of failure (*Antimicrob Agents Chemother 51:3599, 2007*). Flu superior to oral suspension of **nystatin**. **Itra** 100 mg q12h x14d may be effective in pts unresponsive to flu. **Ampho B oral suspension** may be effective for pts refractory to **flu**, but relapse is common. Posa = in OPC (*CID 42:1179, 2006; Cochrane Database Syst Rev 3:CD003940, 2006*).
	Esophageal (14–21d): • **Flu** 100 mg (up to 400mg) po or IV q24h; or • **Itra** oral solution 200 mg po q24h; or • **Vori** 200 mg po q12h; or • **Caspofungin** 50 mg IV q24h; or • **Anidulafungin** 100 mg IV day 1 followed by 50 mg per day; or • **Micafungin** 150 mg/d	**Fluconazole-refractory esophageal:** • **Caspofungin** 50 mg IV q24h; or • **Vori** 200 mg po or IV q12h; or • **Posaconazole** 400 mg po bid x 3d followed by 400 mg po qd x 25d; or • **Micafungin** 150 mg IV per day; or • **Ampho B** 0.3–0.7 mg/kg IV q24h; or • **Ampho liposomal or lipid complex** 3–5 mg/kg IV q24h	For esophagitis, **caspofungin** as effective as **ampho B IV** but less toxic. Rare resistance & clinical failure to caspo reported (*Pharmaco Therapy 26:877, 2006*). **Voriconazole** as effective as **fluconazole** for esophagitis. **Micafungin** 100 mg or 150 mg IV per day equal to flu 200 mg per day. **Anidulafungin** 100 mg IV day 1 followed by 50 mg per day = to flu 200 mg on day 1 followed by 100 mg per day in 494 pts: cure rate 97% vs 98.8% (*CID 39:770, 2004*), but relapse rate higher (53% vs 19%) with anidulafungin. Posa effective in refractory/azole resistant OP & esophageal candidiasis (*HIV Clin Trials 8:86, 2007; CID 44:607, 2007*).
Vulvovaginitis Common among healthy young females & unrelated to HIV status.	• Topical **azoles** (clotrimazole, buto, mico, tico, or tercon) x3–7d; or • Topical **nystatin** 100,000 units/day as vaginal tablet x14d; or • Oral **itra** 200 mg q12h x1d or 200 mg q24h x3d; or • Oral **flu** 150 mg x1 dose		
Post-treatment chronic suppression (secondary prophylaxis) for disabling recurrent oral, esophageal infection. Authors would dc if sustained CD4 count ↑ to >200/mm³ following ARV RX.	Suppressive rx generally not recommended unless pts have frequent or severe recurrences. • **Oropharyngeal: fluconazole** or **itraconazole** oral solution may be considered. • **Vulvovaginal**: daily **topical azole** for recurrent cases. • **Esophageal: fluconazole** 100–200 mg q24h. Chronic or prolonged use of azoles promotes development of resistance.		Fluconazole 200 mg q24h does reduce risk of candida esophagitis & cryptococcosis. Disadvantages: Risk of emergence of fluconazole (azole)-resistant Candida species.
Coccidioidomycosis (See IDSA guidelines: *CID 41:1217, 2005*)	**Primary prophylaxis:** Not recommended.		

NOTE: All dosage recommendations are for adults (unless otherwise indicated) & assume normal renal function.

TABLE 12 (18)

TYPE OF INFECTION/ORGANISM/ SITE OF INFECTION	SUGGESTED REGIMENS		COMMENTS
	PRIMARY	ALTERNATIVE	
Pulmonary & extrapulmonary (not meningitis). Usually seen in pts with <250 CD4/mm³. Usually involves generalized lymphadenopathy, skin nodules or ulcers, peritonitis, liver abnormalities, & bone/joint involvement. (See Medicine 85:263, 2006 for review of unusual clinical presentations).	**Acute phase (milder disease):** • **Flu** 400–800 mg po q24h; or **itra** 200 mg po q12h **Acute phase (diffuse pulmonary disease):** • **Ampho B** 0.5–1 mg/kg IV q24h, continue until clinical improvement, usually 500–1000mg total dose **Disseminated disease:** • **Ampho B** 0.5–1 mg/kg IV q24h, continue until clinical improvement, usually 500–1000 mg total dose • **Flu** 400 mg/d (up to 2g/d recommended by some) • **Itra** up to 800 mg/d as 200 mg doses	Acute phase (diffuse pulmonary or disseminated disease): Some specialists add azole to ampho B therapy.	Lung infection in 80% of pts. Despite rx with ampho B ± subsequent po azole, mortality reported as 60%. Posaconazole 400 mg twice daily per day effective in 11/15 patients with refractory non-meningeal cocci (*Chest 132:952, 2007*); 400 mg per day effective in 17/20 patients with chronic or desseminated non-meningela disease (*CID 45:562, 2007*).
	Suppression: • **Flu** 400 mg/d (preferred) • **Itra** 200 mg po q12h		In those patients with CD4+ cell counts > 250 μL dc of suppression may be considered if there is clinical evidence of control of infection.
Meningitis **Occurs in 1/10 to 1/3 of pts with disseminated cocci** CSF demonstrates lymphocytic pleocytosis. CSF glucose <50mg/day & normal to mildly ↑ protein.	**Treatment: Fluconazole** 400–800 mg po q24h	IV amphotericin B as for pulmonary + 0.2–0.5 mg intrathecal (intraventricular via reservoir device) 2–3x/wk	Flu effective in up to 80% of cases. Vori successful in high doses (6 mg/kg IV q12h) followed by oral suppression (400 mg po q12h). Itra should not be used for treatment or suppression of meningitis, as it does not penetrate into CSF.
	Suppression: Do not dc for patients with meningits even with robust response to ARV RX **Fluconazole** 400 mg/day po as single dose or 200 mg po q12h	**Amphotericin B** 1 mg/kg IV once/	Relapses are common in both HIV+ & HIV− pts. Lifelong suppression indicated for patients with meningitis.
Cryptococcosis	**Primary prophylaxis:** Not recommended. In review of 1316 pts both flu & itra decreased incidence of crypto meningitis but neither increased survival (*Cochrane Database Syst Rev 3: CD004773, 2005*).		

NOTE: All dosage recommendations are for adults (unless otherwise indicated) & assume normal renal function.

TABLE 12 (19)

FUNGAL INFECTIONS/Cryptococcosis (continued)

TYPE OF INFECTION/ORGANISM/ SITE OF INFECTION	SUGGESTED REGIMENS		COMMENTS
	PRIMARY	**ALTERNATIVE**	
Cryptococcemia &/or Meningitis **Treatment** (also see Table 11A) ↓ in era of ARV RX but still common presenting OI in newly diagnosed AIDS pts. Cryptococcal infection may be manifested by positive blood culture or positive test of serum for cryptococcal antigen (CRAG: >95% sens). CRAG no help in monitoring response to therapy. With ARV RX, symptoms of acute meningitis may return: immune reconstitution inflammatory syndrome (IRIS) ↑ CSF pressure associated with high mortality: lower with CSF removal. If frequent LPs not possible, ventriculoperitoneal shunts an option (Surg Neurol 63:529 & 531, 2005).	**Ampho B** 0.7 mg/kg IV q24h + **flucytosine**[1] 25 mg/kg po q6h x2wks **or** **Liposomal amphotericin B** 4 mg/kg IV q24h + **flucytosine** 25 mg/kg po q6h x2wks **Then** **Consolidation therapy: Fluconazole** 400 mg po q24h to complete a 10-wk course or until CSF culture sterile, then suppression (see below). Start Highly Active Antiretroviral Therapy (ARV RX) if possible.	**Fluconazole** 400–800 mg/day po or IV for less severe disease **or** **Fluconazole** 400–800 mg/day po or IV + **flucytosine** 25 mg/kg po q6h x4–6wks	Outcome of treatment: failure associated with dissemination of infection & high serum antigen titer, indicative of ↑ burden of organisms and lack of 5FC use during inductive Rx, abnormal neurological evaluation & underlying hematological malignancy. Mortality rates still 12% at 3 mos. Early Dx essential for improved outcome (PLOS Medicine 4:e47, 2007). Ampho B + 5FC treatment ↓ crypto CFUs more rapidly than ampho + flu or ampho + 5FC + flu. Ampho B 1 mg/kg/d alone much more rapidly fungical in vivo than flu 400 mg/d (CID 45:76&81, 2007). Monitor 5-FC levels: peak 70–80 mg/L, trough 30–40 mg/L. Higher levels assoc. with bone marrow toxicity. No difference in outcome if given IV or po (AAC Dec 28, 2006). If normal mental status, >20 cells/mm³ CSF, & CSF CRAG <1:1024, flu alone may be reasonable. Failure of flu may rarely be due to resistant organism, especially if burden of organism high at initiation of Rx. Although 200 mg qd = 400 mg qd of flu: median survival 76 & 82 days respectively, authors prefer 400 mg po qd (BMC Infect Dis 18:118, 2006). Role of other azoles uncertain: successful outcomes were observed in 14/29 (48%) subjects with cryptococcal meningitis treated with posaconazole (JAC 56:745, 2005). Voriconazole also may be effective. Survival probably improved with ARV RX, but IRIS may complicate its use. Of 52 patients treated with ARV RX initiated at a median time of 2.6 mo after dx of crypto meningitis, 10 (19%) developed IRIS; median time to onset of IRIS of 9.9 months after initiation of ARV RX (J Acquir Immune Defic Syndr 45:595, 2007). Presentation: aseptic meningitis, high CSF opening pressure, positive CSF CRAG, negative culture; prognosis good. Short course corticosteroids may be beneficial in severe disease (Expert Rev Anti Infect Ther. 4:469, 2006).
Suppression (chronic maintenance therapy)	**Fluconazole** 200 mg/day po. If CD4 count rises to >100/mm³ with effective antiretroviral rx and is sustained for 6 mo, suppressive rx can be discontinued. Some might consider performing a lumbar puncture before discontinuation of maintenance rx.	**Itraconazole** 200 mg po q12h if flu intolerant or failure.	Itraconazole not as effective as fluconazole & not recommended because of higher relapse rate (23% vs 4%). Recurrence rate (95% CI) of 0.4 to 3.9 per 100 patient-years with discontinuation of suppressive therapy in 100 patients on ARV RX with CD4 > >100 cells/mm³ (CID 38:565, 2004); reappearance of pos. serum CRAG may predict relapse.

[1] Flucytosine = 5-FC
NOTE: All dosage recommendations are for adults (unless otherwise indicated) & assume normal renal function.

TABLE 12 (20)

TYPE OF INFECTION/ORGANISM/ SITE OF INFECTION	SUGGESTED REGIMENS		COMMENTS
	PRIMARY	ALTERNATIVE	
FUNGAL INFECTIONS (continued)			
Fusariosis Causes infection in eye, skin, sinus & disseminated diseases—increased in transplant patients. Rare in HIV-infected patients (1 reported case).	• **Ampho B** 1–1.2 mg/kg/d or • **Lipid- ampho B** 5 mg/kg/d or • **Voriconazole** 6 mg/kg IV q12h on day 1, then either 4 mg/kg q12h or 200 mg po q12h for body weight ≥40kg (100 mg po q12h for body weight <40kg)	• **Posaconazole** 400 mg po bid	Optimal therapy unknown. Voriconazole and posaconazole have been successfully used in those failing ampho B (Clin Micro Rev 20: 695, 2007).
Histoplasmosis (IDSA treatment guidelines in CID 45:807, 2007) In a Colombian study comparing 30 pts with AIDS with 20 pts without HIV infection with disseminated histo, the AIDS pts had ↑ numbers of skin lesions, ↑ sed rate, anemia, leucopenia, fungal isolated from multiple sites, had ↓ response to itra which ↑ with ARV RX to non-AIDS levels (Am J Trop Med Hyg 73:576, 2005). Risk factors for death: dyspnea, platelet count <100,000/mm³, & LDH >2x upper limit normal. In 1 study suppression was safely dc after 12mos. of antifungal rx & 6mos. of ARV RX with CD4 >150: 0 relapses after 2yrs followup in 32 pts (CID 38:1485, 2004).	**Primary prophylaxis:** itraconazole (200 mg daily) for patients with CD4 cell counts <150 cells/mm³ in endemic areas where the incidence of histoplasmosis is >10 cases per 100 patient-years.		
	Severe disseminated: Acute phase (1–2 wks): • **Liposomal ampho B** 3 mg/kg/d IV; or • **ABLC** 5 mg/kg/d IV		Institute ARV RX as early as possible. ARV RX improves outcome (Am J Trop Hyg 73:576, 2005) and although immune response inflammatory syndrome occurs, it is rare, usually not severe and easily managed. L-AMB less toxic and more effective than ampho B: higher response rate, lower mortality.
	Continuation phase (12 mos): Itra 200 mg po q12h		Itra is the preferred azole: flu less effective; keto less expensive but has more adverse effects; vori and posa anecdotally effective, but too few patients to recommend. All are second-line agents and if any of these instead of itra is used, reasons for soing so should be documented in the medical record.
	Less severe disseminated: Itra 200 mg po twice daily for 12 mos		Blood levels should be documented during the first month of itra Rx.
	Meningitis: Liposomal ampho B 5 mg/kg/d IV for 4–6 wks; itra 200 mg 2–3 times a day for 12 mos		**Itra is a potent CYP3A4 inhibitor: contraindicated drugs include efavirenz, statins, rifamycins, midazolam, triazolam, cisapride, pimozide, quinidine, dofetilide, or levacetylmethadol. Important drug interactions with antiretroviral agents, PIs in particular.**
			Itra, ~5% relapse rate; 10–20% relapses with ampho B, 60% with ketoconazole.
	Suppression : Itra 200 mg po q24h. Suppressive therapy may be discontinued in pts who have completed 1 yr of therapy, neg. blood cultures, a serum and urinary hosto antigen < 2 ng/mL, CD4>150 cells/mm³, and who are on ARV RX.	**Amphotericin B** 1 mg/kg IV weekly or biweekly	

NOTE: All dosage recommendations are for adults (unless otherwise indicated) & assume normal renal function.

TABLE 12 (21)

TYPE OF INFECTION/ORGANISM/ SITE OF INFECTION	SUGGESTED REGIMENS		COMMENTS
	PRIMARY	ALTERNATIVE	
FUNGAL INFECTIONS (continued)			
Nocardiosis N. asteroides complex, N. farcinica, & N. brasiliensis, numerous other species, varying in susceptibilities; susceptibility testing recommended for all clinically significant isolates (Clin Micro Rev 19:259, 2006). Reference labs: R.J. Wallace (903) 877-7680 or CDC (404) 639-3158			
Cutaneous & lymphocutaneous (sporotrichoid)	**TMP/SMX**: 5–10 mg/kg/day TMP & 25–50 mg/kg/day SMX in 2–4 div. doses/day, po or IV	**Sulfisoxazole** 2 gm po q6h or **minocycline** 100–200mg po q12h	**TMP/SMX** (or other sulfonamide) is drug of choice
Pulmonary, disseminated, brain abscess	**Triple drug regimen for empirical therapy of serious infection pending results of susceptibility testing:** **TMP/SMX**: initially 15 mg/kg/day of TMP & 75 mg/kg/day of SMX IV or po, div. in 2–4 doses plus **IMP** 500 mg IV q6h, plus **Amikacin** 7.5 mg/kg IV q12h After 3–4wks, **TMP/SMX as** 10 mg/kg/day TMP in 2–4 doses po. Do serum level. (See Comment.)	**Ceftriaxone** 2 gm once or twice daily + **amikacin** 7.5 mg/kg IV q12h x 3–4wks & then po regimen	**Linezolid** 600mg po bid for 1.5–12 mos an alternative for TMP/SMX intolerance or salvage: 9/11 non-HIV (5 disseminated, 4 CNS, 1 lung, 1 skin) cured with 1 possible relapse, 1 clinical failure; high adverse events rate with myelosuppression or peripheral neuropathy in 7 (Ann Pharmacother 41:1694, 2007). **Ceftriaxone** & other cephalosporins, minocycline, amoxicillin/clavulanate may also be active, depending on the species (Clin Micro Rev 19:259, 2006). Optimal therapy not established. Duration of therapy based on clinical response but generally 3mos. for immunocompetent host & 6mos. for immuno-compromised (e.g., organ transplant, malignancy, chronic lung disease, diabetes, ETOH use, steroid rx, & AIDS).
Paracoccidioidomycosis (South American blastomycosis)/P. brasiliensis	**Itraconazole** 200 mg/day po x 6mos or **Ketoconazole** 400 mg/day po for 6–18mos	**Ampho B** 0.4–0.5 mg/kg/day IV to total dose of 1.5–2.5 gm or **sulfonamides**	Improvement in >90% pts on itra or keto.[NFDAJ] Sulfa: 4–6gm/day for several weeks, then 500mg/day for 3–5yrs also used. **TMP/SMX ± ampho B** used successfully in AIDS patients (J Infect 51: 248, 2005).
Lobomycosis (keloidal blastomycosis)/P. loboi	Surgical excision, clofazimine or ampho B		Low-dose itra (50–100mg/day), keto (200–400mg/day) & sulfadiazine (up to 6mg/day) showed similar clinical responses in 4–6mos. in a randomized study (Cochrane Database Syst Rev. 2006 Apr 19:CD004967, 2006). **HIV+: TMP/SMX suppressive rx.**
Penicilliosis (Penicillium marneffei) Common disseminated fungal infection in AIDS pts in SE Asia (esp. Thailand & Vietnam). Most occur when CD4 <50/mm³	**Ampho B** 0.5–1 mg/kg/day x2 wks followed by **itraconazole** 400 mg/day for 10 wks Then **suppressive therapy** 200 mg/day po **for HIV-infected pts.**	For less sick pts: **Itra** 200 mg po q8h x3 days, then 200 mg q12h po x12 wks, then 200 mg po q24h (IV if unable to take po); continue as suppressive therapy for HIV-infected pts.	3rd most common OI in AIDS pts in SE Asia following TB & cryptococcal meningitis. May resemble histoplasmosis or TB. Skin nodules are umbilicated (mimic cryptococcal infection or molluscum contagiosum). In AIDS pts. suppression with itra effective in **preventing relapses.** One retrospective study of 33 patients on ARV RX and > 6mos of CD4 > 100 cells/mm³ in whom suppressive therapy was stopped found zero cases of recurrence per 641 person-months (95% confidence interval 0–0.6 cases per person-month) after a median follow-up of 18 months (range 6–45) (AIDS 21:365, 2007).

NOTE: All dosage recommendations are for adults (unless otherwise indicated) & assume normal renal function.

TABLE 12 (22)

TYPE OF INFECTION/ORGANISM/ SITE OF INFECTION	SUGGESTED REGIMENS		COMMENTS
	PRIMARY	ALTERNATIVE	
FUNGAL INFECTIONS (continued)			
Phaeohyphomycosis, Black molds, Dematiaceous fungi (See *Clin Microbiol Rev 21:157, 2008*). Sinuses, skin, bone & joint, brain abscess, endocarditis emerging especially in HSCT pts with disseminated disease (Infect in Medicine 24:45, 2007). **Species: Scedosporium prolificans;** (other genuses): Bipolaris, Wangiella, Curvularia, Exophiala, Phialemonium, Scytalidium, Alternaria.	**Surgery + itraconazole** 400 mg/day po, duration not defined, probably 6mos[NFDAI]	**Voriconazole** 6 mg/kg IV q12h on day 1, then either 4 mg/kg IV q12h or 200mg po q12h for body weight ≥40kg (100 mg po q12h for body weight <40kg). (*JAC 61:6*6, 2008 & AAC 2008 Jan 22 [Epub ahead of print]*). **Itraconazole + terbinafine** synergistic against *S. prolificans.* No clinical data but combination could show ↑ toxicity (see Table 13).	Notoriously resistant to antifungal rx including amphotericin & azoles. Mortality >80%. **Vori** achieved overall 57% favorable response rate in 107 pts with scedosporium infection (70 *S. apiospermum*, 37 *S. prolificans*) (CNS disease, 20%; lungs/sinus, 24%; CNS 20%, disseminated, infection, 21%); pts with CNS or disseminated infection, *S. prolificans,* and severely immunosuppressed did worse (*AAC 2008 Jan 22 [Epub ahead of print]*). Terbinafine + vori or + itra, vori + micafungin synergistic against *S. prolificans* vitro (*Clin Microbiol Rev 21:157, 2008*). Case report of cure of brain abscess with combination of vori + terbinafine *Scand J Infect Dis 39:87-90, 2007*).
Scedosporium apiospermum (Pseudallescheria boydii) (not considered a true dematiaceous mold) Skin, subcutaneous (Madura foot), brain abscess, recurrent meningitis. May appear after near-drowning incidents. Also emerging especially in HSCT pts with disseminated disease.	**Voriconazole** 6 mg/kg IV q12h on day 1, then either (4 mg/kg IV q12h) or (200 mg po q12h for body weight ≥40kg, but 100 mg po q12h for body weight <40kg).	Surgery – **itraconazole** 200 mg po q12h until clinically well.[NFDAI] (Many species r ow resistant or refractory to itra) or **Posa**[NFDAI] 400 mg po bid with meals (If not taking meals, 200 mg po q6h)	Notoriously resistant to antifungal drugs including amphotericin. In vitro voriconazole more active than itra (*JAC 61:616, 2008*). **See comment above** concerning vori for scedosporium infection. Vori or ampho B + micafungin synergistic in vitro (*Clin Microbiol Rev 21:157, 2008*), Posa active in vitro; one report of successful Rx of brain abscess with posa (*Clin Infect Dis 15:1648, 2002*).
Sporotrichosis (See IDSA treatment guidelines: *CID 45:1255, 2007*)			
Cutaneous/Lymphonodular Dissemination is uncommon in immunocompetent pts, but tends to occur in AIDS.	**Itraconazole** 200 mg/day po x3-6mos. For non-responders, use itra 200 mg twice daily; or terbinafine 500 mg twice daily, or saturated solution of potassium iodide (SSKI) 5 drops 3x a day, increasing to 40-50 drops 3x a day as tolerated.	**Fluconazole** 400-800 mg po q24h Only in those unable to tolerate other agents.	SSKI side-effects: nausea, rash, fever, metallic taste, salivary gland swelling. Duration of itra suppressive therapy is indefinite. Based on experience with other fungal infections, it seems reasonable to discontinue suppressive therapy in those treated with itra for at least 1 year and whose CD4+ cell counts have remained > 200 cells/mm³ for >1 year.

NOTE: All dosage recommendations are for adults (unless otherwise indicated) & assume normal renal function.

TABLE 12 (23)

TYPE OF INFECTION/ORGANISM/ SITE OF INFECTION	SUGGESTED REGIMENS		COMMENTS
	PRIMARY	ALTERNATIVE	
FUNGAL INFECTIONS/Sporotrichosis (continued)			
Osteoarticular	**Itraconazole** 200mg po q12h for 12 mos. (IV if unable to take po).	**Lipid-based ampho B** 3-5 mg/kg/d or ampho B 0.7-1.0 mg/kg/d for initial therapy; then after a favorable response **itra** 200 mg q12h to complete 12 mos of therapy.	Determine itra serum concentrations at two weeks of therapy to document adequate levels.
Pulmonary	For more severe disease: **Lipid-based ampho B** 3-5 mg/kg/d OR **Ampho B** 0.7-1.0 mg/kg/d for initial therapy then after a favorable response **itra** 200 mg q12h to complete 12 mos of therapy	For less severe disease **itra** 200mg po q12h for 12 mos. (IV if unable to take po).	Determine itra serum concentrations at two weeks of therapy to document adequate levels. Surgery is recommended for resection of localized disease.
Disseminated	**Lipid-based ampho B** 3-5 mg/kg/d for initial therapy then after a favorable response **itra** 200 mg q12h to complete 12 mos of therapy		Determine itra serum concentrations at two weeks of therapy.
Meningeal	**Lipid-based ampho B** 5 mg/kg/d for 4-6 weeks then **itra** 200 mg q12h to complete 12 mos of therapy		Determine itra serum concentrations at two weeks of therapy.
Suppressive therapy	**Itra** 200 mg once daily		Suppressive therapy is recommended for AIDS and other immunocompromised pts to prevent relapse of meningeal and disseminated disease and, because of propensity for dissemination in AIDS, should be considered for cutaneous, osteoarticular, and pulmonary disease. Duration of suppression is not defined, but may be lifelong in meningeal disease. In disseminated and localized disease discontinuation of itra may be reasonable in the patient treated with itra for at least 1 yr and whose CD4 counts are >100 cells/mm^3 for ≥1 yr.

NOTE: All dosage recommendations are for adults (unless otherwise indicated) & assume normal renal function.

TABLE 12 (24)

FUNGAL INFECTIONS (continued)

TYPE OF INFECTION/ORGANISM/ SITE OF INFECTION	SUGGESTED REGIMENS		COMMENTS
	PRIMARY	ALTERNATIVE	
Zygomycosis, Mucormycosis—Rhizopus, Rhizomucor, Absidia. (CID 41:521, 2005) Rhinocerebral, pulmonary, pulmonary, gastrointestinal forms; invasive. Key to successful rx: early dx with symptoms suggestive of sinusitis (or lateral facial pain or numbness): think mucor with palatal ulcers, &/or black eschars, onset unilateral blindness in immunocompromised or diabetic p. Rapidly fatal without rx. Dx by culture of tissue or stain: wide ribbon-like, non-septated with variation in diameter & right angle branching (ClinMicro&Infect 12.7, 2006).	**Liposomal Ampho B** 5-10 mg/kg/day (optimal dose not defined) **Or** **Posaconazole** 400 mg po bid with meals (if not taking meals, 200 mg qid).		Cure dependent on: (1) surgical debridement, (2) rx of hyperglycemia, correction of neutropenia, or reduction in immunosuppression; (3) antifungal rx: liposomal amphotericin (J Clin Micro 43:2012, 2005) or **posaconazole**. Complete or partial response rates of 60-80% in posaconazole salvage protocols (JAC 61, Suppl. 1, i35, 2008). Resistant to voriconazole; prolonged use of voriconazole prophylaxis predisposes to zygomycetes infections (Lancet ID 5:594, 2005).

PARASITIC INFECTIONS. Reference with pediatric dosages: Medical Letter online version: *Drugs for Parasitic Infections (Suppl), 2007*

Protozoan—Intestinal

CAUSATIVE AGENT/DISEASE	MODIFYING CIRCUMSTANCES	SUGGESTED REGIMENS		COMMENTS
		PRIMARY	ALTERNATIVE	
Blastocystis hominis	Role as pathogen supported by one controlled rx trial: metro vs placebo	**Nitazoxanide** 500 mg q12h x 3d.	**Metronidazole** 1.5 gm po once daily x10d; **Iodoquinol** 650 mg po q8h x20d or **TMP/SMX-DS**, 1 po q12h x7d	**Nitazoxanide**: Approved in liquid formulation for rx of children & 500 mg tabs for adults. Ref.: CID 40:1173, 2005. In AIDS pts, infection of respiratory and biliary tracts recognized.
Cryptosporidium parvum & C. hominis Ref.: CID 39:504, 2004	Effective ARV RX best therapy	**Immunocompetent —no HIV:** **Nitazoxanide** 500 mg po q12h x3d	**HIV with immunodeficiency:** **Nitazoxanide** 500 mg po q12h x14d in adults (60% response.) No response in HIV+ children.	
Cyclospora cayetanensis		Immunocompetent pts: **TMP/SMX-DS** tab 1 po q12h x7d	AIDS pts: **TMP/SMX-DS** 1 po q6h x10d; then tab 1 po 3x/wk.	If sulfa-allergic: **CIP** 500mg po q12h x7d & then 1 tab po 3x/wk x2 wks or **Nitazoxanide** 500 mg po q12h x 7 days (CID 44:466, 2007).
Entamoeba histolytica Refs.: Ln 361:1025, 2003; NEJM 348:1563, 2003	Asymptomatic cyst passer	**Paromomycin**[NUS] (aminosidine in U.K.) 500 mg po q8h x7d OR **iodoquinol** (Yodoxin) 650 mg po q8h x20 days	**Diloxanide furoate**[NUS] (Furamide) 500 mg po q8h x10 days (Source: Panorama Compound Pharm., 800-247-9767)	Metronidazole not effective vs cysts.

NOTE: All dosage recommendations are for adults (unless otherwise indicated) & assume normal renal function.

145

TABLE 12 (25)

CAUSATIVE AGENT/DISEASE	MODIFYING CIRCUMSTANCES	SUGGESTED REGIMENS		COMMENTS
		PRIMARY	ALTERNATIVE	
PARASITIC INFECTIONS/Protozoan—Intestinal *(continued)*				
	Patient with diarrhea/dysentery; mild/moderate disease. Oral rx possible	**Metronidazole** 500–750 mg po q8h x10d or **tinidazole** 2gm po q24h x3d, followed by: Either [**iodoquinol** (was diiodohydroxyquin) 650mg po q8h x20d] or [**paromomycin**^{NUS} 500mg po q8h x7d]	**Ornidazole**^{NUS} 500 mg po q12h x5d followed by:	Colitis can mimic ulcerative colitis; ameboma can mimic adenocarcinoma of colon. **Dx:** Antigen detection and PCR better than O&P. Watch out for non-pathogenic but morphologically identical *E. dispar* (CID 29:1117, 1999. Another alternative: **nitazoxanide** 500 mg po bid x 3 days (*Trans R Soc Trop Med & Hyg* 101:1025, 2007).
	Extraintestinal infection, e.g., hepatic abscess	**Metronidazole** 750 mg IV/po q8h x10d OR **tinidazole** 800 mg po q8h x20d followed by **paromomycin** 500mg po q8h x7d		**Serology positive with extraintestinal disease.**
Giardia lamblia Ref.: *MMWR* 49:55, 2000	Epigastric-ulcer-like symptoms	**Tinidazole** 2 gm po x1 **OR Nitazoxanide** 500 mg po q12h x3d	**Metronidazole** 500–750 mg po q8h x5d (high frequency of GI side-effects). See *Comment*. Rx if pregnant: **Paromomycin**^{NUS} 500 mg 4x/day x7d.	**Refractory pts: (Metro** 750 mg po + **quinacrine** 100 mg po)—both 3x/day x3wks. Ref.: *CID* 33:22, 2001. **Nitazoxanide** ref.: *CID* 40:1173, 2007.
Isospora belli		**TMP/SMX-DS** tab 1 po q12h x10d; if AIDS pt, then TMP-SMX-DS q6h x10d & then q12h x3wks	[(**Pyrimethamine** 75 mg/day po + **folinic acid** 10 mg/day po) x14 days] **or CIP** 500 mg po q12h x7d (*AnIM* 132:885, 2000)	Chronic suppression in AIDS pts; either 1 **TMP/SMX-DS** tab 3x/wk OR (**pyrimethamine** 25 mg/day po + **folinic acid** 5mg/day po)
Microsporidiosis (Ref.: *MMWR* 53:RR-15, 2004). *Effective ARV RX is main therapy.*				
Ocular: Encephalitozoon hellum or cuniculi, Vittaforma (Nosema) corneae or Nosema sp.		**Albendazole** 400 mg po q12h x3wks	In HIV+ pts, reports of response of E. hellum to **fumagillin** eyedrops. For V. corneae, may need keratoplasty.	To obtain fumagillin: 1-800-292-6773 or www.leiterrx.com. Neutropenia/thrombocytopenia serious side effects. **Dx:** Most labs use modified trichrome stain. Need electron micrographs for species identification. FA & PCR methods in development.
Intestinal (diarrhea): Enterocytozoon bieneusi; Encephalitozoon (Septata) intestinalis		**Albendazole** 400 mg po q12h x3wks. Peds dose: 15 mg/kg per day divided bid x 7d (*PIDJ* 23:915, 2004).	Fumagillin 20 mg po q8h reported effective for E. bieneusi (*NEJM* 346:1963, 2002)	To obtain fumagillin: 800-292-6773 or www.leiterrx.com. Neutropenia/thrombocytopenia serious side effects.
Disseminated: E. hellum, cuniculi or intestinalis; Pleistophora sp. Ref.: *NEJM* 351:42, 2004		**Albendazole** 400 mg po q12h x3wks	No established rx for Pleistophora sp.	For Trachipleistophora sp., try itraconazole + albendazole (*NEJM* 351:42, 2004).
Protozoan—Extraintestinal				
Babesiosis (B. microti) Refs.: *CID* 32:1117, 2001	Treatment: Exchange transfusion if >10% parasitemia & hemolysis.	**Atovaquone** 750 mg po bid x7–10d + **azithro** 500 mg po x1d, then 250 mg/day x 7d. (*NEJM* 343:1454, 2000)	(**Clinda** 600 mg po tid) + (**quinine** 650 mg po tid) x7d. For adults, can give **clinda** IV as 1.2 gm q12h.	Long-term suppressive rx in AIDS pts: clindamycin + doxycycline + azithro (2 gm po q24h) has been used (*CID* 22:809, 1996).
Pneumocystis carinii pneumonia (PCP) New name: **Pneumocystis jiroveci** (yee-row-vek-ee)	**Not acutely ill,** able to take po meds. PaO$_2$ >70 mmHg	**TMP/SMX-DS,** 2 tabs po q8h x21d) OR (**Dapsone** 100 mg po q24h + TMP 5 mg/kg po q8h x21d)	[**Clinda** (600 mg IV or 300–450 mg po) q6h + **primaquine** 15 mg base po q24h] OR **atovaquone suspension** 750 mg po bid with food x21d	Mutations in gene of the target enzyme of sulfamethoxazole identified; relationship to clinical resistance unclear (*EID* 10:1721, 2004). **After 21 days of therapy, then chronic suppression in AIDS pts** (see next page).

NOTE: Concomitant use of corticosteroids usually reserved for sicker pts with PaO$_2$ <70 (see below)

NOTE: All dosage recommendations are for adults (unless otherwise indicated) & assume normal renal function.

TABLE 12 (26)

CAUSATIVE AGENT/DISEASE	MODIFYING CIRCUMSTANCES	SUGGESTED REGIMENS PRIMARY	SUGGESTED REGIMENS ALTERNATIVE	COMMENTS
PARASITIC INFECTIONS/Protozoan—Extraintestinal/Pneumocystis carinii pneumonia (PCP) *(continued)*				
Refs: *NEJM* 350:2487, 2004; *CID* 40 (suppl 3):S131, 2005; *CID* 41:1752 & 1756, 2005; *CID* 42:1208, 2006	**Acutely ill,** po therapy not possible. PaO₂ <70 mmHg	[**Prednisone** 15–30min. before TMP/SMX—start with 40 mg po q12h x5d, then 40 mg po q24h x5d, then 20 mg po q24h x11d] + [**TMP/SMX** (15 mg of TMP component/kg/day) IV div. q6–8h x21d]	**Prednisone** as in primary rx PLUS [(**Clinda** 600 mg IV q8h) + (**primaquine** 15 mg base po q24h) x21d OR **Pentamidine** 4 mg/kg/day IV x21d	After 21 days of therapy, then chronic suppression (see below). Clinical failure defined as absence of clinical response after 4–8 days; then switch to another regimen. Optimal alternative drug is unclear. **Caspofungin** active in animal models: *CID* 36:1445, 2003.
	Primary prophylaxis & post-treatment suppression Ref *CID* 40 (suppl 3), 2005	Can substitute IV predniso one (reduce dose 25%) for po prednisone (**TMP/SMX-DS,** 1 tab po q24h or 3x/wk) OR (**dapsone** 100 mg po q24h) OR (**TMP/SMX-SS,** 1 tab po q24h) DC when CD4 >200 x3 mos.	(**Pentamidine** 300 mg in 6 mL sterile water by aerosol q4wks) OR (**dapsone** 200 mg po + **pyrimethamine** 75 mg po + **folinic acid** 25 mg po—all once a week); OR **atovaquone** 1500 mg po q24h with food.	TMP/SMX-DS regimen also provides cross-protection vs toxo & other bacterial infections. Dapsone + pyrimethamine protects vs toxo. Atovaquone refs.: *JID* 180:369, 1999; *NEJM* 339:1889, 1998.
Toxoplasma gondii (*Ln* 363:1965, 2004; *MMWR* 53:RR-15, 2004; *CID* 40 (suppl 3):S131, 2005)				
Cerebral toxoplasmosis (Toxoplasma encephalitis) IgG toxo antibody positive in approx. 84% (*NEJM* 327: 1643, 1992).		**Pyrimethamine** (pyri) 200 mg x1 po, then 50–75 mg/day po] + (**sulfadiazine** 1–1.5 gm po q6h) + (**folinic acid** 10–20 mg/day po) x 4–6 wks after resolution of signs/symptoms, & then suppressive rx (*see below*) OR **TMP/SMX** 10/50 mg/kg/day po or IV div. q12h x6 wks)	[**Pyri + folinic acid** (as in primary regimen)] plus one of the following: (1) **Clinda** 600 mg po/IV q6h or (2) **Atovaquone** 750 mg po q6h or (3) **Azithro** 1.2–1.5 gm po q24h. (4) **Clarithro** 1 gm po bid. All above for 4–6 weeks after resolution of signs & symptoms, then suppression.	Use alternative regimen for pts with severe sulfa allergy. If multiple ring-enhancing brain lesions (CT or MRI), >85% of pts respond to 7–10days of empiric rx; if no response, suggest brain biopsy. **Pyri**. Dose weight based: <60kg: 500 mg/day; ≥60 kg: 75mg/day. Folinic acid prevents hematologic toxicity.
	Primary prophylaxis, AIDS pts—IgG toxo antibody + CD4 count <100/μl	(**TMP/SMX-DS,** 1 tab po q24h) or (**TMP/SMX-SS,** 1 tab po q24h)	[(**Dapsone** 50 mg po q24h) + (**pyri** 50 mg po q week)] + (**folinic acid** 25 mg po q week)] **or** [**atovaquone** 1500 mg po q24h]	Prophylaxis for pneumocystis with TMP/SMX also effective vs toxo. Refs.: *CID* 25(Suppl.3):S299, 1997.
	Suppression after rx of cerebral toxo Ref.: *CID* 40 (suppl.3), 2005	(**Sulfadiazine** 500–1000mg po ≤x/day) + (**pyri** 25–50 po q24h) + (**folinic acid** 10–25 mg po q24h)	**Clinda** 300–450 mg po q6–8h) + (**pyri** 25–50 mg po q24h) + (**folinic acid** 10–25 mg po q6–12h).	(**Pyri + sulfa**) prevents PCP & toxo; (**clinda + pyri**) prevents toxo only.
Vaginitis—*MMWR* 55(RR-11), 2006				
Bacterial vaginosis Polymicrobic: associated with Gardnerella vaginalis, Mobiluncus, Mycoplasma hominis, Prevotella sp., Atopobium sp., et al. Etiology unclear. Malodorous vaginal discharge, pH >4.5 Ref: *JID* 193:1475, 2006		**Metronidazole** (0.5 gm po bid x7d) OR **metronidazole vaginal gel** (1 applicator intravaginally) once daily x5d (avoid in 1st trimester pregnancy) OR **tinidazole** (2 gm po once daily x 2 days) OR (1 gm po once daily x 5 days).	**Clinda** (0.3 gm po bid x7d) or 2% **clinda vaginal cream** 5 gm intravaginally at bedtime x7d OR **clinda ovules** 100 mg intravaginally at bedtime x3d	50% increase in cure rate with condoms or if abstain from sex (*CID*:44:213 & 20, 2007). **Rx of male sex partner not indicated unless balanitis present.** Metronidazole: 2gm po single dose not as effective as 5–7d course (*JAMA* 268:92, 1992). **Metro-ER** 750 mg po once daily available, efficacy unclear. **In pregnancy:** Rx same as non-pregnancy, except avoid clindamycin cream (↑ risk premature birth). Atopobium resistant to **metro** in vitro; susceptible to **clinda** (*BMC Inf Dis* 6:51, 2006).

[1] 1 applicator contains 5 gm of gel with 37.5 mg metronidazole
NOTE: All dosage recommendations are for adults (unless otherwise indicated) & assume normal renal function.

TABLE 12 (27)

CAUSATIVE AGENT/DISEASE	MODIFYING CIRCUMSTANCES	SUGGESTED REGIMENS		COMMENTS
		PRIMARY	ALTERNATIVE	
PARASITIC INFECTIONS/Protozoan—Extraintestinal/ Vaginitis (continued)				
Candidiasis, vulvovaginal Pruritus, thick cheesy discharge, pH <4.5	Candida albicans 80–90%. C. glabrata, C. tropicalis may be increasing—less suscept. to azoles.	**Fluconazole** 150 mg single dose po or **itraconazole** 200 mg po q12h x1d	**Intravaginal azoles:** Variety of strengths. Regimens vary from 1 dose to 7–14d. Examples (all end in -azole): butocon, clotrim, micon, tiocon, tercon	**Intravaginal azoles available both OTC & by prescription.** Nystatin vaginal tabs x 14 days less effective than azoles. Other rx for azole-resistant strains: gentian violet, boric acid. With normal CD4 lymphocyte count, usual duration of rx; if AIDS pt, treat for 10–14d. If 4 or more episodes/year: 6 mos suppression with fluconazole 150 mg po once weekly.
Trichomoniasis Copious foamy discharge, pH >4.5	Trichomonas vaginalis	**Metronidazole** (2 gm as single dose) (contraindicated in 1st trimester of pregnancy) OR **Tinidazole** 2 gm po x1 dose **Pregnancy:** See Comment	**For rx failure:** Re-treat with metro 500 mg po q12h x7d; if 2nd failure: metro 2 gm po q24h x3–5d. If still failure, suggest ID consultation &/or contact CDC: 770-488-4115 or www.cdc.gov/std	**Treat male sexual partners (2gm metronidazole po as single dose).** Nearly 20% of men with NGU infected with trichomonas (JID 188:465, 2003). **Pregnancy: Metro is not mutagenic or teratogenic.**
Nematode infections **Strongyloides stercoralis (strongyloidiasis)**		**Ivermectin** 200 mcg/kg po q24h x2d	**Albendazole** 400 mg po bid x2d or 7–10d for hyperinfection syndrome	Retreatment often required. Long-term suppressive rx likely to be necessary in AIDS pts.
Ectoparasites. Refs.: CID 36:1355, 2003; Ln 363:889, 2004. **NOTE: Due to potential neurotoxicity, use lindane products only as last resort.**				
Pediculus humanus corporis **(body lice)** For use of ivermectin in outbreak see JID 193:474, 2006.		Treat the clothing. Organism lives in, deposits eggs in seams of clothing. Discard clothing; if not possible, treat clothing with 1% malathion powder or 10% DDT powder.		Body louse leaves clothing only for blood meal. Nits in clothing viable for 1 month.
P. humanus var. capitis **(head louse,** nits**)** Ref.: Med Lett 47:68, 2005 Phthirus pubis (crabs)		**Permethrin,** 1% generic lotion or cream rinse (NIX): Apply to shampooed dry hair for 10min; repeat in one week **OR** **Ivermectin** 200-400 mcg/kg po once (report that 3 doses at 7 day intervals works (JID 193:474, 2006)); does not affect nits. **OR** **Malathion 0.5% lotion** (Ovide). Apply to dry hair for 8–12hrs, then shampoo. Repeat 7 days.		**Permethrin:** Success in 78%. Extra nit combing of no benefit. Resistance increasing. No advantage to 5% permethrin. Treat sex partners if body or pubic lice. **Malathion:** 98% effective. In alcohol—potentially flammable. Ref: Ped Derm 21:670, 2004.
Sarcoptes scabiei **(scabies)** (mites) Immunocompetent patients Refs: LnID 6:769, 2006; NEJM 354:1718, 2006.		**Primary: Permethrin** 5% cream (ELIMITE). Apply entire skin from chin to toes. Leave on 8–10hrs. Repeat in 1wk. Safe for children >2mos. old. **Alternatives: Ivermectin** 200 mcg/kg po, repeat in 14 days OR **crotamiton** 10% cream topically q24h x2d.		Trim fingernails. Reapply to hands after handwashing. Pruritus may persist x2wks after mites gone. **Do not use lindane in pregnancy or in young children**—absorbed through skin; can use 6–10% precipitated sulfur in petrolatum q24h x3d. Norwegian scabies in AIDS pts: Extensive, crusted. Can mimic psoriasis. Not pruritic. **Highly contagious—isolate!**
AIDS patients, CD4 <150/ mm³ **(Norwegian scabies**—See Comments)		For Norwegian scabies: **Permethrin** 5% as above on day 1, then repeat x several weeks. **Ivermectin** 200 mcg/kg x1 reported effective.		

NOTE: All dosage recommendations are for adults (unless otherwise indicated) & assume normal renal function.

TABLE 12 (28)
FIGURE 4 - ACTIVITY OF ANTIVIRAL AGENTS AGAINST TREATABLE PATHOGENIC VIRUSES

Virus	Acyclovir	Amantadine	Adefovir Entecavir Lamivudine	Cidofovir	Famciclovir	Foscarnet	Ganciclovir	αInterferon Or PEG INF	Oseltamivir	Ribavirin	Rimantidine	Valacyclovir	Valganciclovir	Zanamivir
Adenovirus	-	-	-	+	-	-	±	-	-	-	-	-	±	-
BK virus	-	-	-	+	-	-	-	-	-	-	-	-	-	-
Cytomegalovirus	±	-	-	+++	±	+++	+++	-	-	-	-	±	+++	-
Hepatitis B	-	-	+++	-	-	-	-	++	-	±	-	-	-	-
Hepatitis C	-	-	-	-	-	-	-	++++*	-	++++*	-	-	-	-
Herpes simplex virus	+++	-	-	++	+++	++	++	-	-	-	-	+++	++	-
Influenza A	-	±**	-	-	-	-	-	-	+++	-	±**	-	-	+++
Influenza B	-	-	-	-	-	-	-	-	++	-	-	-	-	++
Respiratory Syncytial Virus	-	-	-	-	-	-	-	-	-	+	-	-	-	-
Varicella-zoster virus	++	-	-	+	++	++	+	-	-	-	-	++	+	-

* 1st line rx = an IFN + Ribavirin   ** not CDC recommended

- = no activity; ± = possible activity; + = active, 3rd line therapy (least active clinically)
++ = Active, 2nd line therapy (less active clinically); +++ = Active, 1st line therapy (usually active clinically)

NOTE: All dosage recommendations are for adults (unless otherwise indicated) & assume normal renal function.

TABLE 12 (29)

TYPE OF INFECTION/ORGANISM/ SITE OF INFECTION	SUGGESTED REGIMENS		COMMENTS
	PRIMARY	ALTERNATIVE	
VIRAL INFECTIONS			
Cytomegalovirus (CMV) Marked ↓ in CMV infections & death from CMV with Highly Active Antiretroviral Rx: there is a progressive ↓ in CMV DNA & most pts actually become neg. after a median time of 3mos (JID 180:847, 1999; JAC 54:582, 2004; EJCMID 23:550, 2004). Initial rx for CMV infections should include optimization of ARV RX.	**Primary prophylaxis** not generally recommended; preemptive rx in pts with ↑ CMV DNA titers in plasma & CD4 <100/mm³. Recommended by some: **valganciclovir** 900 mg po q24h (CID 32: 783, 2001). Authors rec. primary prophylaxis be dc if response to ARV RX ↑ CD4 >100 for 6mos. (MMWR 53:98, 2004).		Risk for developing CMV disease correlates with quantity of CMV DNA in plasma: +DNAα ↑ 3.4-fold & each log₁₀ ↑ associated with 3.1-fold ↑ in disease (JCI 101:497, 1998; CID 28:758, 1999).
Colitis, esophagitis Dx best by biopsy of ulcer base/edge (Clin Gastro Hepatol 2:564, 2004)	**Ganciclovir** as with retinitis except induction period extended for 3-6wks. No agreement on use of maintenance; may not be necessary except after relapse (ArIM 158:957, 1998). Responses less predictable than for retinitis (AJM 98:109, 1995). **Foscarnet** 90mg/kg q12h effective in 9/10 pts (AAC 41:1226, 1997). **Valganciclovir also likely effective.** Switch to oral valganciclovir when po tolerated & when symptoms not severe enough to interfere with absorption.		
CMV of the nervous system: Encephalitis & ventriculitis. Treatment not defined, but should be considered the same as retinitis. Disease may develop while taking ganciclovir as suppressive therapy. [See Herpes 11(Suppl.12):95A, 2004]. Optimize ARV RX! Most would use combination of ganciclovir & foscarnet, but high dose valganciclovir (900 mg po bid) successful in single case (AIDS Reader 17:133, 2007).			
Lumbosacral polyradiculopathy	**Ganciclovir**, as with retinitis. Consider combination of ganciclovir & foscarnet, esp. if prior CMV rx used. Switch to **valganciclovir** when possible. Suppression continued until CD4 remains >100/mm³ for 6mos.		About 50% will respond (CID 20:747, 1995), survival ↑ (5.4wks to 14.6wks) (CID 27:345, 1998).
Mononeuritis multiplex	Not defined		Due to vasculitis & may not be responsive to antiviral rx (AnNeurol 29:139, 1991).
CMV pneumonia—seen predominantly in transplants (esp. bone marrow), **rare in HIV** Rx only when histological evidence present in AIDS pts & other pathogens not identified.	**Ganciclovir/valganciclovir**, as with retinitis. Many transplant units also use IVIG or CMV specific immune globulin as adjunctive Rx (no studies).		11/16 pts showed initial improvement with either ganciclovir or foscarnet but disease eventually progressed despite maintenance (CID 23:76, 1996). In BMT recipients, serial measure of pp65 antigen was useful in establishing early dx of CMV interstitial pneumonia with good results if GCV was initiated within 6 days of antigen positivity (Bone Marrow Transplant 26:413, 2000). For preventive therapy, see Table 10.

TABLE 12 (30)

TYPE OF INFECTION/ORGANISM/ SITE OF INFECTION	SUGGESTED REGIMENS		COMMENTS
	PRIMARY	ALTERNATIVE	

VIRAL INFECTIONS (continued)

Retinitis (most common in AIDS) Still the most common cause of blindness in AIDS patients with <50/mm3 CD4 counts. Differential dx: HIV retinopathy, herpes simplex retinitis (Arch Ophthal 114: 834, 1996), varicella-zoster retinitis (rare, hard to diagnose). 11.6% of 374 pts followed with CMV retinitis who responded to ARV RX (↑ of ≥50 CD4 cells/ ml) developed immune recovery vitreitis (vision ↓ & floaters with posterior segment inflammation —vitreitis, papillitis & macular changes) (Ophthal 113:684, 2006). Risk for IRV were large CMV retinitis lesions and use of intravitreus cidofovir. Another reported 8/21 pts receiving ARV RX had inflammatory complications (AIDS 14: 1163, 2000). Corticosteroid rx ↓ inflammatory reaction of immune recovery vitreitis without reactivation of CMV retinitis, either periocular corticosteroids or short course of systemic steroid.	**Treatment:** • **For immediate sight-threatening lesions:** **Ganciclovir** intraocular implant & **Valganciclovir** 900 mg po q24h. • **For peripheral lesions:** **Valganciclovir** 900 mg po q12h x14–21d, then 900 mg po q24h **Suppression:** • **Chronic maintenance Rx or secondary prophylaxis:** **Valganciclovir** 900 mg po q24h OR **Foscarnet** 90 mg/kg IV q24h Dc with CD4 >100 x 6 mos.	**Ganciclovir** 200 to 400 μgm/0.1 mL (of 4 mgm/ml solution) by intravitreal injection every other week until retinitis inactive: ↓ cost and useful in resource restricted regions (J Med Assoc Thai 88:Suppl9:S63, 2005). OR **Ganciclovir** 5 mg/kg IV q12h x14–21d, then **valganciclovir** 900 mg po q24h OR **Foscarnet** 60 mg/kg IV q12h x14–21d, or 90 mg/kg IV q8h x14–21d, then 90–120 mg/kg IV q24h OR **Cidofovir** 5 mg/kg IV x2wks, then 5 mg/kg every other wk; each dose should be administered with IV saline hydration & oral probenecid OR Repeated intravitreal injections with **fomivirsen** (for relapses only, not as initial therapy, active against resistant strains) **Suppression, 2°:** Chronic maintenance therapy: **Cidofovir** 5 mg/kg IV every other week with **probenecid** 2 gm po 3hrs before the dose followed by 1gm po 2hrs after the dose, & 1 gm by mouth 8hrs after the dose (total of 4 gm); OR **fomivirsen**1 vial (330 mg) injected into the vitreous, then repeated every 2–4 wks	Valganciclovir po equal to GCV IV in induction of remission: 7/71 progressed on Val & 7/70 on GCV during 1st 4wks & 72% of Val- & 77% of GCV-treated pts had satisfactory responses to induction rx. Adverse events were similar (NEJM 346:1119, 2002). Valganciclovir 900mg q24h has similar efficacy (17% progressed over 1 year) & toxicity profile as IV ganciclovir but with fewer IV-related events (J AIDS 30:392, 2002). There is also a significant ↓ in cost with oral vs IV rx (J AIDS 36:972, 2004). Cannot use GCV ocular implant alone as approx. 50% risk of CMV retinitis other eye at 6 mos. & 31% risk visceral disease. When contralateral retinitis does occur, ganciclovir-resistant mutation often present (JID 189:611, 2004). **Concurrent systemic rx recommended which reduce risk!** Complications related to implant occurred at rate of 0.064 events per pt yr and ↓ with time (Ophthal 113:683e1-8, 2006) Intravitreal ganciclovir qow effective in 827 pts with active retinitis also receiving ARV RX in Thailand. A mean of 5 cc injections necessary and no relapses but follow up only 5 mos. Complications in 7 of 51 eyes (14%) included vitreous haze, retinal detachment, endoophthalmitis & immune recovery vitreitis (J Med Assoc Thai 88:Suppl9:S63, 2005). Retinal detachments 50–60% within 1yr of dx of retinitis. In 271 AIDS pts with CMV retinitis, both 2nd eye involvement & retinal detachment markedly ↓ with ARV RX but only if good CD4 cell response (Ophthal 111:2232, 2004). Equal efficacy of IV GCV & FOS. GCV avoids nephrotoxicity of FOS; FOS avoids bone marrow suppression of GCV. (**Oral valganciclovir should replace both**) although bone marrow toxicity may be similar to ganciclovir. A single report indicates success of combination rx with GCV at ½ dose 5mg/kg/day q24h & FOS up to 125mg/kg/day for GCV-resistant isolates in solid organ transplants (CID 34:1337, 2002). Hypomagnesemia common complication. Potential emergence of resistant CMV. 27.5% pts treated 9mos developed CMV isolates resistant to GCV (JID 177:770, 1998), hence may be reason for clinical failure.
Maintenance can be discontinued if CD4 >100/mm³ x6mos. Pts who discontinue maintenance rx should undergo regular eye examination for early detection of relapses! Risk for reactivation very low 0.016 per person yr of follow up (HIV CLin Trials 7:1, 2006).			

NOTE: All dosage recommendations are for adults (unless otherwise indicated) & assume normal renal function.

TABLE 12 (31)

TYPE OF INFECTION/ORGANISM/ SITE OF INFECTION	SUGGESTED REGIMENS		COMMENTS
	PRIMARY	ALTERNATIVE	
VIRAL INFECTIONS/Retinitis *(continued)*			
Hairy leukoplakia (Epstein Barr virus, EBV)	Usually asymptomatic & no treatment indicated	**Acyclovir** (800 mg po 5x/day) or topical podophyllin resin (one application) (not currently FDA-approved for this indication)	Patients usually asymptomatic, lesions respond to rx but recur.
Hepatitis A (*Ln 351:1643, 1998*)	No therapy recommended. If within 2wks of exposure, gamma globulin 0.02 ml/kg IM injection x1 is protective.		For vaccine recommendations, see Table 19 (*MMWR 48:RR-12, 1999*). Based on increased severity of acute hepatitis A superimposed on chronic liver disease, HAV vaccine recommended for all patients with chronic liver disease (*Am J Med 118:21S, 2005*).
Hepatitis B (*see Ln 362:2089, 2003*)			
Acute	No therapy recommended		Most common cause of death from acute hepatitis in Italy (*Dig Liver Dis 35:404, 2003*)
Chronic (*AnIM 132:326, 2000*) Prevalence of post-exposure to HBV (presence of anti-HBs) is high (90–95%) in HIV+ individuals; active infection only occurs in 10–15%. Prevalence of triple infection with HIV/HCV/ HBV estimated at 1–5%. Incidence of acute HBV was 12.2 cases/1000 person-yrs in HIV-infected CDC cohort (16,248 cases). Risk factors were black race (RR 1.4), alcoholism (RR 1.7), recent injection drug use (1.6%), & history of AIDS (RR 1.5) but risk ↓ with those taking ARV RX (RR 0.6). Prevalence of chronic HBV was 7.6% (*JID 188:571, 2003*).	(See *MMWR 53:100, 2004*) For HBV in non-HIV/HBV co-infected pts, see the *Sanford Guide to Antimicrobial Therapy*. Because of lack of controlled studies, it is difficult to make specific recommendations; however, the following seem reasonable: **When ART not indicated** (*see Table 6A*): **Adefovir** (ADV) 10 mg po q24h OR **Entecavir** (ETV) 0.5 mg po fasting q24h. If previous LAM treatment or known YMDD mutation, use 1 mg q24h. Treat 1yr or min. 6mos. after seroconversion. OR **PEG INF alfa 2a** 180 mcg subcut		**ADV:** Has no activity against HIV at this dose & unlikely to generate resistant mutations. Active against HBV (and YMDD LAM mutants) in HIV co-infected pts: ↓ of 4 log$_{10}$ HBV DNA & normalization of ALT levels at 48 wks in 11 pts (*Ln 358:718, 2001*). Long-term safety not established in HIV+ pts **ETV:** Min. toxicity. Active vs YMDD LAM mutants & ADV-resistant strains. Headache & fatigue in 3–4%. (*CID 42:126, 2006*). More effective with less toxicity than lamivudine in HBeAg-positive & negative HBV. (*NEJM 354;1001, 1011 2006*). May generate nucleoside resistant mutants in HIV (*CROI #1366D, 2007*) and HBV resistance in lamivudine experienced pts! Do not use as initial rx in HIV/HBV coinfected pts. **PEG INF alfa 2a** may be superior to standard INF in HIV/HBV co-infection (*J Viral Hepat 10:298, 2003*).

NOTE: All dosage recommendations are for adults (unless otherwise indicated) & assume normal renal function.

TABLE 12 (32)

TYPE OF INFECTION/ORGANISM/ SITE OF INFECTION	SUGGESTED REGIMENS		COMMENTS
	PRIMARY	ALTERNATIVE	

VIRAL INFECTIONS/Hepatitis B (continued)

HIV infection assoc. with ↑ risk for development of chronic Hep B, ↑ HBV DNA levels, ↑ likelihood of having detectable HBeAg, ↑ in liver fibrosis/cirrhosis & ↑ risk of liver-related mortality (*Ln* 360:194, 2002). Goal of rx is to reduce HBV-related morbidity & mortality. Surrogate endpoints include sustained suppression of HBV DNA, prevention of liver disease progression & clearance of HBeAg (treated HIV+ pts rarely become HBsAg−). Rx likely ↓ risk of HCC. Occult HBV infection was present in 20% of HIV+ pts and associated with ↑ in – of hepatitis In general, **consider rx in pts with persistent ↑ of aminotransferase; detectable levels of HBsAg & HBV DNA in serum (levels >10^5 copies/ml) for at least 6mos; hepatitis on liver bx; & compensated liver disease.** **Always treat HBV if treating HIV!** **New DHHS Guidelines recommend treating HBV as an indication for ARV Rx.**	**Lamivudine-naïve pts requiring ART:** OR **Tenofovir** 300 mg + **emtricitabine** 200 mg as Truvada^{NFDA-1} po q24h looks promising, plus additional agents to achieve ARV RX OR **Entecavir** (ETV) 0.5 mg po fasting q24h OR	**Lamivudine** (LAM) 150 mg po q12h + **Tenofovir** (TDF) 300 mg po q24h + Additional agents to achieve ARV RX	When selecting antiretroviral drugs for HIV, it is critical to also consider the effect of the drugs on Hep B virus. It is now possible to effectively treat both infections with the same drug combinations (*AIDS Res Hum Retrovir* 22:842, 2006; *CID* 43:904, 2006). Tenofovir (TDF) effective in ↓ HBV DNA in retroviral rx-experienced: ↓ 4.9 log$_{10}$ (10 pts) after 10wks vs ↑ 1.2 log$_{10}$ in placebo (2 pts) (p .041). Retroviral rx-naive: 4.7 log$_{10}$ ↓ with tenofovir + lamivudine (5 pts) vs 3.0 log$_{10}$ ↓ with lamivudine (6 pts) (p .055) (*JID* 189: 1185, 2004). In another retrospective study, simultaneous therapy with LAM and TDF more effective in ↓ HBV DNA than LAM alone or whe TDF added to LAM (*J Viral Hepat* 14:176, 2007). Some reports of renal toxicity & hypophosphatemia with tenofovir in HIV co-infected pts. Long term effects on HBV resistance unknown. In non-HIV infected, lamivudine alone effective until YMDD mutations arise; rate of development is approx. 20%/year among HIV/HBV co-infected pts receiving lamivudine alone (*Hepatol* 30:1320, 1999). Hepatitis flares & occ. hepatic decompensation may occur when YMDD mutations "break through" (*NEJM* 351:1521, 2004). Rx with lamivudine for 1 year resulted in seroconversion of HBeAg+ to HBeAb+ in 22% (*JID* 180:609, 1999).
	OR Add **PEG INF alfa 2a** 180 mcg subQ/wk to ARV RX **Lamivudine-experienced pts requiring ART:** **Tenofovir** 300 mg + **emtricitabine** 200 mg as Truvada^{NFDA-1} po q24h looks promising, plus additional agents to achieve ARV RX OR **Tenofovir** 300 mg po q24h as part of ART regimen ± lamivudine		Duration of INF alfa rx: HBeAg+ 16–24wks, HBeAg− min 12mos See *Comments* above for lamivudine-naive pts. Addition of lamivudine continued but unlikely to add much when YMDD mutations present (>90% with 4yrs 3TC rx) (*Antiviral Therapy* 8:257, 2004). TDF alone as effective in Rx of HBV as TDF + LAM in LAM failures in 75 HIV/HBV co-infected pts (*AIDS* 20:1951, 2006). Both TDF and ADV effective in ARV experienced pts albeit TDF had greater reduction in HBV DNS (-4.4 vs 3.2 log)(*Hepatol* 44:1110, 2006). ADV resistant mutations emerged in LAM experienced pts: after ADV Rx at 6 mos—0%, 12 mos—6.5%, 18 mos—24.6%, 24 mos—38.3%. Emergence of ADV resistance associated with ↓ effectiveness of Rx and ↑ rates of cirrhosis (*Antivir Ther* 11:771, 2006). Actual rate of emergence of ADV resistance overall still unclear. Truvada effective in pts failing to respond to ADV-containing regimens (*Eur J Gastroenterol Hepat* 18:1247, 2006). ARV RX should always include HBV therapy to minimize immune reconstitution flares.

NOTE: All dosage recommendations are for adults (unless otherwise indicated) & assume normal renal function.

TABLE 12 (33)

TYPE OF INFECTION/ORGANISM/ SITE OF INFECTION	SUGGESTED REGIMENS		COMMENTS
	PRIMARY	ALTERNATIVE	

VIRAL INFECTIONS (continued)

Hepatitis C (up to 3% of world infected, 4 million in U.S.) See *NEJM 345:41, 2001; CID 33:1728, 2001; AnIM 136:747, 2002*

Acute: Most pts asymptomatic (>75%), occasionally non-specific complaints such as fatigue.	PEG INF + ribavirin, *as below*, but remains controversial; requires confirmation (*NEJM 346:1091, 2002*).		Data emerging that early rx of acute hepatitis C with INF alfa 2b may reduce progression to chronic Hep C infection: 43/44 pts in Germany with pos. HCV RNA (mean 54 days to signs/symptoms of hepatitis & mean 89 days to start of rx after exposure/infection) had neg. HCV RNA & normal ALT after 24wks of INF alfa 2b rx (*NEJM 345:1452, 2001*). A review of published trials (206 pts) concluded that SVR following rx of acute Hep C with INF alfa 2b was 32% vs 4% with placebo (p=0.00007) (*Cochrane Database Sys & Rev:CD000369, 2002*). No data available in HCV/HIV co-infected pts.

Chronic: see 2002 NIH consensus statement, http://consensus.nih.gov/cons/116/116cdc_intro.htm.
Genotype 1 is most common in U.S. (>75%), & least responsive to rx in HIV/HCV co-infected pts (*CID 34:831, 2002*).

Hepatitis C & HIV are closely linked conditions & frequently occur in the same pts; >80% of IVDUs & 8–10% of men who have sex with men have HCV compared to 0.4% of routine blood donors in the U.S. Overall 37% of HIV+ persons in the U.S. are also infected with HCV (*CID 34:831, 2002*). As CD4 cells ↓, HCV titers ↑, resulting in a ↑ in perinatal & sexual transmission of HCV & an acceleration of HCV disease (cirrhosis); after 20 yrs, 40% of HCV-infected individuals will have developed cirrhosis vs 10% of HIV-infected individuals without HCV (*Hepatology 34: 193, 2001*). The rate of progression to cirrhosis in HCV disease is ↑ by 3.6-fold in HIV-infected individuals (*CID 33:562, 2001; AIDS 17: 1803, 2003*); endstage liver disease has emerged as a common cause of death in co-infected individuals accounting for 11% of deaths in 1991, 14% in 1994 & 50% in 1998 (*AnIM 136:747, 2002 & 138:197, 2003; AIDS 16:813, 2002*). The rate of liver related hospital admissions and deaths peaked in 2002 in Spain and has decreased significantly since (*J Virol Hepat 13:851, 2006*).

The impact of HCV on the course of HIV infection & response to ARV RX remains inconclusive (*Ln 362:1687, 2003*). HCV infection appeared to accelerate HIV progression in 1 study: HR 1.7 for progression to new AIDS-defining event (*CID 36:97, 2003*). However, in another large (1,955 pts) prospective study, no impact of HCV on progression to AIDS, death, or response to ARV RX was found (*CID 33:1579, 2002*).

- Standard HCV antibody testing was falsely negative in 20% of HIV co-infected pts; check HCV RNA by PCR in pts with neg. HCV Ab & ↑ ALT (*Hepatol 36/4, Abst. 746, 53rd AASLD, 2002*). Both HCV & HIV appear to complicate rx of the co-infecting virus. HIV may reduce effectiveness of HCV rx & HCV effectiveness of ARV RX on HIV while significantly ↑ risk of ARV RX hepatotoxicity (↑ X3).
- Therefore, it seems prudent to rx HCV 1st if HIV is not advanced (CD4 >300 & VL <55,000). Pegylated INF itself may ↓ CD4 counts (↓ 194 cells/mm^3) & accelerate HIV (*Int AIDS Conf, Barcelona, 2002, Abst. LB Or 16*). **If ARV RX indicated (CD4 <200–300/mm3), rx HIV 1st; it is clear now that ARV RX improves survival in co-infected pts & even ↓ longterm liver-related mortality from HCV** (*Ln 362: 1708, 2003*). Don't start with both simultaneously—too complicated & ↑ toxicity.
- Equally important is treatment of IVDU & alcoholism; both impact negatively on response to rx & will likely reduce compliance to regimens.

NOTE: All dosage recommendations are for adults (unless otherwise indicated) & assume normal renal function.

TABLE 12 (34)

TYPE OF INFECTION/ORGANISM/ SITE OF INFECTION	SUGGESTED REGIMENS		COMMENTS
	PRIMARY	ALTERNATIVE	

VIRAL INFECTIONS/VIRAL INFECTIONS (continued)

Ref.: www.va.gov/hepatitisc
Rx recommended for all HCV/HIV co-infected pts with persistent elevations ALT, HCV RNA+, & findings of fibrosis & at least moderate inflammation by liver bx.*
	Genotypes 1 & 4 in HIV co-infected patients (AnIM 140:346, 2004):
	
	Pegylated Interferon + Ribavirin
	
	Pegylated INF:
	Either **Alfa 2a (Pegasys)**
	180 mcg subQ q wk
	OR
	Alfa 2b (PEG-Intron)
	1.5 mcg/kg subQ q wk
	
	Weight Ribavirin Dose*
	<75 kg 400 mg am & 600 mg pm
	>75 kg 600 mg am & 600 mg pm
	
	Monitor response by quantification:
	HCV RNA Result Action
	After 4 wks rx: <1 log ↓ Discontinue therapy
	After 12 wks rx: <2 log ↓ Discontinue therapy
	    >2 log ↓ or undetectable Treat 48 wks
	
	Genotype 2 or 3 In HIV co-infected patients:**
	PEG IFN alfa-2a or 2b—dose as types 1 & 4 above + **Ribavirin 400 mg po bid**
	
	Monitor response by quantification:
	HCV RNA Result Action
	After 4 wks rx: <1 log ↓ Discontinue therapy
	After 12 wks rx: <2 log ↓ Discontinue therapy
	    >2 log ↓ or undetectable Treat 48 wks
	
	* Standard ribavirin dose in 3 major clinical trials was 800mg q24h; however, several trials both in HCV/HIV co-infected & HCV alone support higher doses recommended here (ICAAC 2004, Abst. V-1148; AnIM 140: 346, 2004).
	**Some would only rx genotypes 2 & 3 for 24wks, but most studies with HCV/HIV co-infected pts have rx for 48wks (AIDS 19:s3, S166, 2005).
			Obtain baseline CBC & at wks 2 & 4 of rx (see Table 13, page 169); hemolytic anemia very common with ribavirin. In nearly 1500 HCV/HIV co-infected pts, 3 prospective randomized trials reported in late 2004 demonstrated superiority of 48 wks of PEG INF (180mcg q wk) + ribavirin (800mg q24h) over standard INF alfa + ribavirin (NEJM 351:438 & 451, 2004; JAMA 292:2839, 2004; APRICOT, ACTG, RIBAV/C). Sustained viral response (SVR) was lower than previously reported in non-co-infected pts (27%–40% vs 55–60%). SVR was 14–29% for genotype 1 & 44–73% for genotype 2 or 3. As in other trials, lack of response at 12wks predicted failure at 48wks: in ACTG study, 63 pts (59%) who failed to ↓ HCV RNA by 2 logs or to neg, 0 had SVR at 48wks. Of the pts in ACTG study who failed to achieve SVR, 35% did have histological response by liver biopsy. 15 pts developed pancreatitis; all were receiving ddl-containing ARV RX. Don't use ddl with ribavirin! 14/133 cirrhotic pts developed hepatic decompensation during rx & 6 died (APRICOT, AIDS 18:F21, 2004; J AIDS 40:47, 2005). Watch cirrhotic pts carefully during PEG-INF/ribavirin rx.
			African Americans respond less well to INF & RIB compared to Caucasians (Am J Gastroenterol 131:470, 2006).
			Excessive **alcohol consumption** (>5oz/day) **accelerates hepatic fibrosis** from HCV (Ln 349: 825, 1997). Occult HBV or HIV infection might account for lack of response to rx in some pts (NEJM 341:22, 1999; CID 36:1564, 2003).
			Side effects significant: 10–14% receiving PEG INF-Rib dc rx 2° to side effects (flu-like symptoms, hematological & particularly neuropsychiatric abnormalities. **2002 FDA warning:** Intron can cause or aggravate life-threatening neuropsychiatric, autoimmune, ischemic & infectious disorders—monitor closely). See Table 13, page 169. **Ribavirin is teratogenic & must not be used if pregnancy possible in pt or partner.**

NOTE: All dosage recommendations are for adults (unless otherwise indicated) & assume normal renal function.

TABLE 12 (35)

TYPE OF INFECTION/ORGANISM/ SITE OF INFECTION	SUGGESTED REGIMENS		COMMENTS
	PRIMARY	ALTERNATIVE	
VIRAL INFECTIONS/Hepatitis C (continued)			
Prevention **Risk factors:** (1) contaminated blood via transfusion (1/100,000 per unit in U.S.); (2) injection drug use (in IVDU, prevalence of Hep C 79%); (3) occupation exposure—risk of infection from needlestick from HCV+ source is 1.8%, highest from hollow-bore needles; (4) sexual activity risk low but male → female > female → male. HCV recovered from 36.4% cervical secretions in 22 HCV+ women (*CID 35:966, 2002*). Perinatal transmission: infants born to HCV+ mothers have 5–6% risk of infection (when co-infection of HCV + HIV, risk is 14%)			See *MMWR 47(RR-19), Oct. 16, 1998*. Although interferon + ribavirin is now approved for rx of chronic hepatitis C (*see Table 13, page 169*), not recommended for post-exposure prophylaxis. IG not effective. Early treatment of HCV seroconversion in 7 pts (with persistent HCV RNA for 12–20wks following exposure) with INF-alfa alone x1yr achieved sustained response in 7/7 pts (*Gastroenterol 130:632, 2006*). Thus, early rx of acute infection may be advisable but data lacking on optimal regimens & duration.
Herpes simplex virus (HSV) Genital herpes ↑ transmission and acquisition of HIV (See *JAIDS 35:435, 2004; Ln 357:1149, 2001*)			
Mucocutaneous (oral, anal, genital, skin) **Treatment** Mild	Acyclovir 400 mg po q8h x7–14d **OR** Famciclovir 500 mg po q12h x7–14d **OR** Valacyclovir 1000 mg po q12h x7–14d^NFDA No data on treating recurrences in HIV+ pts— use recommendations for treating HIV- pts.	Chronic suppression indicated if frequent recurrences &/or extensive disease. 1% foscarnet cream applied 5x/day in acyclovir-unresponsive ulcers had 65–90% partial to complete response (*J AIDS 21:301, 1999*). Famciclovir approved for "fever blister" at 1500 mg po x 1 dose and for acute exacerbations of genital lesions at 1000 mg po bid x one day for normal hosts. Not yet approved for HIV-infected persons at these doses.	
Severe—extensive disease, systemic toxicity	Acyclovir 5 mg/kg q8h IV x5–10d [For encephalitis, ↑ to 10 mg/kg IV q8h x10 d] After lesions begin to heal, switch to famciclovir 500 mg po q12h or valacyclovir 1000 mg po q12h, or acyclovir 400 mg po q8h. Continue rx until lesions have completely healed.	If acyclovir-resistant: Foscarnet 40–60 mg/kg q8h IV **OR** Cidofovir 5 mg/kg IV q wk until clinical response	Severe disease not responding to acyclovir may represent resistant virus. Acyclovir-resistant HSV occurs, esp. in large ulcers. Most will respond to IV foscarnet, but recur after drug discontinued [median 6wks (*NEJM 325:551, 1991*)]. HSV that becomes resistant to both acyclovir & foscarnet will usually remain sensitive to cidofovir (*JID 180:487, 1999*).
Suppression, post-treatment; only if recurrences are frequent or severe See *CID 39(Suppl.5):S237, 2004*	Acyclovir 400 mg po q12h or 200 mg po q8h indefinitely. [Higher doses 800 mg 4x/d more effective in 1 study (*5th CRV, Abst. 499*)] **OR** Famciclovir 250–500 mg po q12h **OR** Valacyclovir 500 mg po q24h approved for HIV-infected pts with CD4 count ≥100. If acyclovir-resistant: Foscarnet 40 mg/kg IV q24h indefinitely		NOTE: For pts taking acyclovir for chronic suppression who then develop CMV retinitis, stop acyclovir when ganciclovir started—GCV active vs H. simplex. Suppressive rx with famciclovir (500mg po q12h) reduced viral shedding & clinical recurrences (total days with lesions 18% vs 5%) in HIV-infected pts (*AnIM 128:21, 1998*), similar to findings with acyclovir. Valacyclovir (500mg po q12h) rx of HIV-infected pt: at 6mos, 65% were recurrence-free vs 26% receiving placebo (*package insert, Valtrex*). Effective suppression with valacyclovir decreased genital HSV and HIV shedding while also reducing plasma HIV RNA levels. *Will it also reduce HIV transmission?* (*NEJM 356:790, 2007*).
Human herpesvirus 8 (Kaposi's sarcoma-associated herpesvirus) See *JCI 113:21, 2004*	See *Table 18, Treatment of HIV-Associated Malignancies*. Effective suppression of HIV-1 replication with ART has best chance of preventing progression of KS or occurrence of new lesions.		Virus appears to be spread by saliva (*JID 190:199, 2004*). HHV8-associated Castleman disease responds to ARV RX with immune reconstitution, but relapse of disease still occurred. Survival was 48mos. (*CID 35:880, 2002*).

NOTE: All dosage recommendations are for adults (unless otherwise indicated) & assume normal renal function.

TABLE 12 (36)

TYPE OF INFECTION/ORGANISM/ SITE OF INFECTION	SUGGESTED REGIMENS		COMMENTS
	PRIMARY	ALTERNATIVE	
VIRAL INFECTIONS (continued)			
Human papillomavirus (HPV): Condyloma acuminatum (CA) (anogenital warts) (MMWR 53:46, 2004) Progression of disease correlates with ↑ HIV RNA in plasma (JID 179:1405, 1999). Rate of recurrence is high, esp. in HIV+ pts, despite rx. For rx of cervical or anal intraepithelial neoplasia (CIN & AIN), see MMWR 53 (RR-15):46 & 91, 2004.	**Patient-applied:** **Podofilox** 0.5% solution or 0.5% gel. Apply to all lesions q12h x3 consecutive days. Repeat weekly for up to 4wks. OR **Imiquimod** 5% cream; apply to lesions at bedtime & remove in morning on 3 consecutive nights, weekly for up to 16wks.	**Provider-applied:** Liquid nitrogen cryotherapy—apply until each lesion is thoroughly frozen; repeat every 1–2wks x3–4 times **Trichloroacetic acid or bichloracetic acid cauterization 80–95% aqueous solution**—apply to each lesion; repeat weekly for 3–6wks Podophyllin resin 10–25% suspension in tincture of benzoin—apply to area & wash off in a few hrs; repeat weekly for up to 3–6wks Surgical excision or laser surgery	Do not rx cervical warts until results of Pap smear known. Avoid podophyllin & podofilox in pregnant women. Alternatives: cryotherapy with liquid nitrogen, electrocautery. Cidofovir topical gel + surgical excision 100% effective in achieving complete response in 19 pts but 27% relapsed (AIDS 16:447, 2002).
Molluscum contagiosum virus (See Curr Opin Inf Dis 12:185, 1999)	**Treatment:** Usually rx with destructive modalities: cryotherapy with liquid nitrogen, light electrocautery, or curettage. **Suppression:** Retinoic acid (Retin A)' applied once nightly to face may ↓ rate of appearance but does not affect established lesions.	3 pts also responded to either IV or topical cidofovir (1% cream) (5th CRV, Abst. 504; Ln 353:2042, 1999).	Interferon alfa is not effective. Spontaneous resolution observed in pts with good response to combination antiretroviral therapy. Retinoic acid cannot be used on eyelids or genitalia. Lesions in disseminated cryptococcosis, histoplasmosis may resemble molluscum contagiosum.
Parvovirus B-19 "Pure red cell aplasia"	**Immunoglobulin G:** 2gm/kg IVIG given over 2 days. Most pts with <80 CD4/mm³ suffer relapse within 6mos. & require re-rx with IVIG. Maintenance rx with IVIG 0.4gm/kg q4wks effective in preventing relapses; probably not necessary if CD4 count >300/mm³ (Am J Hematol 61:16, 1999).		Persistent parvovirus B-19 infection is a cause of anemia in HIV+ pts. Found in 1/3 HIV+ pts (J Invest Med 45:65A, 1997). Essentially all pts (27) reported have responded to IVIG (Am J Hematol 61:16, 1999).
Progressive multifocal leukoencephalopathy (PML) (JC virus) Usually in pts with advanced HIV disease (see Table 11A, page 79)	ARV RX ↑ survival (545days vs 60days; p < 0.001) & either improved (50%) or stabilized (50%) neurological deficits n 12 pts (AIDS 12:2467, 1999). Pts have experienced ↑ neurological manifestations (including death) after initiating ARV RX—possibly due to IRIS.		Cytarabine of no value in controlled trial (NEJM 338:1345, 1998). Camptothecin, a human topoisomerase I inhibitor, was administered to a single pt with slowing of progression (Ln 349:1366, 1997).
Varicella zoster virus (VZV) ↑ frequency of zoster reported within 2 mos. of starting ARV RX (7% of 193 pts) (5th CRV, Abst. 501). PCR for VZV DNA in CSF for CNS infection helpful for dx (J Neurovirol 15:172, 1999). Herpes zoster (shingles) (CID 44:Suppl:S1, 2007)			Treatment must be begun within 72hrs of onset of vesicles. Chronic post-treatment suppression not required. Acyclovir: adjust dose if renal function ↓. Acyclovir-resistant VZV occurs in HIV pts previously rx with acyclovir & is associated with poor prognosis. However, in 11 pts who failed 10 days acyclovir, only 3 had in vitro resistance (mutation of thymidine kinase gene) & no resistance developed on rx. Authors recommend 21 days of rx in such cases (CID 33:2061, 2001). Foscarnet: 4/5 pts rx responded, although 2 relapsed within 14 days. (An M 115:19, 1991; J AIDS 7:254, 1994).
Not severe (local dermatomal zoster)	**Acyclovir** 800 mg po 5 x/day OR **Famciclovir** 500 mg po tid OR **Valacyclovir** 1 gm po tid^NFDAI All for 7–10 days		
Severe (extensive cutaneous, >1 dermatome, trigeminal nerve or visceral involvement)	**Acyclovir** (Zovirax) 10 mg/kg IV (infuse over 1hr) q8h. Continue until cutaneous & visceral disease clearly resolved.	**Foscarnet** 40mg/kg IV (infuse over 2hrs) q8h or 60mg IV q12h for 14–26 days. *Especially if previous Rx with acyclovir documented acyclovir resistance.*	

NOTE: All dosage recommendations are for adults (unless otherwise indicated) & assume normal renal function.

TABLE 12 (37)

TYPE OF INFECTION/ORGANISM/ SITE OF INFECTION	SUGGESTED REGIMENS		COMMENTS
	PRIMARY	ALTERNATIVE	
VIRAL INFECTIONS / Varicella zoster virus (VZV) *(continued)*			
Varicella (chickenpox) Mortality high (43%) in AIDS pts *(Int J Inf Dis 6:6, 2002)*	Acyclovir 10 mg/kg IV (infuse over 1hr) q8h x7d	Switch to oral rx (acyclovir 800 mg po 5x/day or famciclovir 500 mg po q8h or valacyclovir 1 gm po q8h) after defervescence if no evidence for visceral involvement *(MMWR 53:99, 2004)*.	Adjust dosage if renal function ↓.

CAUSATIVE AGENT/DISEASE	MODIFYING CIRCUMSTANCES	SUGGESTED REGIMENS		COMMENTS
		PRIMARY	ALTERNATIVE	
MISCELLANEOUS CONDITIONS				
Aphthous ulcers, recurrent (RAU)		**Thalidomide** 200 mg po q24h x14–28d or 400 mg po q24h x7d followed by 200 mg q24h x7wks. **CAUTION: Severe teratogenicity—pregnancy category X!** Contraindicated in women who are or have potential to become pregnant. Men must use condoms because drug appears in semen. *Restricted distribution; prescribers must be registered.* Teratogenicity may occur after a single dose. Not an approved indication. Numerous adverse effects including: somnolence, rash (incl. Stevens-Johnson), photosensitivity, neuropathy, ↓ WBC, venous thrombosis.		16/29 pts responded to 200mg q24h vs 2/28 placebo. Side effects: somnolence 7/29 & rash 6/29 *(NEJM 336:1487, 1997)*. In another study, 8/11 responded to 200 q24h; 4 had somnolence, 2 rash *(JID 180:61, 1999)*. 9/10 responded to high-dose (400 mg q24h) but 8/10 developed rash *(CID 28:892, 1999)*.
Gingivitis (periodontitis/stomatitis) (See Table 11A, page 90)		Topical Betadine & chlorhexidine gluconate (Peridex) mouthwash + antibiotics effective vs anaerobes (metronidazole, clindamycin or amoxicillin/clavulanate).[1] Often requires curettage debridement.		
Psoriasis	Mild to moderate	Topical therapy: emollients, steroids + tar products or equivalent		Methotrexate rx has been associated with rapid immune suppression & death *(AnIM 106:19, 1987)*.
	Severe	Skin lesions may improve with initiation of ARV RX *(Lancet ID 7:496, 2007; Skin Ther Lett 12: 1, 2007)*		
Seborrheic dermatitis	Scalp, mild-moderate	Regular use of dandruff shampoo containing selenium sulfide (Selsun), zinc pyrithione (Head & Shoulders, Danex, Zincon) or sulfur/salicylic acid (Vanseb, Sebulex) + medium potency steroid solution (triamcinolone 0.1%), ketoconazole shampoo (2%).		Extremely common in HIV+ patients. Involves hairy areas of scalp, face, chest, back & groin.
	Facial, trunk, &/or groin	Topical imidazole cream (ketoconazole 2%, clotrimazole 1%) + low potency topical steroid (hydrocortisone 1–2.5%, desonide 0.05%) applied 2x q24h		For refractory trunk lesions, ↑ strength of topical steroid. For severe disease, ketoconazole 200–400mg po q24h x2–4wks

[1] This is the regimen used by JS Greenspan, *MEDICAL MANAGEMENT OF AIDS*, 6th Ed. Eds.: MA Sande, PA Volberding. W.B. Saunders & Co., 1999

NOTE: All dosage recommendations are for adults (unless otherwise indicated) & assume normal renal function.

TABLE 13: DRUGS USED IN TREATMENT &/OR CHRONIC SUPPRESSION OF AIDS-RELATED INFECTIONS: ADVERSE EFFECTS, COMMENTS, COST

DRUG NAME, GENERIC (TRADE)/ USUAL DOSAGE	ADVERSE EFFECTS/COMMENTS
ANTIFUNGAL DRUGS	
Non-lipid amphotericin B deoxycholate (Fungizone): 0.3–1 mg/kg/day as single infusion 50 mg Mixing ampho B with lipid emulsion results in precipitation & is discouraged.	**Admin:** Ampho B is a colloidal suspension that must be prepared in electrolyte-free D5W at 0.1 mg/ml to avoid precipitation. No need to protect drug suspensions from light. Ampho B infusions cause chills/fever, myalgia, anorexia, nausea, rarely hemodynamic collapse/hypotension. Postulated due to proinflammatory cytokines but does not appear to be histamine release. Manufacturer recommends a test dose of 1 mg, but often not done (1st few ml of 1st dose is a test dose). Duration of infusion usually 4 or more hrs. No difference found in 1- vs 4-hr infusions except chills/fever occurred sooner with 1-hr. infusion. Febrile reactions decrease with repeated doses. Rare pulmonary reactions (severe dyspnea & focal infiltrates suggesting pulmonary edema) associated with rapid infusion. Severe rigors respond to meperidine (25–50mg IV). Premedication with acetaminophen, diphenhydramine, hydrocortisone (25–50mg) & heparin (1000 units) had no influence on rigors/fever. If cytokine postulate correct, NSAIDs or high-dose steroids may prove efficacious but their use may risk worsening infection under rx or increased risk of nephrotoxicity (i.e., NSAIDs). Clinical side effects ↓ with ↑ age. **Toxicity:** Major concern is nephrotoxicity (15% cf 102 pts surveyed). Manifest initially by kaliuresis & hypokalemia, then fall in serum bicarbonate (may proceed to renal tubular acidosis),↓ in renal erythropoietin & anemia, & rising BUN/serum creatinine. Hypomagnesemia may occur. Can reduce risk of renal injury by **(a) pre- & post-infusion hydration with 500ml saline (if clinical status will allow salt load)**, (b) avoidance of other nephrotoxins, e.g., radiocontrast, aminoglycosides, cis-platinum, (c) use of lipid prep of ampho B. Use of low-dose dopamine did not significantly reduce renal toxicity.
Lipid-based ampho B products:[1,2] Amphotericin B lipid complex (ABLC) (Abelcet): 5 mg/kg/day as single infusion	**Admin:** Consists of ampho B complexed with 2 lipid bilayer ribbons. Compared to standard ampho B, larger volume of distribution, rapid blood clearance & high tissue concentrations (liver, spleen, lung). Dosage: **5mg/kg q24h;** infuse at 2.5mg/kg/hr; adult & ped. dose the same. DO NOT use an in-line filter. Do not dilute with saline or mix with other drugs or electrolytes.[3] **Toxicity:** Fever & chills in 14–18%; nausea 9%, vomiting 8%; serum creatinine ↑ in 11%; renal failure 5%; anemia 4%; ↓ K 5%; rash 4%.
Liposomal amphotericin B (L-AmB, AmBisome): 1–5 mg/kg/day as single infusion.	**Admin:** Consists of vesicular bilayer liposome with ampho B intercalated within the membrane. Dosage: **3–5mg/kg/day** IV as single dose infused over a period of approx. 120min. If infusion is well tolerated, infusion time can be reduced to 60min.[2] 1mg/kg/day was as effective as 4mg/kg/day (6mos. survival rates 43% vs 37%, respectively) in pts with invasive aspergillosis complicating bone marrow transplant &/or neutropenia from malignancy (CID 27:1406, 1998). **Major toxicity:** Generally less than ampho B. Nephrotoxicity 18.7% vs 33.7% for ampho B, chills 47% vs 75%, nausea 39.7% vs 38.7%, vomiting 31.8% vs 43.9%, rash 24% for both, ↓ Ca 18.4% vs 20.9%, ↓ K 20.4% vs 25.6%, ↓ Mg 20.4% vs 25.6%. Acute infusion-related reactions are common with liposomal ampho B, 20–40%. 86% occurred within 5 min. of infusion, including chest pain, dyspnea & hypoxia or severe abdominal, flank or leg pain; 14% developed flushing & urticaria near the end of 4-hr infusion. All responded to diphenhydramine (1mg/kg) & interruption of L-AmB infusion. These reactions may be due to complement activation by the liposome.

[1] Published data from patients intolerant of or refractory to conventional ampho B deoxycholate (Amp B). **In general ampho B lipid formulations are not superior to ampho B in efficacy in prospective trials although they are less nephrotoxic.**

[2] Comparisons between Abelcet & AmBisome suggest higher infusion-assoc. toxicity (rigors) & febrile episodes with Abelcet (70% vs 36%) but a higher frequency of mild hepatic toxicity with AmBisome (59% vs 38%, p=0.05). Mild elevations in serum creatinine were observed in 1/3 of both.

TABLE 13 (2)

DRUG NAME, GENERIC (TRADE)/ USUAL DOSAGE	ADVERSE EFFECTS/COMMENTS
ANTIFUNGAL DRUGS (continued)	
Caspofungin (Cancidas) 70 mg IV on day 1 followed by 50 mg IV q24h (reduce to 35 mg IV q24h with moderate hepatic insufficiency) Ref.: *Ln 362:1142, 2003*	An echinocandin which inhibits synthesis of β-(1,3)-D-glucan, a critical component of fungal cell walls. Fungicidal against candida (MIC <2 mcg/ml) including those resistant to other antifungals & active against aspergillus (MIC 0.4-2.7 mcg/ml). Serum levels on rec. dosages = peak 12, trough 1.3 (24hrs) mcg/ml. Approved for rx of candidemia & other candida infections (intra-abdominal abscess, esophageal peritonitis, pleural sponge infection) & refractory aspergillus infections & was successful as salvage Rx in approx half of pts with invasive aspergillus infections in severely impaired hosts. **Toxicity:** remarkably non-toxic with no nephrotoxicity reported. Only 2% of 263 pts in double-blind trial dc drug due to drug-related adverse event. 14% had ↑ transaminases (similar to triazoles). Most common adverse effect: pruritus at infusion site & headache, fever, chills, vomiting, & diarrhea associated with infusion. Drug metabolized in liver & dosage ↓ to 35mg in moderate to severe hepatic failure. Class C for pregnancy (embryotoxic in rats & rabbits), so only use if potential benefits outweigh risks. See Table 16A *for drug-drug interactions, esp. cyclosporine (hepatic toxicity) & tacrolimus (drug level monitoring recommended).*
Micafungin (Mycamine) 150 mg/day IV for esophageal candidiasis; 100 mg/day IV for candidemia; 50 mg per day for prophylaxis post-bone marrow stem cell transplant	The 2nd echinocandin approved by the FDA (March 2005) for rx of esophageal candidiasis & for prophylaxis against candida infections in HSCT recipients. Active against most strains of candida sp. & aspergillus sp. including those resistant to fluconazole such as *C. glabrata & C. krusei*. No antagonism seen when combined with other antifungal drugs & occ. synergism with ampho B *(AAC 49:2994, 2005)*. No dosage adjustment for severe renal failure or moderate hepatic impairment. Low potential for drug interactions. Micafungin is well tolerated & common adverse events include nausea 7.8%, vomiting 2.4%, & headache 2.4%. Transient ↑ LFTs, BUN, creatinine reported; rare cases of significant hepatitis & renal insufficiency *(package insert for micafungin).*
Anidulafungin (Eraxis) 200 mg IV on day 1 followed by 100 mg/day IV; for esophageal candidiasis 100 mg IV times 1, then 50 mg IV q24h	An echinocandin with antifungal activity (cidal) against candida sp. & aspergillus sp. including ampho B- & triazole-resistant strains. Effective in clinical trials of esophageal candidiasis & in 1 trial was superior to fluconazole in rx of invasive candidiasis/candidemia *(NEJM 356:2472, 2007).* Like other echinocandins, remarkably non-toxic; most common side effects: nausea, vomiting, ↓ Mg, ↓ K & headache in 11–13% of pts. No dose adjustments for renal or hepatic insufficiency. Few drug-drug interactions.
Fluconazole (Diflucan) (available generically) 100 mg tabs 150 mg tabs 200 mg tabs 400 mg IV Oral suspension: 50 mg/5ml	IV=oral dose because of excellent bioavailability. Pharmacology: absorbed po, water solubility enables IV. Peak serum levels *(see Table 14).* T½ 30 hrs (range 20–50hrs). 12% protein bound. **CSF levels 50–90% of serum in normals,** ↑ in meningitis. No effect on mammalian steroid metabolism. **Drug-drug interactions common, see Table 16A.** Side effects overall 16% [more common in HIV+ pts (21%)]. Nausea 3.7%, headache 1.9%, skin rash 1.8%, abdominal pain 1.7%, vomiting 1.7%, diarrhea 1.5%, ↑ SGOT 20%. Alopecia (scalp, pubic crest) in 12–20% pts on ≥400 mg po q24h after median of 3mos (reversible in approx. 6mo). Rare: severe hepatotoxicity, exfoliative dermatitis. Anaphylaxis, thrombocytopenia, leukopenia.
Flucytosine (Ancobon) 500 mg cap	AEs: Overall 30%. GI 6% (diarrhea, anorexia, nausea, vomiting); hematologic 22% [leukopenia, thrombocytopenia, when serum level > 100mcg/ml (esp. in azotemic pts)]; hepatotoxicity (asymptomatic ↑ SGOT, reversible); skin rash 7%; aplastic anemia (rare—2 or 3 cases). False ↑ in serum creatinine on EKTACHEM analyzer.

TABLE 13 (3)

DRUG NAME, GENERIC (TRADE)/ USUAL DOSAGE	ADVERSE EFFECTS/COMMENTS
ANTIFUNGAL DRUGS *(continued)*	
Griseofulvin (Fulvicin, Grifulvin, Grisactin) 500 mg tab; Susp 125 mg/mL	Photosensitivity, urticaria, GI upset, fatigue, leukopenia (rare). Interferes with warfarin drugs. Increases blood & urine porphyrins, should not be used in patients with porphyria. Minor disulfiram-like reactions. Exacerbation of systemic lupus erythematosus.
Imidazoles, topical — For vaginal &/or skin use	Not recommended in 1st trimester of pregnancy. Local reactions: 0.5-1.5%: dyspareunia, mild vaginal or vulvar erythema, burning, pruritus, urticaria, rash. Rarely similar symptoms in sexual partner.
Itraconazole (Sporanox) 100 mg cap; 10 mg/mL oral solution (fasting state)	**Itraconazole tablet & solution forms are not interchangeable, solution preferred.** Many authorities recommend measuring drug serum concentration after 2 wks on prolonged rx to ensured satisfactory absorption. To obtain the highest plasma concentration, the tablet is given with food & acidic drinks (e.g., cola) while the solution is taken in the fasted state; under these conditions, the peak conc. of the capsule is approx. 3 μg/ml & of the solution 5.4mcg/ml. Peak levels are reached faster (2.2 vs 5hrs) with the solution. **Peak plasma concentrations after IV injection (200mg) compared to oral capsule (200mg): 2.8 μg/ml (on day 7 of rx) vs 2 μg/ml (on day 35 of rx).** Protein-binding for both preparations is over 99%, which explains the virtual absence of penetration into the CSF **(do not use to treat meningitis)**. Most common adverse effects are dose-related nausea 10%, diarrhea 8%, vomiting 6%, & abdominal discomfort 5.7%. Allergic rash 8.6%, ↑ bilirubin 6%, edema 3.5%, & hepatitis 2.7% reported. ↑ doses may produce hypokalemia 8% & ↑ blood pressure 3.2%. Thrombocytopenia & leukopenia reported. Delirium reported *(Psychosomatics 44:260, 2003)*. Hypokalemia & rhabdomyolysis reported. **Reported to produce impairment in cardiac function.** Potential for significant **drug-drug interactions (see Table 16A) which can be** life-threatening.
IV usual dose 200 mg q12h x4 doses followed by 200 mg q24h for a maximum of 14 days	
Ketoconazole (Nizoral) 200 mg tab	Gastric acid required for absorption—cimetidine, omeprazole, antacids block absorption. In achlorhydria, dissolve tablet in 4 ml 0.2N HCl, drink with a straw. Coca-Cola ↑ absorption by 65% *(AAC 39:1671, 1995)*. CSF levels "none". **Drug-drug interactions important,** see *Table 16A*. Some interactions can be life-threatening. Dose- dependent nausea & vomiting. Liver toxicity of hepatocellular type reported in about 1:10,000 exposed pts—usually after several days to weeks of exposure. At doses of ≥800mg/day serum testosterone & plasma cortisol levels fall. With high doses, adrenal (Addisonian) crisis reported.
Miconazole (Monistat IV) 200 mg—*not available in U.S.*	IV miconazole indicated in patient critically ill with Pseudallescheria boydii. Very toxic due to vehicle needed to get drug into solution.
Nystatin (Mycostatin) 30 gm cream; 500,000 units oral tab	Topical: virtually no adverse effects. Less effective than imidazoles & triazoles. PO: large doses give occasional GI distress & diarrhea.
Posaconazole *(Noxafil)* 400 mg po bid with meals (if not taking meals, 200 mg qid). No cost data available. (See *Drugs 65:1552, 2005*) 200 mg po tid (with food) for prophylaxis	An oral triazole with activity against a wide range of fungi refractory to other antifungal rx including: aspergillosis, zygomycosis, fusariosis, Scedosporium (Pseudallescheria), phaeohyphomycosis, histoplasmosis, refractory candidiasis, refractory coccidioidomycosis, refractory cryptococcosis, & refractory chromoblastomycosis. Approved for prophylaxis. Posaconazole has similar toxicities as other triazoles: nausea 9%, vomiting 6%, abd. pain 5%, headache 5%, diarrhea, ↑ALT, AST, & rash (3% each). In pts rx for >6 mos., serious side-effects have included adrenal insufficiency, nephrotoxicity, & QTc interval prolongation. Significant drug-drug interactions; inhibits CYP3A4
Terbinafine (Lamisil) 250 mg tab	Rare cases (8) of idiosyncratic & symptomatic hepatic injury & more rarely liver failure leading to death or liver transplantation reported in pts receiving terbinafine for onychomycosis. Therefore, the drug is **not recommended** for pts **with chronic or active liver disease** although hepatotoxicity may occur in pts with or without pre-existing disease. Pretreatment screening of serum transaminases (ALT & AST) is advised & alternate rx used for those with abnormal levels. Pts started on terbinafine should be warned about symptoms suggesting liver dysfunction (persistent nausea, anorexia, fatigue, vomiting, RUQ pain, jaundice, dark urine or pale stools). If symptoms develop, drug should be discontinued & liver function immediately evaluated. In controlled trials, changes in ocular lens & retina reported—clinical significance unknown. Major drug-drug interaction is 100% ↑ in rate of clearance by rifampin. AEs: usually mild, transient & rarely caused discontinuation of rx. % with AE, terbinafine vs placebo: nausea/diarrhea 2.6–5.6 vs 2.9; rash 5.6 vs 2.2; taste abnormality 2.8 vs 0.7. Inhibits CYP2D6 enzymes.

TABLE 13 (4)

DRUG NAME, GENERIC (TRADE)/ USUAL DOSAGE	ADVERSE EFFECTS/COMMENTS
ANTIFUNGAL DRUGS (continued)	
Voriconazole (Vfend) IV: Loading dose 6 mg/kg q12h x 1 day, then 4 mg/kg q12h IV for invasive aspergillus & serious mold infections; 3 mg/kg q12h IV for serious candida infections **Oral: >40kg body weight:** 400 mg po q12h x1 day, then 200 mg po q12h; **<40kg body weight:** 200 mg po q12h x1 day, then 100 mg po q12h **Take oral dose 1hr before or 1hr after eating.** Oral suspension (40 mg/mL) Oral suspension dosing: Same as for oral tabs. Reduce to ½ maintenance dose for moderate hepatic insufficiency.	A triazole with activity against Aspergillus sp., including Ampho resistant strains of A. terreus. Active vs Candida sp. (including krusei), Fusarium sp., & various molds. Steady state serum levels reach 2.5–4 µg/ml. Toxicity similar to other azoles/triazoles including uncommon serious hepatic toxicity (hepatitis, cholestasis & fulminant hepatic failure. Liver function tests should be monitored during rx & drug dc' if abnormalities develop. Rash reported in up to 20%, occ. photosensitivity & rare Stevens-Johnson, hallucinations, & anaphylactoid infusion reactions with fever & hypertension. 1 case of QT prolongation with ventricular tachycardia in a 15 y/o pt with ALL reported. **Approx. 30% experience a transient visual disturbance** following IV or po ("altered/enhanced visual perception", blurred or colored visual change or photophobia) within 30–60 minutes. Visual changes resolve within 30-60min. after administration & are attenuated with repeated doses **(do not drive at night for outpatient rx).** No persistence of effect reported. Cause unknown. In patients with ClCr <50 ml/min., the drug should be given orally, not IV, since the intravenous vehicle (SBECD-sulfobutylether-B cyclodextrin) may accumulate. Potential for drug-drug interactions high—see Table 16A. **NOTE:** Not in urine in active form.
ANTIMYCOBACTERIAL DRUGS	
FIRST LINE DRUGS	
Isoniazid (INH) (Nydrazid, Laniazid, Teebaconin) 300 mg/day po 300 mg tab 100 mg/mL in 10 ml vials (IM) (Nydrazid, Apothecon)	**Adverse effects:** Overall ~1%. **Peripheral neuropathy** (<1.0%); pyridoxine 25mg q24h will ↓ incidence; other neurologic sequelae, convulsions, optic neuritis, toxic encephalopathy, psychosis, muscle twitching, dizziness & alterations of sensorium, coma (all rare); allergic skin rashes, lymphadenopathy & vasculitis (SLE-like syndrome), fever, minor disulfiram-like reaction, flushing after Swiss cheese, constipation, **hepatitis** (children 10% mild ↑ SGOT, normalizes with continued rx, age <20yrs rare, 20–34yrs 0.3%, 35–40yrs 1.2%, ≥50yrs 2.3%) (also ↑ with daily alcohol); acute liver failure (fatal or requiring transplantation) (Lancet 345:555, 1995); blood dyscrasias (rare); + antinuclear antibody 20%.
Rifampin (Rifadin, Rimactane, Rifocin) 600 mg/day po 300 mg cap (IV available, Aventis, 600mg)	**Adverse effects:** Produces an orange-brown discoloration of urine, tears (can stain contact lens), semen, & sweat. Can falsely elevate lab measurements of bilirubin. **Drug-drug interactions:** Many (see Table 16A): induces liver cytochrome P450 system (CYP3A) to ↑ drug metabolism, e.g., ↑ Coumadin requirement, ↑ steroid dosage in pts with Addison's disease or asthmatics, ↓ effectiveness of oral contraceptives (uterine bleeding, pregnancies), methadone less effective, reduced levels of azole antifungals, e.g., fluconazole. "Flu syndrome": Manifest as fever/chills, headache, bone pain, dyspnea if rifampin ingestion irregular. Hepatotoxicity: 16 deaths reported in 500,000 recipients. Minor enzyme changes common & resolve while continuing the drug. Alcoholics with pre-existing liver disease prone to rifampin-induced toxicity. Interstitial nephritis reported.
Ethambutol (Myambutol) 15–25 mg/kg/day po 400 mg tab	**Adverse effects: Optic neuritis** with decreased visual acuity, central scotomata, & loss of green & red perception at 25mg/kg/day, not at 15mg/kg/day; peripheral neuropathy & headache (~1%), rashes (rare), arthralgia (rare), hyperuricemia (rare). Monthly evaluation of visual acuity (>10% loss considered significant), red/green color discrimination; usually reversible if drug discontinued. Anaphylactoid reaction. **Comment:** Disrupts outer cell membrane in M. avium with ↑ activity of other drugs.
Pyrazinamide (PZA) 25 mg/kg/day po 500 mg tab	**Adverse effects: Arthralgia; hyperuricemia** (with or without symptoms); hepatitis (not over 2% if recommended dose not exceeded); gastric irritation; photosensitivity (rare). Serum uric acid if symptomatic gouty attack occurs. **Comment:** Maximum dose 2gm/day.

TABLE 13 (5)

DRUG NAME, GENERIC (TRADE)/ USUAL DOSAGE	ADVERSE EFFECTS/COMMENTS
ANTIMYCOBACTERIAL DRUGS/FIRST LINE DRUGS *(continued)*	
Streptomycin 0.75–1 gm/day IM (or IV) 1gm	**Adverse effects:** Overall 8%. **Ototoxicity,** vestibular dysfunction (vertigo); paresthesias; dizziness & nausea (all less in pts receiving 2–3 doses/wk); tinnitus & high frequency loss 1%; nephrotoxicity (rare); peripheral neuropathy (rare); allergic skin rashes 4–5%; drug fever. Available from Pfizer/Roerig 1-800-254-4445. Reference for IV use: *CID* 19:1150, 1994.
Rifamate® *(See Comment for content)* 2 tablets single dose po q24h (1hr before meal). 1 tab	**Adverse effects:** Same as individual components. **Comments:** 1 tablet contains 150mg INH, 300mg RIF
Rifater® *(See Comment for content)* If pt not >55kg: 6 tablets single dose po q24h (1hr before meal). 1 tab	**Adverse effects:** Same as individual components. **Comments:** 1 tablet contains 50mg INH, 120mg RIF, 300mg PZA. Used in 1st 2mos of rx (PZA 25mg/kg). Purpose is convenience in dosing, ↑ compliance (*AnIM* 122:951, 1995) but costs 1.5x more.
SECOND LINE DRUGS	
Para-aminosalicylic acid (PAS) (Na⁺ or K⁺ salt) (Paser) 4–6 gm po q12h (200 mg/kg/day) 450 mg tab	**Adverse effects: Gastrointestinal irritation** 10–15%; goitrogenic action (rare); depressed prothrombin activity (rare); G6PD-mediated hemolytic anemia (rare), drug fever, rashes, hepatitis, myalgia, arthralgia. Retards hepatic enzyme induction, may ↓ INH hepatotoxicity. Available from Jacobus Pharm. Co. (609) 921-7447; CDC (404) 639-3670.
Ethionamide (Trecator-SC) 500–1000 mg/day (15–20mg/kg/day) po as 1–3 doses. 250 mg tab	**Adverse effects: Gastrointestinal irritation** (up to 50% on large dose); goiter; peripheral neuropathy (rare); convulsions (rare); changes in affect (rare); difficulty in diabetes control; rashes; hepatitis; purpura; stomatitis; gynecomastia; menstrual irregularity. Give drug with meals or antacids; 50–100mg pyridoxine per day concomitantly; SGOT monthly. Possibly teratogenic.
Cycloserine (Seromycin) 750–1000 mg/day (15mg/kg/day) po as 2–4 doses. 250 mg cap	**Adverse effects:** Convulsions, **psychoses** (5–10% of those receiving 1gm/day); headache; somnolence; hyperreflexia; increased CSF protein & pressure, peripheral neuropathy; contraindicated in epileptics & active alcoholics; 50mg pyridoxine for every 250mg cycloserine should be given concomitantly.
Amikacin (Amikin) 7.5–10 mg/kg/day IV or IM 500 mg vial	**Adverse effects:** Nephrotoxicity; **ototoxicity** [usually high frequency loss—especially with larger total dose (>10gm), longer duration (>10 days), prior aminoglycosides, pos. family history, assoc. renal impairment & rising trough level (>10µg/ml). All aminoglycosides may cause or ↑ neuromuscular blockade. Use with caution in pts with myasthenia gravis, Parkinsonism, botulism, with neuromuscular blocking drugs *(Table 16A)*, or with massive transfusion of citrated blood. Avoid concurrent use with ethacrynic acid, furosemide or methoxyflurane. ↑ risk of nephrotoxicity with cis platinum, vancomycin, radiocontrast agents. **Comments:** With edema, ascites, &/or obesity, base calculation of est. creatinine clearance on ean body mass & ideal body weight. For dosing with renal impairment, see *Table 15A*.
Capreomycin sulfate (Capastat sulfate) 1 gm/day (15 mg/kg/day) as 1 dose IM	**Adverse effects: Nephrotoxicity** 36%, **ototoxicity** (auditory 11%), eosinophilia, leucopenia, skin rash, fever, hypokalemia, neuromuscular blockade. Abnormal liver function tests.
Amithiozone (Thiacetazone, Tibione, Thioparamizone) (NOT MARKETED IN U.S.) 150 mg/day po	**Adverse effects:** Common: nausea, vomiting, skin rash, dizziness. Uncommon: bone marrow depression, jaundice 0.2%, & renal toxicity. Marked differences in frequency of side effects between racial groups noted, Asia > Africa. Total incidence 21–38%, ½ in 1st 4 weeks, ½ mild. **Comments: Skin reactions** reported in 20% of HV+ pts. Felt to be responsible for a 3% **mortality** (*Lancet 1:627, 1991*). In trial comparing RIF/INH/PZA (RHZ) with SM/thiacetazone/INH (STH), relative risk of death with STH 1.6, drug reactions 11.7 & sputum negative at 2mos RHZ 74% vs 37% in STH (*Lancet 344:323, 1994; ibid, 345:62, 1995*).

163

TABLE 13 (6)

DRUG NAME, GENERIC (TRADE)/ USUAL DOSAGE	ADVERSE EFFECTS/COMMENTS
Antimycobacterial Drugs/SECOND LINE DRUGS *(continued)*	
Clofazimine (Lamprene) 50 mg/day po (with meals) 50 mg	**Adverse effects:** Skin: **pigmentation (pink-brownish black)** 75–100%, dryness 20%, pruritus 5%. GI: abdominal pain 50% (rarely severe leading to exploratory laparoscopy), splenic infarction (very rare), bowel obstruction (very rare), GI bleeding (very rare). Eye: conjunctival irritation, retinal crystal deposition.
Rifabutin (Mycobutin) 300 mg/day po (prophylaxis or treatment) 150 mg	**Adverse effects:** In an anti-MAI trial, rifabutin-related adverse effects occurred in 77% of pts receiving 600mg (high dose) rifabutin with either clarithro or azithro. Most common was a fall in WBC, then nausea/vomiting/diarrhea in 42%, diffuse polyarthralgia in 19%, & anterior uveitis in 8% (*CID* 21:594, 1995). Uveitis responds to topical steroids & cycloplegics [*CID* 22(Suppl. 1):S43, 1996]. Subsequently, max. dose of rifabutin reduced to 300 mg. Other adverse effects similar to rifampin: skin rash 11%, orange-tan to brown skin pigmentation (*CID* 21:1515, 1995). Discolored (reddish) urine 30%. Lab: ↑ SGOT/SGPT 8%.
Rifapentine (Priftin) 600 mg po twice weekly for first 2mos., then 600mg po q week 150 mg tabs	**Adverse effects:** Similar to other rifamycins (see *RIF, RFB*). Hyperuricemia seen in 21%. Causes red-orange discoloration of body fluids. Note ↑ prevalence of RIF resistance in pts on weekly rx (*Ln* 353:1843, 1999).
Fluoroquinolones	**Review drug-drug interactions.**
Ciprofloxacin (Cipro) & **Ciprofloxacin-extended release** (Cipro XR) **500–750 mg po q12h.** **Urinary tract infection: 250 mg po q12h or Cipro XR 500 mg q24h.** Parenteral rx 200–400 mg IV q12h. 500 mg po, Cipro XR 500 mg, 400 mg IV	**Children:** No FQ approved for use under age 16 based on joint cartilage injury in immature animals. Articular SEs in children est. at 2–3% (*Ln ID* 3:537, 2003). **CNS toxicity:** Poorly understood. Varies from mild (lightheadedness) to moderate (confusion) to severe (seizures). May be aggravated by NSAIDs. **Gatifloxacin:** Due to documented hypo- and hyperglycemic reactions (*NEJM* 354:1352, 2006), U.S. distribution of gati ceased in Jun 2006. Gati ophthalmic solution remains available. **Opiate screen false-positives:** FQs can cause **false-positive urine assay for opiates** (*JAMA* 286:3115, 2001). **Photosensitivity** **QT$_c$ (corrected QT) interval prolongation:** ↑ QT$_c$ (>500 msec or >60 msec from baseline) is considered possible with any FQ. ↑ QT$_c$ can lead to torsades de pointes & ventricular fibrillation. Risk low with current marketed drugs. Risk ↑: women, ↓ K$^+$, ↓ Mg^{++}, bradycardia. (Refs.: *NEJM* 351:1053 & 1089, 2004). **Avoid concomitant drugs with potential to prolong QTc:** For list of such drugs, see SANFORD GUIDE TO ANTIMICROBIAL THERAPY, Table 10C, fluoroquinolones, or www.qtdrugs.org.
Gemifloxacin (Factive) 320 mg po q24h 320 mg	**Skin rash with gemifloxacin.** Macular rash after 8–10 d of Rx. Highest frequency in females <age 40 treated for 14 d (22.6%). Mechanism unclear. Self-limited. No known cross-reactivity with other FQs. **Tendinopathy:** Over age 60, approx. 2–6% of all Achilles tendon ruptures attributable to use of FQ (*ArIM* 163:1801, 2003). ↑ risk with concomitant steroid or renal disease (*CID* 36:1404, 2003).
Levofloxacin (Levaquin) 250–750 mg po/IV q24h. 750 mg po; 750mg IV	
Moxifloxacin (Avelox) 400 mg po/IV q24h 400 mg po/IV	
Ofloxacin (Floxin) 200–400 mg po q12h. 400 mg po	
Clarithromycin (Biaxin) 500 mg po q12h or extended release (Biaxin XL) 2 x 500 mg q24h 500 mg; 500 mg ER (FDA approved for MAC; investigational for other atypical mycobacteria, not effective vs M. tuberculosis)	**Adverse effects:** Overall ~13%, ~3% discontinued drug secondary to side effects. GI ~13%: diarrhea 3%, nausea 3%, abnormal taste 3%, abdominal pain 2%, dyspepsia 2%. CNS: headache 2%. Lab (each <1%): ↑ SGOT, alk p'tase, ↓ WBC, ↑ prothrombin time 1%, ↑ BUN 4%, ↑ creatinine <1%. Should not be used in pregnant women, has demonstrated adverse effects in animals at blood levels 2–17x higher than achieved in humans. **Check drug-drug interactions, Table 16A.** **Remember** potential prolongation of QTc interval by clarithro, erythro & other macrolides, esp. in combination with other drugs capable of prolonged QTc (*NEJM* 312:301, 2005). For list of worrisome drugs: www.qtdrugs.org

TABLE 13 (7)

DRUG NAME, GENERIC (TRADE)/ USUAL DOSAGE	ADVERSE EFFECTS/COMMENTS
Antimycobacterial Drugs/SECOND LINE DRUGS *(continued)*	
Azithromycin (Zithromax) 250–500 mg po q24h, 1200 mg po once weekly 250 mg; 600 mg *(Investigational in T. gondii, not effective vs M. tuberculosis)*	**Adverse effects:** Overall 12%, 0.7% discontinued drug secondary to side effects. GI 12.8%: diarrhea 4%, nausea 3%, abdominal pain 2%, vomiting 1%. CNS 1%, ototoxicity (3/21 pts 30–90 days after 500 mg/day, *Lancet* 343:241, 1994). Lab: ↑ SGOT 1.5%, WBC ↓ or ↑ 1%, others <1%. Has not been studied in pregnant women. In rats no embryopathy a: dose of 60x human total dose.
Imipenem-cilastatin (Primaxin) 500 mg q6h IV 500 mg	Active in vitro vs M. tuberculosis. Being used in some trials. **Adverse effects:** Local: phlebitis 3%. Hypersensitivity 2.5%: rash, pruritus, eosinophilia <1%. Blood: + Coombs <1%, neutropenia <1%. Renal: oliguria <0.2%. Hepatic: ↑ SGOT, SGPT, alk p'tase <1%. CNS (0.2%): confusion, seizures (with 0.5 gm q6h 0.5–1.0% but with 1 gm q6h ~10%). GI: nausea 2%, vomiting 2% especially with too rapid IV, diarrhea 3%. **Comment:** Tbc treatment is not an FDA-approved indication, i.e., use is investigational.
ANTIPARASITIC DRUGS	
Albendazole (Albenza) Doses vary with indication, 200–400 mg po q12h 200 mg tab	**Adverse effects: Teratogenic, Pregnancy Cat. C.** Give after negative pregnancy test. Abdominal pain, nausea/vomiting, alopecia, ↑ serum transaminase. Rare reports of bone marrow suppression.
Atovaquone (Mepron) 750 mg po q12h x21 days for PCP rx, 1500 mg po q24h for PCP prophylaxis 750 mg/5ml suspension, cost 210 mL Ref.: *AAC 46:1163, 2002*	**Adverse effects:** Discontinuation rate 9%. Skin rash 23%, only 4% required discontinuation of rx, pruritus 5%. GI: nausea 21%, diarrhea 19%, vomiting 14%, abdominal pain 4%. CNS: headache 16%, insomnia 13%, dizziness 3%. General: fever 14%. Lab: anemia (Hgb <8.0gm/day, 6%), neutropenia (<750/mm³, 3%), ↑ AST 4%, ↑ amylase 7%. **Comments:** Has not been evaluated in severe PCP. Better absorbed with meals. Plasma concentration 3x higher when taken with fatty (>23 gm) meal.
Clindamycin (Cleocin) 600 mg po or IV q6h 300 mg cap 600 mg IV NB	**Adverse effects:** Diarrhea ± C. difficile toxin, nausea, rash, neutropenia, eosinophilia
Dapsone (Dapsone USP) 100 mg po q24h or 2x weekly 100 mg Ref.: *CID 27:191, 1998*	**Adverse effects:** Nausea, vomiting, rash, & oral lesions (*CID 18:630, 1994*). Hemolytic anemia if G6PD deficient, methemoglobinemia (usually asymptomatic but if pt has dyspnea, O₂ saturation disproportionately low to pO₂; check for methemoglobinemia—if >10–15%, discontinue dapsone). Peripheral neuropathy (rare). **Comment:** Usually tolerated even if rash after TMP/SMX.
Iodoquinol (Yodoxin) 650 mg	**Adverse effects:** Nausea, abdominal cramps, rash, acne, increase in thyroid size & PBI. Optic atrophy risk if daily dose over 2 gm. Contraindicated if iodine intolerant.
Ivermectin (Stromectol) Strongyloidiasis: 200 mcg/kg x1 dose po Onchocerciasis: 150 mcg/kg x1 po Scabies: 200 mcg/kg x1 po 3 mg tabs	**Adverse effects:** Mild side-effects—fever, pruritus, rash. Host may experience inflammatory reaction due to death of adult worms (Mazzotti reaction): fever, urticaria, asthma, GI upset.

TABLE 13 (8)

DRUG NAME, GENERIC (TRADE)/ USUAL DOSAGE	ADVERSE EFFECTS/COMMENTS
ANTIPARASITIC DRUGS (continued)	
Metronidazole (Flagyl) 500–750 mg po q12h–q8h 500 mg	**Adverse effects:** GI: nausea, vomiting, metallic taste. Neuro: headache, paresthesias, avoid alcohol during & 48 hours post-rx (disulfiram-like reaction). Peripheral neuropathy possible.
Nitazoxanide (Alinia) Ages 1–4: 100 mg po q12h x3 days Ages 4–11: 200 mg po q12h x3 days Adults: 500 mg po q12h 500 mg	**Adverse effects:** Only approved for otherwise healthy children with infection due to Giardia lamblia or Cryptosporidium parvum. Caution in diabetics: 5 ml suspension contains 1.5gm sucrose. AEs in <1%. Discolored eyes & urine. Ref: CID 40:1173, 2005.
Paromomycin (Humatin)^{NUS} 500 mg q8h or q6h po 250 mg caps	**Adverse effects:** GI: doses of >3gm, nausea, abdominal cramps, diarrhea. Skin: rash. **Comment:** This is an aminoglycoside similar to neomycin ("non-absorbed", ~3% of dose is absorbed). Discontinue promptly if patient complains of tinnitus, ↓ in hearing, or vertigo.
Pentamidine isethionate IV) (Pentam 300) 4 mg/kg/day IV 300 mg	**Adverse effects:** Hypotension with rapid IV administration, rash, nausea, vomiting, nephrotoxicity, cardiac arrhythmia (ventricular tachycardias including torsade de pointes), neutropenia (15%), thrombocytopenia, pancreatitis, hypocalcemia, hypoglycemia followed by hyperglycemia. Sterile abscesses after IM administration. **Comments:** Pentamidine inhibits distal nephron absorption of Na^+ with resultant hyperkalemia similar to K-sparing diuretics (AnIM 122:103, 1995).
Pentamidine (aerosol) (NebuPent) 300 mg/month (prophylaxis) 300 mg	**Adverse effects:** Cough may respond to bronchodilator, upper lobe pneumocystis may occur if given with patient sitting. **Comment:** Risk of extrapulmonary pneumocystis & pneumothorax greater than with systemic prophylaxis. Use aerosol only in patients intolerant of oral drugs.
Primaquine: Primaquine phosphate 26.3mg = 15mg of base 15 mg (base) po q24h 26.3 mg	**Adverse effects:** Hemolytic anemia if G6PD deficient; may cause clinically significant methemoglobinemia; nausea/abdominal pain if taken on empty stomach.
Pyrimethamine (Daraprim, Malocide) 50–75 mg po q24h; 25 mg with Leucovorin, tablet 5 mg —see Comments	**Adverse effects:** Major problem hematologic: megaloblastic anemia, ↓ WBC, ↓ platelets. PO folinic acid, 5mg/day, will ↓ heme adverse effects & not interfere with efficacy of rx. If high-dose pyrimethamine, ↑ folinic acid to 10–50 mg/day. Pyri + sulfadiazine can cause mental changes due to carnitine deficiency (AJM 95:112, 1993). Other: rash, vomiting, diarrhea, xerostomia
Sulfadiazine 1–1.5 gm po q6h 500 mg tablet	**Adverse effects:** Compared to non-HIV pts, dramatic ↑ in incidence of pruritus, rash, Stevens-Johnson syndrome, myalgia/arthralgia in AIDS pts. Traditionally thought on hypersensitivity basis. New data support postulate of dose-dependent accumulation of toxic sulfonamide metabolites that fail to clear due to concomitant glutathione deficiency in the AIDS pt (Brit J Pharm 39:621, 1995; JAC 34:1, 1994). In addition, can cause hemolytic anemia in G6PD-def. pts. All sulfonamides can cause crystalluria. Do not use in newborns or late stages of pregnancy.
Trimethoprim (Proloprim) 5 mg/kg po q6h 100 mg tabs	**Adverse effects:** Rash, pruritus, marrow suppression rare. Rare cases of aseptic meningitis [fever, headache, CSF ↑ cells (monos), ↑ protein] reported (CID 19:431, 1994). **Comment:** Fewer reactions than TMP/SMX.
Trimethoprim (TMP)-sulfamethoxazole (SMX) (Cotrim, Bactrim, Septra) (Dosage depends on indication) 1 double-strength tab (160 TMP/ 800 mg SMX); 160/800 mg IV	**Adverse effects:** Compared to non-AIDS pts, dramatic dose-dependent ↑ in pruritus, skin rash, Stevens-Johnson syndrome. In pts given TMP/SMX + steroids for PCP, % skin reactions ↓ from 47 to 13 (CID 18:319, 1994). Initially thought hypersensitivity was reason; accumulating data support hypothesis of dose-dependent accumulation of toxic sulfonamide metabolites (hydroxylamine). Clearance of metabolites requires glutathione & AIDS pts are deficient (Brit J Pharm 39:621, 1995; JAC 34:1, 1994). May explain ability 2/3 of time to rx through rash (Arch Derm 130:1383, 1994). Beware progressive exanthem— some pts progress to exfoliation &/or Stevens-Johnson syndrome. Tremors associated with high dose (CID 22:598, 1996). **TMP** competes with creatinine for tubular secretion & **can** ↑ **serum creatinine (reversible); TMP** also blocks distal renal tubular reabsorption of Na^+ & secretion of K^+; ↑ **serum K^+** in 21% of pts (AnIM 124:316, 1996).

TABLE 13 (9)

DRUG NAME(S) GENERIC (TRADE)	DOSAGE/ROUTE	COMMENTS/ADVERSE EFFECTS
ANTIVIRAL DRUGS (other than retroviral)		
CMV		
Cidofovir (Vistide)	5 mg/kg IV q week x2 weeks, then once weekly every 2wks. Properly timed IV prehydration with normal saline & oral probenecid **must be used with each cidofovir infusion** (see *pkg insert for details*). Renal function (serum creatinine & urine protein) must be monitored prior to each dose (see *pkg insert for details*).	**Adverse effects: Nephrotoxicity;** dose-dependent proximal tubular injury (Fanconi-like syndrome): proteinuria, glycosuria, bicarbonaturia, phosphaturia, polyuria (nephrogenic diabetic insipidus now reported, *Ln 350:413, 1997*), ↑ creatinine. Concomitant saline prehydration, probenecid, extended dosing intervals allowed use. 25% of pts dc IV cidofovir due to nephrotoxicity. Other toxicities: nausea 48%, fever 31%, alopecia 16%, myalgia 16%, probenecid hypersensitivity 16%, neutropenia 29%. No effect on hematocrit, platelets, LFTs. Other **Black Box** warnings: contraindicated with concomitant nephrotoxic agents, ↓WBC, carcinogenic/teratogenic & ↓sperm in animals, only indicated for rx of CMV retinitis. Contraindicated with serum creatinine > 1.5 mg/dL, Ccr ≤ 55 mL/min or urine protein ≥ 100 mg/dL. **Comment:** Recommended dosage, frequency or infusion rate of cidofovir must not be exceeded. Dose must be reduced or discontinued if changes in renal function occur during rx. For ↑ of 0.3–0.4mg/dl in serum creatinine, cidofovir dose must be ↓ from 5 to 3 mg/kg; discontinue cidofovir if ↑ of 0.5mg/dl above baseline or 3+ proteinuria develops (for 2+ proteinuria, observe pts carefully & consider discontinuation).
Foscarnet (Foscavir)	90 mg/kg q12h IV (induction) 90 mg/kg q24h (maintenance) Dosage adjustment with renal dysfunction (see *Table 15A*)	**Adverse effects: Major clinical toxicity is renal impairment (1/3 of patients)**—↑ creatinine, proteinuria, nephrogenic diabetes insipidus, ↓ K⁺, ↓ Ca⁺⁺, ↓ Mg⁺⁺, ↓ or ↑ phosphate. Other **Black Box** warnings: hydration & frequent monitoring imperative; dose adjustment for renal function (see *label and Table 15A*); **seizures** related to electrolyte/mineral abnormalities. Infusion rate must be controlled: administer by infusion pump over 1.5 to 2 hrs. Prehydrate to establish diuresis before first dose and hydrate concomitantly with subsequent doses. Toxicity ↑ with other nephrotoxic drugs [amphotericin B, aminoglycosides or pentamidine (especially severe ↓ Ca⁺⁺)]. Other: headache, mild (100%); fatigue (100%); nausea (80%), fever (25%). CNS: seizures. Hematol.: ↓ WBC, ↓ Hgb. Hepatic: liver function tests ↑. Neuropathy. Penile ulcers.
Ganciclovir (Cytovene)	IV: 5 mg/kg q12h x14 days (induction) 5 mg/kg IV q24h daily or 6mg/kg q24h 5 days per/wk (maintenance) Dosage adjustment with renal dysfunction (see *Table 15A*) Oral: 1 gm q8h with food (fatty meal)	**Adverse effects: Black Box** warnings: cytopenias, carcinogenicity/teratogenicity & aspermia in animals. Absolute neutrophil count d'opped below 500/mm³ in 15%, thrombocytopenia 21%, anemia 6%. Fever 48%. GI 50%: nausea, vomiting, diarrhea abdominal pain 19%, rash 10%. Retinal detachment 11%. **(Likely related to underlying disease, not drug)**. Confusion, headache, psychiatric disturbances & seizures. Neutropenia may respond to granulocyte colony stimulating factor (G-CSF or GM-CSF). Severe myelosuppression may be ↑ with coadministration of zidovudine or azathioprine. 32% dc/interrupted rx, principally for neutropenia. Avoid extravasation. Hematologic less frequent than with IV. Granulocytopenia 18%, anemia 12%, thrombocytopenia 6%. GI, skin same as with IV. Retinal detach ment 8%.
Ganciclovir (Vitrasert)	Intraocular implant (~$5000/device + cost of surgery)	**Adverse effects:** Late retinal detachment (7/30 eyes). Does not prevent CMV retinitis in good eye or visceral dissemination. **Comment:** Replacement every 6mos recommended.
Valganciclovir (Valcyte)	900 mg (two 450mg tabs) po q12h x 21 days for induction, followed by 900 mg po q24h for maintenance. Take with food. Dosage adjustment with renal dysfunction (see *Table 15A*)	A prodrug of ganciclovir with better bioavailability than oral ganciclovir: 60% with food. **Adverse effects:** Similar to ganciclovir.

167

TABLE 13 (10)

DRUG NAME(S) GENERIC (TRADE)	DOSAGE/ROUTE	COMMENTS/ADVERSE EFFECTS
ANTIVIRAL DRUGS (other than retroviral) *(continued)*		
Herpesvirus (Non-CMV)		
Acyclovir (Zovirax)	Doses: see *Table 12* 200 mg caps, 400 mg and 800 mg tabs IV injection (multiple) Oral suspension 200mg/5ml Topical: 5% cream and 5% ointment Dosage adjustment with renal dysfunction (see *Table 15A*).	**Oral:** Generally well-tolerated with occ. diarrhea, vertigo, arthralgia. Less frequent rash, fatigue, insomnia, fever, menstrual abnormalities, acne, sore throat, muscle cramps, lymphadenopathy. **IV:** Phlebitis, caustic with vesicular lesions with IV infiltration, CNS (1%): lethargy, tremors, confusion, hallucinations, delirium, seizures, coma (*CID 21:435, 1995*). Improve 1–2wks after rx stopped. Renal (5%): ↑ creatinine, hematuria. With high doses may crystallize in renal tubules → obstructive uropathy (rapid infusion, dehydration, renal insufficiency & ↑ dose ↑ risk). Adequate pre-hydration may prevent such nephrotoxicity. Hepatic: ↑ ALT, AST. Uncommon: neutropenia (*CID 20: 1557, 1995*), rash, diaphoresis, hypotension, headache, nausea.
Famciclovir (Famvir)	Doses: see *Table 12* Tabs: 125 mg, 250 mg, 500 mg.	Pro-drug of penciclovir. **Adverse effects:** similar to acyclovir, included headache, nausea, diarrhea, & dizziness but incidence did not differ from placebo (*JAMA 276:47, 1996*). May be taken without regard to meals. Dose should be reduced if CrCl <60 ml/min (see package insert & *Table 12, page 156 & Table 15A, page 178*).
Penciclovir (Denavir)	Topical 1% cream (1.5gm tubes)	Apply to area of recurrence of herpes labialis with start of sx, then q2h while awake x 4 days. Well tolerated.
Trifluridine (Vioptic)	Topical 1% solution :1 drop q2h (max. 9 drops/day) until corneal re-epithelialization, then dose is reduced for 7 additional days (one drop q4h for at least 5 drops/day), not to exceed 21 days total rx.	For HSV keratoconjunctivitis or recurrent epithelial keratitis. **Adverse effects:** Mild burning (5%), palpebral edema (3%), punctate keratopathy, stromal edema
Valacyclovir (Valtrex)	Doses: see *Table 12*. 500 mg tabs and 1 gm caplets. Dosage adjustment with renal dysfunction (see *Table 15A*).	An ester pro-drug of acyclovir that is well-absorbed, bioavailability 3–5x greater than acyclovir. Can take without regard to meals. **Adverse effects** similar to acyclovir (see *JID 186:S40, 2002*). Thrombotic thrombocytopenic purpura/hemolytic uremic syndrome reported in pts with advanced HIV disease & transplant recipients participating in clinical trials at doses of 8gm/day.
Hepatitis		
Adefovir dipivoxil (Hepsera)	10 mg po q24h (with normal CrCl) 20–49 CrCl: 10mg q48h 10–19 CrCl: 10mg q72h Hemodialysis: 10mg q7 days following dialysis. Each tab contains 10mg	Adefovir dipivoxil is a prodrug of the active moiety adefovir. It is an acyclic nucleotide analog with activity against hepatitis B (HBV) at 0.2–2.5mM (IC$_{50}$). Peak plasma concentration after 10mg po was 18.4 ± 6.26ng/ml, 1–4hrs after dose. Terminal elimination t½ was 7.48 ± 1.65hrs. Primarily renal excretion—adjust dose. No food interactions. Remarkably few side effects. Nephrotoxicity found in early studies with 30 mg/d.; at 10 mg/d there is potential for delayed nephrotoxicity. Monitor renal function, esp. with pts with pre-existing or other risks for renal impairment. Lactic acidosis reported with nucleoside analogs, esp. in women. Pregnancy Category C. Hepatitis may exacerbate when rx dc. 6–25% of pts developed ALT ↑ 10x normal within 12 wks; usually responds to re-treatment or self-limited, but hepatic decompensation has occurred.
Emtricitabine/tenofovir disoproxil fumerate (Truvada)	See *Table 6B*	Treatment of hepB is not an FDA approved indication, but drug is used in HIV/HBV co-infected patients requiring therapy for both.
Entecavir (Baraclude)	0.5 mg q24h. If refractory to lamivudine: 1mg per day Tabs: 0.5 mg and 1 mg Oral solution: 0.05 mg/mL	A nucleoside analog active against HBV including some lamivudine-resistant mutants. Minimal adverse effects reported: headache, fatigue, dizziness, & nausea reported in 22% of pts. Potential for lactic acidosis, exacerbation of hepB at discontinuation, and HIV resistance (see *Black Box warning*). Adjust dosage in renal impairment (see *Table 15A*). Do not use as single anti-retroviral agent in co-infected pts. HIV resistant mutation M134V will emerge (*NEJM 356:2614, 2007*).

TABLE 13 (11)

DRUG NAME(S) GENERIC (TRADE)	DOSAGE/ROUTE	COMMENTS/ADVERSE EFFECTS
ANTIVIRAL DRUGS (other than retroviral)/Hepatitis *(continued)*		
Interferon alfa is available as alfa-2a (Roferon-A), alfa-2b (Intron-A)	For HepC, usual Roferon-A and Intron-A doses are 3 million international units thrice weekly subQ. Depending on agent, available in pre-filled syringes, vials of solution, or powder.	**Black Box warnings:** include possibility of serious neuropsychiatric effects, autoimmune disorders, ischemic events, infection. **Adverse effects:** Flu-like syndrome is common, esp. during 1st wk of rx: fever 98%, fatigue 89%, myalgia 73%, headache 71%. GI: anorexia 46%, diarrhea 29%. CNS: dizziness 21%. Rash 18%, later profound fatigue & psychiatric symptoms in up to ½ of pts (*J Clin Psych* 64:708, 2003) (depression, anxiety, emotional lability & agitation), alopecia, ↑ TSH, autoimmune thyroid disorders with hypo- or hyperthyroidism. Hematol.: ↓ WBC 49%, ↓ Hgb 27%, ↓ platelets 35%. Consider prophylactic antidepressant in pts with history. Acute reversible hearing loss &/or tinnitus in up to 1/3 (*Ln* 343:1134, 1994). Optic neuropathy (retinal hemorrhage, cotton wool spots, ↓ in color vision) reported (*AIDS* 18:1805, 2004). Side-effects ↑ with ↑ doses & dose reduction necessary in up to 46% receiving chronic rx for HBV.
PEG interferon alfa-2b (PEG-Intron)	0.5–1.5 mcg/kg subQ q wk	Attachment of INF to polyethylene glycol (PEG) prolongs half-life & allows weekly dosing. Better efficacy data with similar adverse effects profile compared to regular formulation. Doses may require adjustment (or dc) based on individual response or adverse events, and can vary by product, indication (eg, HCV or HBV) and mode of use (mono- or combination-rx). *(Refer to labels of individual products.)*
Pegylated-40k interferon alfa-2a (Pegasys)	180 mcg subQ q wk	
Lamivudine (3TC) (Epivir-HBV)	Hepatitis B dose: 100 mg po q24h Dosage adjustment with renal dysfunction (see label). Tabs 100 mg and oral solution 5 mg/mL.	**Black Box warnings:** caution that this dose is lower than HIV dose, so must exclude co-infection with HIV before using this formulation; lactic acidosis/hepatic steatosis; severe exacerbation of liver disease can occur on dc; YMDD-mutants resistant to lamivudine may emerge on treatment. **Adverse effects:** See Table 6B.
Ribavirin (Rebetol, Copegus)	For use with an interferon for hepatitis C. Available as 200 mg caps and 40 mg/mL oral solution (Rebetol) or 200 mg tabs (Copegus) *(See Comments regarding dosage)*	**Black Box warnings:** ribavirin monotherapy of HCV is ineffective; hemolytic anemia may precipitate cardiac events—use with caution; teratogenic/embryocidal (**Preg Category X**). Drug may persist for 6 mo, avoid pregnancy for at least 6 mo after end of rx of women *or their partners*. Only approved for pts with Ccr > 50 mL/min. Also should not be used in pts with severe heart disease or some hemoglobinopathies. ARDS reported (*Chest* 124:406, 2003). **Adverse effects:** hemolytic anemia (may require dose reduction or dc), dental/periodontal disorders, and all adverse effects of concomitant interferon used (see above). See Table 12 for specific regimens, but dosing depends on: interferon used, weight, HCV genotype, and is modified (or dc) based on side effects (especially degree of hemolysis, with different criteria in those with/without cardiac disease). For example, initial Rebetrol dose with Intron A (interferon alfa-2b) is wt-based: 400 mg am & 600 mg pm for ≤ 75 kg, and 600 mg pm for wt > 75 kg, but with Pegintron approved dose is 400 mg am & 400 mg pm with meals. Doses and duration of Copegus with peg-interferon alfa-2a are less in pts with genotype 2 or 3 (800 mg per day divided into 2 doses, for 24 wks) than with genotypes 1 or 4 (1000 mg per day divided into 2 doses for wt < 75 kg and 1200 mg per day divided into 2 doses for ≥ 75 kg for 48 wks). *(See individual labels for details, including initial dosing and criteria for dose modification in those with/without cardiac disease.)*
Telbivudine (Tyzeka)	One 600 mg tab orally q24h, without regard to food. Dosage adjustment with renal dysfunction, Ccr < 50 mL/min *(see label)*.	An oral nucleoside analog approved for Rx of Hep B. It has demonstrated higher rates of response and superior viral suppression than lamivudine. **Black Box** warnings regarding lactic acidosis/hepatic steatosis with nucleosides and potential for severe exacerbation of HepB on dc. Generally well-tolerated with reduced mitochondrial toxicity vs other nucleosides and no dose limiting toxicity observed (*Ann Pharmacother* 40:472, 2006; *Medical Letter* 49:11, 2007). Myalgias and myopathy reported. The genotype resistance rate was 4.7 by one yr increasing to 21.5% by 2 yrs of treatment. It selects for YMDD mutation like lamivudine. Combination with lamivudine was inferior to monotherapy (*Hepatology* 45:507, 2007).
Tenofovir (TDF)(Viread)	See Table 6B	Treatment of hepB is not an FDA approved indication, but drug is used in HIV/HBV co-infected patients requiring therapy for both.

TABLE 13 (12)

DRUG NAME(S) GENERIC (TRADE)	DOSAGE/ROUTE	COMMENTS/ADVERSE EFFECTS
ANTIVIRAL DRUGS (other than retroviral) *(continued)*		
Warts (See *CID* 28:S37, 1999) Regimens are from drug labels specific for external genital and/or perianal condylomata acuminata only *(see specific labels for indications, regimens, age limits)*.		
Interferon alfa-2b (IntronA)	Injection of 1 million international units into base of lesion, thrice weekly on alternate days for up to 3 wks. Maximum 5 lesions per course.	Interferons may cause "flu-like" illness and other systemic effects. 88% had at least one adverse effect.
Interferon alfa-N3 (Alferon N)	Injection of 0.05 mL into base of each wart, up to 0.5 mL total per session, twice weekly for up to 8 weeks.	Flu-like syndrome and hypersensitivity reactions. Contraindicated with allergy to mouse IgG, egg proteins, or neomycin.
Imiquimod (Aldara)	5% cream. Thin layer applied at bedtime, washing off after 6-10 hr, thrice weekly to maximum of 16wks.	Erythema, itching & burning, erosions. Flu-like syndrome, increased susceptibility to sunburn (avoid UV).
Podofilox (Condylox)	0.5% gel or solution twice daily for 3 days, no therapy for 4 days; can use up to 4 such cycles.	Local reactions—pain, burning, inflammation in 50%. Can ulcerate. Limit surface area treated as per label.
Sinecatechins (Veregen)	15% ointment. Apply 0.5 cm strand to each wart three times per day until healing but not more than 16 weeks.	Application site reactions, which may result in ulcerations, phimosis, meatal stenosis, superinfection.

TABLE 14: SELECTED PHARMACOLOGIC FEATURES OF ANTIMICROBIAL AGENTS USED IN HIV-ASSOCIATED INFECTIONS IN ADULTS*

Drug	Dose, Route of Administration	For PO Dosing—Take Drug[1]			% AB[3]	Peak Serum Level mcg/ml[4]	Protein Binding, %	Serum T½, Hours[5]	Biliary Excretion, %[6]	CSF[7]/Blood, %	CSF Level Potentially Therapeutic[8]
		With Food	Without Food[2]	With/Without Food							
ANTIFUNGALS											
Amphotericin B											
Standard: 0.4–0.7 mg/kg IV						0.5–3.5		24		0	
Ampho B lipid complex (ABLC): 5 mg/kg IV						1–2.5		173			
Ampho B cholesteryl complex: 4 mg/kg IV						2.9		39			
Liposomal ampho B: 5 mg/kg IV						83		6.8 ± 2.1			
Anidulafungin	200 mg IV x 1, then 100 mg IV q24h					7.2	84	26.5			No
Caspofungin	70 mg IV x1, then 50mg IV q24h					9.9	97	9–11			No
Micafungin	150 mg IV					16.4	>99	15–17			Yes
Flucytosine	2.5 gm po			X	78–90	30–40		3–6		60–100	Yes
Azoles											
Fluconazole	400 mg po/IV		X		90	6.7		20–50		50–94	Yes
	800 mg po/IV		X		90	Approx. 14		20–50			
Itraconazole	Oral soln 200 mg po		X		Low	0.3–0.7	99.8	35		0	
Posaconazole	200 mg po	X				0.2–1.0	98–99	20–66			Yes (JAC 56:745, 2005)
Voriconazole	200 mg po		X		96	3	58	6		22–100	Yes (CID 37:728, 2003)
ANTIMYCOBACTERIALS											
Ethambutol	25 mg/kg po	X			80	2–6	10–30	4		25–50	Probably
Isoniazid	300 mg po		X		100	3–5		0.7–4		90	Yes
Pyrazinamide	20–25 mg/kg po			X	95	30–50	5–10	10–16		100	Yes
Rifampin	600 mg po		X		70–90	4–32	80	1.5–5	10,000	7–56	Yes
Streptomycin	1 gm IV (see Table 13, page 163)					25–50	0–10	2.5	10–60	0–30	No; Intrathecal: 5–10 mg
ANTIPARASITICS											
Albendazole	400 mg po	X				0.5–1.6	70	4			
Atovaquone suspension: 750 mg po		X			47	15	99.9	67		<1	No
Dapsone	100 mg po			X	100	1.1		10–50			
Ivermectin	12 mg po		X			0.05–0.08					
Mefloquine	1.25 gm po	X				0.5–1.2	98	13–24 days			
Nitazoxanide	200 mg po	X				3	99				
Proguanil[9]		X					75				
Pyrimethamine	25 mg po			X	"High"	0.1–0.3	87	96			
Praziquantel	20 mg/kg po	X			80	0.2–2.0		0.8–1.5			
Tinidazole	2 gm po	X			48		12	13		Chemically similar to metronidazole	

See next page for footnotes

* See SANFORD GUIDE TO ANTIMICROBIAL THERAPY for data for antibacterial drugs

TABLE 14 (2)

ANTIVIRAL DRUGS—NOT HIV

Drug	Dose, Route of Administration	For PO Dosing—Take Drug[1]			% AB[3]	Peak Serum Level mcg/ml[4]	Protein Binding, %	Serum T½, Hours[5]	Biliary Excretion, %[6]	CSF[7]/ Blood, %	CSF Level Potentially Therapeutic[8]
		With Food	Without Food[2]	With/Without Food							
Acyclovir	400 mg po			X	10–20	1.21	9–33	2.5–3.5			
Adefovir	10 mg po			X	59	0.02	≤4	7.5			
Entecavir	0.5 mg po		X		100	4.2 ng/ml	13	128–149			
Famciclovir	500 mg po			X	77	3–4	<20	2–3			
Foscarnet	60 mg/kg IV					155		4		<1	No
Ganciclovir	5 mg/kg IV					8.3	1–2	3.5			
Oseltamivir	75 mg po			X	75	0.65/3.5[10]	3	1–3			
Ribavirin	600 mg po			X	64	0.8		44			
Rimantadine	100 mg po			X		0.1–0.4		25			
Telbivudine	600 mg po			X		3.7	3.3	~15 hrs			
Valacyclovir	1000 mg po			X	55	5.6	13–18	3			
Valganciclovir	900 mg po	X			59	5.6	1–2	4			

Drug	Dose, Route of Administration	For PO Dosing—Take Drug[1]			% AB[3]	Peak Serum Level mcg/ml[4]	Protein Binding, %	Intracellular T½, Hours (See footnote[11])	Serum T½, Hours[5]	Cytochrome P450	CSF/ Blood, %[13]
		With Food	Without Food[2]	With/ W/O Food							

ANTIRETROVIRAL DRUGS

Drug	Dose, Route of Administration	With Food	Without Food[2]	With/W/O Food	% AB[3]	Peak Serum Level mcg/ml[4]	Protein Binding, %	Intracellular T½, Hours	Serum T½, Hours[5]	Cytochrome P450	CSF/Blood, %[13]
Abacavir	600 mg po			X	83	3.0	50	20.6	1.5		36
Atazanavir	400 mg po	X			"Good"	2.3	86		7		
Darunavir	600 mg po + 100 mg ritonavir	X			82	3.5	95				
Delavirdine	400 mg po			X	85	19 ± 11	98		5.8	Inhibitor	0
Didanosine	400 mg EC[12] po		X		30–40	1.18–2.13	<5	25–40	1.4		
Efavirenz	600 mg po		X		42	13 μM	99		52–76	Inducer/ inhibitor	0
Emtricitabine	200 mg po			X	93	1.8	<4		10		
Enfuvirtide	90 mg subQ				84	5	92		4		
Etravirine	200 mg po	X					99.9	3.8	41		
Fosamprenavir	1400 mg w/100 mg ritonavir po			X	No data	7.9	90	No data	7.7		
Indinavir	800 mg po		X		65	12.6 μM	60		1.2–2	Inhibitor	11
Lamivudine	300 mg po			X	86	2.6	<36	16	5–7		23
Lopinavir	400 mg po	X			No data	9.6	98–99		5–6	Inhibitor	
Maraviroc	300 mg po			X	33	0.3–0.9	76	14–18			

See next page for footnotes

* See SANFORD GUIDE TO ANTIMICROBIAL THERAPY for data for antibacterial drugs

TABLE 14 (3)

Drug	Dose, Route of Administration	For PO Dosing—Take Drug[1]		% AB[3]	Peak Serum Level mcg/ml[4]	Protein Binding, %	Intracellular T½, Hours (See footnote[11])	Serum T½, Hours[5]	Cytochrome P450	CSF/Blood, %[13]
		With Food	Without Food / With/W/O Food							
ANTIRETROVIRAL DRUGS *(continued)*										
Nelfinavir[14]	1250 mg po	X		20–80	3–4	98		3.5–5	Inhibitor	0
Nevirapine	200 mg po		X	>90	2	60		25–30	Inducer	63
Raltegravir	400 mg po		X	32		83	Alpha 1, beta 9			
Ritonavir	300 mg po	X		65	7.8	98–99		3–5	Potent inhibitor	0
Saquinavir (gel)	1000 mg po (with ritonavir 100 mg)	X		4	3.1	97		1–2	Inhibitor	
Stavudine	40 mg po		X	86	1.4	<5	3.5	1		20
Tenofovir	300 mg po		X	39	0.12	<7	10–>60	17		
Tipranavir	500 mg po + 200 mg ritonavir	X			95 µM	99.9		5.5–6		
Zidovudine	300 mg po		X	60	1–2	<38	11	1.1		2

FOOTNOTES:
1. For adult oral preps; not applicable for peds suspension
2. Food decreases rate &/or extent of absorption
3. % absorbed under optimal conditions
4. Total drug; adjust for protein binding to determine free drug concentration
5. Assumes CrCl >80 mg/min.
6. Peak concentration in bile/peak concentration in serum x 100. If blank, no data.
7. CSF levels with inflammation
8. Judgment based on drug dose & organ susceptibility. CSF concentration ideally ≥10 above MIC
9. Given with atovaquone as Malarone for malaria prophylaxis
10. Oseltamivir/oseltamivir carboxylate
11. Methods for calculating intracellular concentration not standardized. Based on in vitro & in vivo studies, hierarchy of ratio of intracellular/extracellular concentrations of protease inhibitors is: nelfinavir > saquinavir > fosamprenavir > lopinavir ≥ritonavir > indinavir (JAC 54:982, 2004).
12. EC = enteric coated
13. CID 41:1787, 2005; abacavir (AAC 49:2504, 2500)
14. Data based on 250 mg tab

TABLE 15A: DOSAGE OF ANTIMICROBIAL DRUGS IN ADULT PATIENTS WITH RENAL IMPAIRMENT

Adapted from a combination of *Drug Prescribing in Renal Failure*, 5th Ed., Aronoff et al (Eds.), American College of Physicians, 2007, & Selected package inserts. For review of continuous renal replacement therapy see: *CID 41:1159, 2005*.

UNLESS STATED, ADJUSTED DOSES ARE % OF DOSE FOR NORMAL RENAL FUNCTION.

Drug adjustments are based on the patient's estimated endogenous creatinine clearance, which can be calculated as:

$\frac{(140-\text{age})(\text{ideal body weight in kg})}{(72)(\text{serum creatinine, mg/dl})}$	for men (x 0.85 for women)	Ideal body weight for men: 50.0kg + 2.3kg per inch over 5ft Ideal body weight for women: 45.5kg + 2.3kg per inch over 5ft

For alternative method to estimate CrCl, see NEJM 354:2473, 2006

NOTE: For summary of drugs that do not require dosage adjustment with renal failure, see Table 15B

The following is a selected list of drugs commonly used in the care of HIV-infected patients. For data on additional antimicrobials, see *Table 17 of The Sanford Guide to Antimicrobial Therapy 2008*.

ANTIMICROBIAL	HALF-LIFE (NORMAL/ESRD) hr	DOSE FOR NORMAL RENAL FUNCTION§	METHOD* (see footnote)	ADJUSTMENT FOR RENAL FAILURE Estimated creatinine clearance (CrCl), ml/min			HEMODIALYSIS, CAPD+ (see footnote)		COMMENTS & DOSAGE FOR CRRT‡
				>50–90	10–50	<10			
ANTIBACTERIAL ANTIBIOTICS									
Aminoglycoside Antibiotics: Traditional multiple daily doses—adjustment for renal disease									
Amikacin	1.4–2.3/17–150	7.5 mg/kg q12h	D&I	60–90% q12h	30–70% q12–18h **Same dose for CRRT‡**	20–30% q24–48h	HEMO:	Extra 3.8mg/kg after dialysis	High flux hemodialysis membranes lead to unpredictable aminoglycoside clearance, measure post-dialysis drug levels for efficacy & toxicity. With CAPD, pharmacokinetics highly variable—**check serum levels.** Usual method for CAPD: 2 liters of dialysis fluid placed qid or 8 liters/day (Example of how much amikacin is lost per day: give 8Lx20mg lost/L = 160mg of amikacin, so give extra 160 mg of amikacin IV). Adjust dosing weight for obesity: [ideal body weight + 0.4 (actual body weight – ideal body weight)] (*CID 25:112, 1997*).
							CAPD:	15–20mg lost/L dialysate/day (see Comment)	
Gentamicin, Tobramycin	2–3/20–60	1.7 mg/kg q8h	D&I	60–90% q8–12h	30–70% q12h **Same dose for CRRT‡**	20–30% q24–48h	HEMO:	Extra 0.9mg/kg after dialysis	
							CAPD:	3–4mg lost/L dialysate/day	
Netilmicin^NUS	2–3/35–72	2 mg/kg q8h	D&I	50–90% q8–12h	20–60% q12h **Same dose for CRRT‡**	10–20% q24–48h	HEMO:	Extra 1mg/kg after dialysis	
							CAPD:	3–4mg lost/L dialysate/day	
Streptomycin	2–3/30–80	15 mg/kg (max. of 1 gm) q24h	I	50% q24h	q24–72h **Same dose for CRRT‡**	q72–96h	HEMO:	Extra 7.5mg/kg after dialysis	
							CAPD:	20–40mg lost/L dialysate/day	

§, *, ** See notes on page 180

‡ **CRRT** = continuous renal replacement therapy. Usually results in CrCl of approx. 30 mL/min.   + **AD** = after dialysis. "**Dose AD**" refers only to timing of dose.   **CAPD** = Continuous ambulatory peritoneal dialysis.

TABLE 15A (2)

ANTIMICROBIAL	HALF-LIFE (NORMAL/ESRD) hr	DOSE FOR NORMAL RENAL FUNCTION[§]	METHOD* (see footnote)	ADJUSTMENT FOR RENAL FAILURE Estimated creatinine clearance (CrCl), ml/min				HEMODIALYSIS, CAPD[+] (see footnote)	COMMENTS & DOSAGE FOR CRRT[‡]
				>50–90	30–40	20–30	<10		

ANTIBACTERIAL ANTIBIOTICS (continued)

ONCE-DAILY AMINOGLYCOSIDE THERAPY: ADJUSTMENT IN RENAL INSUFFICIENCY

Creatinine Clearance (ml/min.)	>80	60–80	40–60	30–40	20–30	10–20	<10
Drug	Dose q24h (mg/kg)					Dose q48h (mg/kg)	
Gentamicin/Tobramycin	5.1	4	3.5	2.5	4	3	2
Amikacin/kanamycin/streptomycin	15	12	7.5	4	7.5	4	3
Isepamicin[NUS]	8	8	8	8 q48h	8	8 q72h	8 q96h
Netilmicin	6.5	5	4	2	3	2.5	2

Cephalosporins; Penicillins; Beta-lactam/beta-lactamase inhibitors; Carbapenems—see Table 17, Sanford Guide to Antimicrobial Therapy 2007

Fluoroquinolone Antibiotics: adjust dosage of trovafloxacin in patients with hepatic insufficiency (see package inserts)

Ciprofloxacin	3–6/6–9	500–750 mg po (or 400 mg IV) q12h	D	100%		50–75% CRRT[‡]: 400 mg IV q24h	50%	HEMO: 250mg po or 200mg IV q12h CAPD: 250mg po or 200mg IV q8h	
Gatifloxacin[NUS]	7–14/36	400 mg po/IV q24h	D	400 mg q24h		200 mg q24h Same dose for CRRT[‡]	400 mg once, then 200mg q24h	HEMO: 200mg q24h AD[+] CAPD: 200mg q24h	
Gemifloxacin	7/>7	320 mg po q24h	D	320 mg q24h		160mg q24h	160 mg q24h	HEMO: 160mg q24h AD[+] CAPD: 160mg q24h	
Levofloxacin	4–8/76	750 mg IV, PO q24h	D&I[1]	750 mg q24h		20–49: 750 mg q48h <20: 750 mg once, then 500 mg q48h	750 mg x1, then 500 mg q48h	HEMO/CAPD: Dose for CrCl <20	CRRT[‡]: 750 mg once, then 500 mg q48h. As for CrCl 10–50

Macrolide Antibiotics: adjust dose of azithromycin in patients with hepatic insufficiency (see package insert)

| Clarithromycin | 5–7/22 | 0.5–1 gm q12h | D | 100% | | 75% | 50–75% | HEMO: Dose AD[1]
CAPD: None | CRRT: as for CrCl 10–50 |
| Erythromycin | 1.4/5–6 | 250–500 mg q6h | D | 100% | | 100% | 50–75% | HEMO/CAPD/CRRT[‡]: None | Ototoxicity with high doses in ESRD. Vol. of distribution increases in ESRD. |

Tetracycline Antibiotics

| Tetracycline | 6–10/57–108 | 250–500 mg qid | I | q8–12h | | q12–24h Same dose for CRRT[‡] | q24h | HEMO/CAPD/CRRT[‡]: None | Avoid in ESRD |

[1] Regardless of CrCl, 1st dose is 500mg, then adjust dose & interval.

[‡] **CRRT** = continuous renal replacement therapy. Usually results in CrCl of approx. 30 mL/min.   [+] **AD** = after dialysis. **"Dose AD"** refers only to timing of dose. **CAPD** = Continuous ambulatory peritoneal dialysis.

TABLE 15A (3)

ANTIMICROBIAL	HALF-LIFE (NORMAL/ESRD) hr	DOSE FOR NORMAL RENAL FUNCTION§	METHOD* (see footnote)	ADJUSTMENT FOR RENAL FAILURE Estimated creatinine clearance (CrCl), ml/min			HEMODIALYSIS, CAPD+ (see footnote)	COMMENTS & DOSAGE FOR CRRT‡
				>50–90	10–50	<10		
ANTIBACTERIAL ANTIBIOTICS *(continued)*								
Miscellaneous Antibacterial Antibiotics								
Linezolid	5-6/6-8	600 mg po/IV q12h	None	600 mg q12h	600mg q12h Same dose for CRRT‡	600 mg q12h, AD+	HEMO: As for CrCl <10 CAPD/CRRT‡: No dose adjustment	If high ultrafiltration rate, might need 600 mg q8h (CID 42:435, 2006) Accumulation of 2 metabolites—risk unknown (JAC 56:172, 2005).
Metronidazole	6–14/7–21	7.5 mg/kg q6h	D	100%	100%	50%	HEMO: Dose AD+ CAPD: Dose for CrCl <10	
Sulfadiazine	17/34	1 gm q6h	I	q8–12h	q24h	q48–72h or avoid	HEMO/CAPD: No data	
Sulfamethoxazole	10/20–50	1 gm q8h	I	q12h	q18h Same dose for CRRT‡	q24h	HEMO: 1gm AD+ CAPD: 1gm q24h	
Trimethoprim	11/20–49	100–200 mg q12h	I	q12h	q18h Same dose for CRRT‡	q24h	HEMO: Dose AD+ CAPD: q24h	CAVH‡: q18h
TMP/SMX-DS Treatment	As above	5 mg/kg IV q8h	D	100%	50%	Not recommended		
Prophylaxis	As above	tab 1 q24h or 3x/wk po	No change	100%	100%	100%		
Vancomycin[1]	6/200–250	1 gm q12h	D&I	1 gm q12h	1 gm q24–96h	1 gm q4–7 days	HEMO/CAPD: Dose for CrCl <10	CRRT‡: 500 mg q24–48h. New dialysis membranes ↑ clearance; **check levels.**
ANTIFUNGAL ANTIBIOTICS								
Amphotericin B & ampho B lipid complexes	24 hrs – 15 days/unchanged	Non-lipid: 0.4-1.0 mg/kg/day; ABCC:[2] 3–6 mg/kg/day; ABLC:[2] 5 mg/kg/day; LAB:[2] 3–5 mg/kg/day	I	q24h	q24h **Same dose for CRRT‡**	q24–48h	For non-lipid ampho B: HEMO/CAPD/CRRT‡: No dose adjustment	Toxicity lessened by saline loading; risk amplified by concomitant cyclosporine A, aminoglycosides, or pentamidine

[1] Vancomycin serum levels may be overestimated in renal failure if measured by either fluorescence polarization immunoassay or radioimmunoassay; vanco breakdown products interfere. EMIT method OK.
[2] **ABCC** = ampho B cholesteryl complex; **ABLC** = ampho B lipid complex; **LAB** = liposomal ampho B

‡ **CRRT** = continuous renal replacement therapy. Usually results in CrCl of approx. 30 mL/min. + **AD** = after dialysis. "**Dose AD**" refers only to timing of dose. **CAPD** = Continuous ambulatory peritoneal dialysis.

TABLE 15A (4)

ANTIMICROBIAL	HALF-LIFE (NORMAL/ESRD) hr	DOSE FOR NORMAL RENAL FUNCTION§	METHOD* (see footnote)	ADJUSTMENT FOR RENAL FAILURE Estimated creatinine clearance (CrCl), ml/min			HEMODIALYSIS, CAPD+ (see footnote)	COMMENTS & DOSAGE FOR CRRT‡
				>50-90	10-50	<10		
ANTIFUNGAL ANTIBIOTICS (continued)								
Fluconazole	37/100	200-400 mg q24h	D	100%	50%‡	50%	HEMO: 100% of normal renal function dose AD+ CAPD: Dose for CrCl <10	CRRT‡: 200-400 mg q24h
Flucytosine¹	3-6/75-200	37.5 mg/kg q6h	I	q12h	q12-24h **Same dose for CRRT‡**	q24h	HEMO: Dose AD+ CAPD: 0.5-1 gm q24h	Goal is peak serum level >25 mcg/ml and <100 mcg/ml¹.
Itraconazole solution, po	21/25	100-200 mg q12h	D	100%	100% **Same dose for CRRT‡**	50%	HEMO/CAPD: oral solution: 100 mg q12-24h No adjustment	
Itraconazole, IV	21/25	200 mg IV q12h	—	200 mg IV q12h			Do not use if CrCl <30 due to accumulation of cyclodextrin carrier	
Voriconazole, IV	Non-linear kinetics	6 mg/kg IV q12h x2, then 4mg/kg q12h	—	No change			If CrCl <50 ml/min, accumulation of IV vehicle (cyclodextrin); switch to po or dc For CRRT‡: 4 mg/kg po q12h	
ANTIPARASITIC ANTIBIOTICS								
Atovaquone	No data	750 mg po q12h					No data in patients with renal or hepatic impairment	
Dapsone	No data	100 mg po/day					No data in patients with renal or hepatic impairment	
Pentamidine	3-12/73-118	4 mg/kg/day	I	q24h	q24 **Same dose for CRRT‡**	q24-36h	HEMO: As for CrCl<10 plus 0.75 gm AD CAPD: As for CrCl<10	
Pyrimethamine	96/96	50-75 mg/day	No change	100%	100%	100%	HEMO/CAPD/CAVH: None	
ANTITUBERCULOUS ANTIBIOTICS (Excellent review: Nephron 64:169, 1993)								
Ethambutol	4/7-15	15-25 mg/kg q24h	I	q24h	q24-36h **Same dose for CRRT‡**	q48h	HEMO: Dose AD+ CAPD: Dose for CrCl <10	25 mg/kg 4-6hr prior to dialysis for usual 3x/wk dialysis. Streptomycin recommended in lieu of ethambutol in renal failure.
Ethionamide	2.1/unknown	250-500 mg q12h	D	100%	100%	50%	HEMO/CAPD/CRRT‡: None	
Isoniazid	0.7-4/8-17	5 mg/kg/day (max. 300mg)	D	100%	100% **Same dose for CRRT‡**	100%	HEMO: Dose AD+ CAPD: Dose for CrCl <10	
Pyrazinamide	9/26	25 mg/kg q24h (max. dose 2.5gm q24h)	D	100%	100% **Same dose for CRRT‡**	12-25 mg/kg q24h	HEMO: 40 mg/kg 24 hrs prior to each 3x/wk dialysis CAPD: No reduction	

[1] Concentrations <25 mcg/ml should be avoided to prevent development of resistance, while >100 mcg/ml avoided because of toxicity (JAC 35:241, 1995)

‡ **CRRT** = continuous renal replacement therapy. Usually results in CrCl of approx. 30 mL/min.   + **AD** = after dialysis. "**Dose AD**" refers only to timing of dose. **CAPD** = Continuous ambulatory peritoneal dialysis.

TABLE 15A (5)

ANTIMICROBIAL	HALF-LIFE (NORMAL/ESRD) hr	DOSE FOR NORMAL RENAL FUNCTION§	METHOD* (see footnote)	ADJUSTMENT FOR RENAL FAILURE Estimated creatinine clearanc (CrCl), ml/min			HEMODIALYSIS, CAPD+ (see footnote)	COMMENTS & DOSAGE FOR CRRT‡
				>50–90	10–50	<10		
ANTITUBERCULOUS ANTIBIOTICS (continued)								
Rifabutin	No data	300 mg/day po					No data available	
Rifampin	1.5–5/1.8–11	600 mg/day	D	600 mg q24h	300–600 mg q24h Same dose for CRRT‡	300–600 mg q24h	HEMO: None CAPD/ CAVH‡: Dose for CrCl <10	Biologically active metabolite
ANTIVIRAL AGENTS								
Acyclovir	2–4/20	5–12.4 mg/kg q8h	D&I	100% q8h	100% q12–24h	50% q24h	HEMO: Dose AD+ CAPD: Dose for CrCl <10	Rapid IV infusion can cause renal failure. CRRT‡ dose: 5-10 mg/kg q24h
Adefovir	7.5/15	10 mg po q24h	I	10 mg q24h	10 mg q48–72h	10 mg q7 days	HEMO: 10 mg q7 days AD+	CAPD: No data CRRT‡: No data
Atripla	See each drug	200 mg emtracitabine + 300 mg tenofovir + 600 mg efavirenz	I	Do not use if CrCl<50				
Cidofovir: **Complicated dosing—see package insert**								
Induction	2.5/unknown	5 mg/kg 1x/wk for 2 wks	—	5 mg/kg 1x/wk	0.5–2 mg/kg 1x/wk	0.5 mg/kg 1x/wk	No data–avoid	Major toxicity is renal. No efficacy, safety, or pharmacokinetic data in pts with moderate/severe renal disease.
Maintenance	2.5/unknown	5 mg/kg q2wks	—	5 mg/kg q2wks	0.5–2 mg/kg q2wks	0.5 mg/kg q2wks	No data–avoid	
Didanosine tablets	0.6–1.6/4.5	125–200 mg q12h buffered tabs	D	200 mg q12h	200 mg q24h	<60 kg: 150 mg q24h >60 kg: 100 mg q24h	HEMO: Dose CAPD/CAVH/CRRT‡: Dose for CrCl <10	Based on incomplete data. Data are estimates.
		400 mg q24h, enteric-coated tabs	D	400 mg q24h	125–200 mg q24h	Do not use EC tabs	HEMO/CAPD: Dose for CrCl <10	If <60kg & CrCl <10 ml per min, do not use EC tabs
Emtricitabine	10/>10	200 mg q24h	I	200 mg q24h	200 mg q48–72h	200 mg q96h	HEMO: Dose for CrCl <10	
Emtracitabine + tenofovir	See each drug	200 mg emtracitabine + 300 mg tenofovir q24h	I	No change	1 tab q48h	Do not use		
Entecavir	128-149/prolonged	0.5 mg q24h	D	0.5 mg q24h	0.15–0.25 mg q24h	0.05 mg q24h	HEMO/CAPD: 0.05 mg q24h	Give after dialysis on dialysis days
Famciclovir	2.3–3.0/10–22	500 mg q8h	D&I	500 mg q8h	500 mg q12–24h	250 mg q24h	HEMO: 250 mg AD+ CAPD: No data	CRRT‡: Not applicable

‡ **CRRT** = continuous renal replacement therapy. Usually results in CrCl of approx. 30 mL/min.   + **AD** = after dialysis.   "**Dose AD**" refers only to timing of dose.   **CAPD** = Continuous ambulatory peritoneal dialysis.

TABLE 15A (6)

ANTIMICROBIAL	HALF-LIFE (NORMAL/ESRD) hr	DOSE FOR NORMAL RENAL FUNCTION§	METHOD* (see footnote)	ADJUSTMENT FOR RENAL FAILURE Estimated creatinine clearance (CrCl), ml/min					HEMODIALYSIS, CAPD+ (see footnote)				COMMENTS & DOSAGE FOR CRRT‡
				CrCl as ml/min²/kg body weight—ONLY FOR FOSCARNET									
				>1.4	>1.0–1.4 / >50–90	>0.8–1.0 / 10–50	>0.6–0.8 / <10	>0.5–0.6	>0.4–0.5	<0.4			

ANTIVIRAL AGENTS (continued)

ANTIMICROBIAL	HALF-LIFE	DOSE FOR NORMAL RENAL FUNCTION	METHOD	>1.4	>1.0–1.4	>0.8–1.0	>0.6–0.8	>0.5–0.6	>0.4–0.5	<0.4	HEMO/CAPD	COMMENTS & DOSAGE FOR CRRT
Foscarnet (CMV dosage) Dosage adjustment based on est. CrCl (ml/min)	Normal half-life (T½) 3hrs with terminal T½ of 18–88hrs. T½ very long with ESRD	Induction: 60mg/kg q8h x2–3wks IV		60 q8h	45 q8h	50 q12h	40 q12h	60 q24h	50 q24h	Do not use		See package insert for further details
		Maintenance: 90–120mg/kg/day IV		120 q24h	90 q24h	65 q24h	105 q48h	80 q48h	65 q48h	Do not use		
Ganciclovir	3.6/30	IV: Induction 5 mg/kg q12h IV	D&I	5mg/kg q12h	2.5–5mg/kg q24h	1.25–2.5mg/kg q24h	1.25 mg/kg 3x/wk		HEMO: Dose AD+ CAPD: Dose for CrCl <10			
		Maintenance 5 mg/kg q24h IV	D&I			0.6–1.25mg/kg q24h	0.625 mg/kg 3x/week		HEMO: 0.6 mg/kg AD+ CAPD: Dose for CrCl <10			
		po: 1 gm po q8h	D&I		0.5–1gm q8h	0.5–1gm q24h	0.5 gm 3x/wk		HEMO: 0.5 gm AD+			
Indinavir/ nelfinavir/ nevirapine	No data			No data with renal insufficiency. Less than 20% renal excretion. Probably no dose reduction.								
Lamivudine	5–7/15–35	300 mg po q24h	D&I	300mg q24h		50–150 mg q24h	25–50 mg q24h		HEMO: Dose AD+; CAPD : No data; CRRT‡:100 mg 1st day, then 50 mg/day			
Maraviroc	14–18/unknown	300 mg bid		300 mg bid		No data	No data		Increased risk of side effects if maraviroc + CYP3A inhibitor and CrCl <50 mL/min			
Ritonavir & saquinavir				Negligible renal clearance. At present, no patient data								
Stavudine, po	1–1.4/5.5–8	30–40 mg q12h	D/I	100%		50% q12–24h Same dose for CRRT	≥60 kg: 20 mg/day <60 kg: 15 mg/day		HEMO: Dose as for CrCl <AD+ 10 CAPD: No data			CRRT‡: Full dose
Tenofovir	8–12/very prolonged	300 mg po q24h	—	300 mg q24h		Avoid if CrCl <60	No data		HEMO: 300 mg po after every 3rd dialysis or every 7 days if no dialysis			

‡ **CRRT** = continuous renal replacement therapy. Usually results in CrCl of approx. 30 mL/min. + **AD** = after dialysis. "**Dose AD**" refers only to timing of dose. **CAPD** = Continuous ambulatory peritoneal dialysis.

TABLE 15A (7)

ANTIMICROBIAL	HALF-LIFE (NORMAL/ESRD) hr	DOSE FOR NORMAL RENAL FUNCTION[§]	METHOD* (see footnote)	ADJUSTMENT FOR RENAL FAILURE Estimated creatinine clearance (CrCl), ml/min			HEMODIALYSIS, CAPD[+] (see footnote)	COMMENTS & DOSAGE FOR CRRT[‡]
				>50–90	10–50	<10		
ANTIVIRAL AGENTS (continued)								
Valacyclovir	2.5–3.3/14	1 gm q8h (for H. zoster in healthy pts)	D&I	1 gm q8h	1 gm q12–24h **Same dose for CRRT**[‡]	0.5 gm q24h	HEMO: Dose AD[+] CAPD: Dose for CrCl <10	
Valganciclovir	4/67	900 mg po q12h	D&I	900 mg po q12h	450 mg q24h to 450 mg every other day	Do not use	see package insert	
Zalcitabine	2.0/>8	0.75 mg q8h	D&I	0.75 mg q8h	0.75 mg q12h **Same dose for CRRT**[‡]	0.75 mg q24h	HEMO: Dose AD[+] CAPD: No data	
Zidovudine	1.1–1.4/1.4–3	300 mg q12h	D&I	300 mg q12h	300 mg q12h **Same dose for CRRT**[‡]	100 mg q6-8h	HEMO: Dose for CrCl <10 AD[+] CAPD: Dose for CrCl <10	

[§] Dosages are for life-threatening infections; *D = dosage reduction, I = interval extension; ** Per cent refers to % change from dose for normal renal function. **Abbreviations: HEMO** = hemodialysis; **CAPD** = chronic ambulatory peritoneal dialysis; **ESRD** = endstage renal disease; **NUS** = not available in the U.S. [+] **AD** = after dialysis. **"Dose AD"** refers only to timing of dose. **CAPD** = Continuous ambulatory peritoneal dialysis.

[‡] **CRRT** = continuous renal replacement therapy. Usually results in CrCl of approx. 30 mL/min.

TABLE 15B: NO DOSAGE ADJUSTMENT WITH RENAL INSUFFICIENCY, BY CATEGORY

Antibacterials		Antifungals	Anti-TBc	Antivirals	
Azithromycin	Linezolid	Amphotericin B	Rifabutin	Abacavir	Indinavir
Ceftriaxone	Minocycline	Anidulafungin	Rifapentine	Atazanavir	Lopinavir
Chloramphenicol	Moxifloxacin	Caspofungin		Darunavir	Nelfinavir
Ciprofloxacin XL	Nafcillin	Itraconazole (oral soln)		Delavirdine	Nevirapine
Clindamycin	Pyrimethamine	Micafungin		Efavirenz	Raltegravir
Dirithromycin	Rifaximin	Posaconazole		Enfuvirtide[1]	Ribavirin
Doxycycline	Tigecycline	Voriconazole, po only		Etravirine	Saquinavir
				Fosamprenavir	Tipranavir

TABLE 15C: DOSAGE OF ANTIRETROVIRAL DRUGS IN PATIENTS WITH IMPAIRED HEPATIC FUNCTION
(See CID 40:174, 2005)

DRUG GENERIC (TRADE)	STANDARD DOSE	DOSING IF HEPATIC IMPAIRMENT CHILD-PUGH SCORE*	ADJUSTED DOSE	COMMENTS
Protease inhibitors				
Amprenavir (Agenerase)	1200 mg po q24h	5–8 / 9–12	450 mg q12h / 300 mg q12h	
Atazanavir (Reyataz)	300–400 mg po q24h	7–9 / >9	300 mg q24h / Do not use	
Darunavir	600 mg po bid with ritonavir	Use with caution. No specific dose suggested		
Fosamprenavir (Lexiva)	1400 mg po q12h	5–9 / 10–12	700 mg q12h / 350 mg bid	
Indinavir (Crixivan)	800 mg po q8h	Mild to moderate hepatic insufficiency	600 mg q8h	
Lopinavir/ritonavir (Kaletra)	400 mg / 100 mg po q12h	No dosage recommendations; use with caution if hepatic impairment		
Nelfinavir (Viracept)	1250 mg po q12h	No dosage recommendations; use with caution if hepatic impairment		
Ritonavir (Norvir)	600 mg po q12h	No dosage recommendations; use with caution if hepatic impairment		
Saquinavir (Invirase)	1000 mg po + 100 mg ritonavir bid	No dosage recommendations; use with caution if hepatic impairment		
Tipranavir	500 mg + 200 mg ritonavir po bid	5-9 / >9	No dosage adjustment / No data	
Fusion & Entry Inhibitors				
Enfuvirtide (Fuzeon)	90 mg subQ q12h	No dosage adjustment recommendations		
Maraviroc (Selzentry)	300 mg po bid; See page 36	No dosage recommendations; use caution if hepatic impairment		

*CALCULATION OF CHILD-PUGH SCORE—Classification below

CLINICAL FEATURE	SCORE GIVEN		
	1	2	3
Encephalopathy (see below)**	None	Grade 1–2	Grade 3–4
Albumin	>3.5 gm/dl	2.8–3.5 gm/dl	<2.8 gm/dl
Total bilirubin	<2 mg/dl	2–3 mg/dl	>3 mg/dl
If taking indinavir or if Gilbert's syndrome	<4 mg/dl	4–7 mg/dl	>7 mg/dl
Prothrombin time	<4	4–6	>6
or INR	<1.7	1.7–2.3	>2.3

CLASSIFICATION

Score	Class
5–6	A
7–9	B
>9	C

**GRADE OF ENCEPHALOPATHY

Grade	Clinical Criteria
1	Mild confusion, anxiety, restlessness, fine tremor, slow coordination
2	Drowsiness, asterixis
3	Somnolent but arousable, marked confusion, speech incomprehensible, incontinent, hyperventilation
4	Coma, decerebrate posturing, flaccidity

---

[1] Enfuvirtide not studied in patients with CrCl<35 ml/min. **DO NOT USE.**

TABLE 16A: DRUG/DRUG INTERACTIONS: ANTIRETROVIRAL DRUGS & DRUGS USED IN TREATMENT OF HIV-ASSOCIATED INFECTIONS & MALIGNANCIES

This is a selected list. For drug-drug interactions of other antimicrobials, please refer to Table 22 of the SANFORD GUIDE TO ANTIMICROBIAL THERAPY 2007 & NEJM 344:985, 2001.

Significance/Certainty: ± = theory/anecdotal; + = of probable clinical import; ++ = of definite clinical import

ANTI-INFECTIVE AGENT (A)	OTHER DRUG (B)	EFFECT	SIGNIFICANCE/ CERTAINTY
Aminoglycosides— parenteral (amikacin, gentamicin, kanamycin, netilmicin, sisomicin, streptomycin, tobramycin) NOTE: Capreomycin is an aminoglycoside, used as alternative drug to treat mycobacterial infections.	Amphotericin B	↑ nephrotoxicity	++
	Cis platinum (Platinol)	↑ nephro & ototoxicity	+
	Cyclosporine	↑ nephrotoxicity	+
	Neuromuscular blocking agents	↑ apnea or respiratory paralysis	+
	Loop diuretics (e.g., furosemide)	↑ ototoxicity	++
	NSAIDs	↑ nephrotoxicity	+
	Non-polarizing muscle relaxants	↑ apnea	+
	Radiographic contrast	↑ nephrotoxicity	+
	Vancomycin	↑ nephrotoxicity	+
Aminoglycosides— oral (kanamycin, neomycin)	Oral anticoagulants (dicumarol, phenindione, warfarin)	↑ prothrombin time	+
Amphotericin B & ampho B lipid formulations	**Antineoplastic drugs**	**↑ nephrotoxicity risk**	+
	Digitalis	↑ toxicity of B if hypokalemia	+
	Nephrotoxic drugs: aminoglycosides, cidofovir, cyclosporin, foscarnet, pentamidine	↑ nephrotoxicity of A	++
Fosamprenavir	Antiretrovirals—see *Table 16B* & *Table 16C*		
	Contraceptives, oral	↓ levels of A & B; **use other contraception**	++
	Lovastatin/simvastatin	↑ levels of B—**avoid**	++
	Methadone	↓ levels of B	++
	Rifabutin	↑ levels of B (↓ dose by 50–75%)	++
	Rifampin	↓ levels of A—**avoid**	++
Atazanavir	See Protease inhibitors & *Table 16B* & *Table 16C*		
Atovaquone	Rifampin (perhaps rifabutin)	↓ serum levels of A; ↑ levels of B	+
	Metoclopramide	↓ levels of A	+
	Tetracycline	↓ levels of A	++

Azole Antifungal Agents[1] [**Flu** = fluconazole, **Itr** = itraconazole, **Ket** = ketoconazole, **Posa** = posaconazole, **Vor** = voriconazole, **+** = occurs, **blank space** = either studied & no interaction OR no data found (may be in pharm. co. databases)]

Posa	Flu	Itr	Ket	Vor	Drug B	Effect	Significance
	+	+			Amitriptyline	↑ levels of B	+
	+	+	+	+	Calcium channel blockers	↑ levels of B	++
		+		+	Carbamazepine (vori contraindicated)	↓ levels of A	++
+	+	+	+	+	Cyclosporine	↑ levels of B, ↑ risk of nephrotoxicity	+
		+	+		Didanosine	↓ absorption of A	
+		+	+		Efavirenz	↓ levels of A, ↑ levels of B	++ (avoid)
+		+	+		H₂ blockers, antacids, sucralfate	↓ absorption of A	+
+	+	+	+	+	Hydantoins (phenytoin, Dilantin)	↑ levels of B, ↓ levels of A	++
	+	+			Isoniazid	↓ levels of A	+
		+		+	Lovastatin/simvastatin	Rhabdomyolysis reported; ↑ levels of B	++
+	+	+	+	+	Midazolam/triazolam, po	↑ levels of B	++
+	+	+	+		Oral anticoagulants	↑ effect of B	++
+		+	+	+	Oral hypoglycemics	↑ levels of B	++
		+			Pimozide	↑ levels of B	++
	+	+	+		Protease inhibitors	↑ levels of B	++
	+	+	+		Proton pump inhibitors	↓ absorption of A, ↑ levels of B	++
+	+	+	+	+	Rifampin/rifabutin (vori contraindicated)	↑ levels of B, ↓ serum levels of A	++
				+	Sirolimus (vori contraindicated)	↑ levels of B	++
+	+		+		Tacrolimus	↑ levels of B with toxicity	++
	+		+		Theophyllines	↑ levels of B	+
		+			Trazodone	↑ levels of B	++
+					Zidovudine	↑ levels of B	+
Caspofungin	Cyclosporine	↑ levels of A	++
	Tacrolimus	↓ levels of B	++
	Carbamazepine, dexamethasone, efavirenz, nelfinavir, nevirapine, phenytoin, rifamycin	↓ levels of A; ↑ dose of caspofungin to 70 mg/day	++

[1] Major interactions given; **unusual or minor interactions** manifest as toxicity of non-azole drug due to ↑ serum levels: Caffeine (Flu), digoxin (Itr), felodipine (Itr), fluoxetine (Itr), indinavir (Ket), lovastatin/simvastatin, quinidine (Ket), tricyclics (Flu), & ↓ effectiveness of oral contraceptives.

TABLE 16A (2)

ANTI-INFECTIVE AGENT (A)	OTHER DRUG (B)	EFFECT	SIGNIFICANCE/ CERTAINTY
Clindamycin (Cleocin)	Kaolin	↓ absorption of A	+
	Muscle relaxants, e.g., atracurium, baclofen, diazepam	↑ frequency/duration of respiratory paralysis	+
Cycloserine	Ethanol	↑ frequency of seizures	+
	INH, ethionamide	↑ frequency of drowsiness/dizziness	+
Dapsone	Didanosine	↓ absorption of A	+
	Oral contraceptives	↓ effectiveness of B	+
	Pyrimethamine	↑ in marrow toxicity	+
	Rifampin/Rifabutin	↓ serum levels of A	+
	Trimethoprim	↑ levels of A & B (methemoglobinemia)	+
	Zidovudine	May ↑ marrow toxicity	+
Delavirdine (Rescriptor)	See Non-nucleoside reverse transcriptase inhibitors (NNRTIs) & TABLE 16C		
Didanosine (ddI) (Videx) NOTE: ddI & tenofovir can ↓ CD4 count without increase in viral "load"	Allopurinol	↑ level of A – **AVOID**	++
	Cisplatin, dapsone, INH, metronidazole, nitrofurantoin, stavudine, vincristine, zalcitabine	↑ risk of peripheral neuropathy	+
	Ethanol, lamivudine, pentamidine	↑ risk of pancreatitis	+
	Fluoroquinolones	↓ absorption 2° to chelation	+
	Ganciclovir	↑ levels of A	+
	Drugs that need low pH for absorption: dapsone, indinavir, itra/ketoconazole, pyrimethamine, rifampin, trimethoprim	↓ absorption	+
	Methadone	↓ levels of A	++
	Ribavirin	↑ levels of ddI metabolite—**avoid**	++
	Tenofovir	↑ levels of A (**reduce dose of A**)	++
Efavirenz (Sustiva)	See Non-nucleoside reverse transcriptase inhibitors (NNRTIs) & TABLE 16C		
Ethambutol (Myambutol)	Aluminum salts (includes didanosine buffer)	↓ absorption of A & B	+
Etravirine (Intelence)	See Non-nucleoside reverse transcriptase inhibitors (NNRTIs) & TABLE 16C		
Fluoroquinolones	(**Cipro** = ciprofloxacin; **Gati** = gatifloxacin; **Gemi** = gemifloxacin, **Levo** = levofloxacin; **Moxi** = moxifloxacin; **Oflox** = ofloxacin)		

Cipro	Gati[1]	Gemi	Levo	Moxi	Oflox	Other Drug (B)	Effect	Sig/Cert
						NOTE: Blank space = either studied & no interaction OR no data found (pharmaceutical company may have data)		
	+		+	+		**Antiarrhythmics (procainamide, amiodarone)**	↑ Q-T interval (torsade)	++
+	+		+	+	+	Insulin, oral hypoglycemics	↑ & ↓ blood sugar	++
+						Caffeine	↑ levels of B	+
+				+		Cimetidine	↑ levels of A	+
+				+		Cyclosporine	↑ levels of B	±
+	+		+	+	+	Didanosine	↓ absorption of A	++
+	+	+	+	+	+	**Cations: Al^{+++}, Ca^{++1}, Fe^{++}, Mg^{++}, Zn^{++} (antacids, vitamins, dairy products), citrate/citric acid**	↓ absorption of A (some variability between drugs)	++
+						Foscarnet	↑ risk of seizures	+
+						Methadone	↑ levels of B	++
+		+		+		NSAIDs	↑ risk CNS stimulation/seizures	++
+						Phenytoin	↑ or ↓ levels of B	+
+	+	+		+		Probenecid	↓ renal clearance of A	+
+						Rasagiline	↑ levels of B	++
			+			Rifampin	↓ levels of A	++
+	+	+	+	+		Sucralfate	↓ absorption of A	++
+						Theophylline	↑ levels of B	++
+						Thyroid hormone	↓ levels of B	++
+						Tizanidine	↑ levels of B	++
+		+		+		Warfarin	↑ prothrombin time	+

ANTI-INFECTIVE AGENT (A)	OTHER DRUG (B)	EFFECT	SIGNIFICANCE/CERTAINTY
Foscarnet (Foscavir)	Ciprofloxacin	↑ risk of seizures	+
	Nephrotoxic drugs: aminoglycosides, ampho B, cis-platinum, cyclosporine	↑ risk of nephrotoxicity	+
	Pentamidine IV	↑ risk of severe hypocalcemia	++
Ganciclovir (Cytovene) & **Valganciclovir**	Imipenem	↑ risk of seizures reported	+
	Probenecid	↑ levels of A	+
	Zidovudine	↓ levels of A, ↑ levels of B	+
Gentamicin	See Aminoglycosides—parenteral		
Indinavir	See Protease Inhibitors & Table 16B & C		

[1] Neither Gati, Gemi, nor Moxi interacts with calcium but may interact with other multi-valent cations.

TABLE 16A (3)

ANTI-INFECTIVE AGENT (A)	OTHER DRUG (B)	EFFECT	SIGNIFICANCE/ CERTAINTY
Isoniazid	**Alcohol, rifampin**	**↑ risk of hepatic injury**	++
	Aluminum salts	↓ absorption (take fasting)	++
	Carbamazepine, phenytoin	↑ levels of B with nausea, vomiting, nystagmus, ataxia	++
Isoniazid (continued)	Itraconazole, ketoconazole	↓ levels of B	+
	Oral hypoglycemics	↓ effects of B	+
Lamivudine	Zalcitabine + emtricitabine	**Mutual interference—do not combine**	++
Linezolid (Zyvox)	Adrenergic agents	Risk of hypertension	++
	Aged, fermented, pickled or smoked foods—↑ tyramine	Risk of hypertension	+
	Rifampin	↓ levels of A	++
	Serotonergic drugs (SSRIs)	Risk of serotonin syndrome	+
Lopinavir	*See Protease inhibitors*		

Macrolides (**Ery** = erythromycin, **Dir** = dirithromycin, **Azi** = azithromycin, **Clr** = clarithromycin; **+** = occurs, **blank space** = either studied & no interaction OR no data (pharmaceutical company may have data)

Ery	Dir	Azi	Clr	Other Drug (B)	EFFECT	SIGNIFICANCE/CERTAINTY
+	+		+	Carbamazepine	↑ serum levels of B, nystagmus, nausea, vomiting, ataxia	++ (avoid with erythro)
+			+	Cimetidine, **ritonavir**	↑ levels of B	+
+				Clozapine	↑ serum levels of B, CNS toxicity	+
				Colchicine	**↑ levels of B (Potent. Fatal)**	++ (avoid)
+				Corticosteroids	↑ effects of B	+
+	+	+	+	Cyclosporine	↑ serum levels of B with toxicity	+
+	+	+	+	Digoxin, digitoxin	↑ serum levels of B (10% of cases)	+
			+	Efavirenz	↓ levels of A	++
+	+		+	Ergot alkaloids	↑ levels of B	++
+	+		+	Lovastatin/simvastatin	↑ levels of B, rhabdomyolysis	++
+				Midazolam, triazolam	↑ levels of B, ↑ sedative effects	+
+	+		+	Phenytoin	↑ levels of B	+
+	+	+	+	Pimozide	**↑ Q-T interval**	++
+			+	Rifampin, rifabutin	↓ levels of A	+
+			+	Tacrolimus	↑ levels of B	++
+			+	Theophyllines	↑ serum levels of B with nausea, vomiting, seizures, apnea	++
+	+		+	Valproic acid	↑ levels of B	+
+	+		+	Warfarin	May ↑ prothrombin time	+
			+	Zidovudine	↓ levels of B	+

ANTI-INFECTIVE AGENT (A)	OTHER DRUG (B)	EFFECT	SIGNIFICANCE/CERTAINTY
Maraviroc	Clarithromycin	↑ serum levels of A	++
	Delavirdine	↑ levels of A	++
	Itraconazole, ketoconazole	↑ levels of A	++
	Nefazodine	↑ levels of A	++
	Protease Inhibitors (not tipranavir/ritonavir)	↑ levels of A	++
	Anticonvulsants: carbamamzepine, phenobarbitol, phenytoin	↓ levels of A	++
	Efavirenz	↓ levels of A	++
	Rifampin	↓ levels of A	++
Metronidazole	**Alcohol**	Disulfiram-like reaction	+
	Cyclosporin	↑ levels of B	++
	Disulfiram (Antabuse)	Acute toxic psychosis	+
	Lithium	↑ levels of B	++
	Oral anticoagulants	↑ anticoagulant effect	++
	Phenobarbital, hydantoins	↑ levels of B	++
Micafungin	Nifedipine	↑ levels of B	+
	Sirolimus	↑ levels of B	+
Nelfinavir	*See Protease inhibitors & Table 16B & Table 16C*		
Nevirapine (Viramune)	*See Non-nucleoside reverse transcriptase inhibitors (NNRTIs) & Table 16C*		

Non-nucleoside reverse transcriptase inhibitors (NNRTIs): For interactions with protease inhibitors, see *Table 16C*.
Del = delavirdine, **Efa** = efavirenz, **Etr** = etravirine, **Nev** = nevirapine

Del	Efa	Etr	Nev	Co-administration contraindicated (CAC):		
+				Anticonvulsants: carbamazepine, phenobarbital, phenytoin		++
+				Antimycobacterials: rifabutin, rifampin		++
+				Antipsychotics: pimozide		++
+	+			Benzodiazepines: alprazolam, midazolam, triazolam		++
+	+			Ergotamine		++
+	+			HMG-CoA inhibitors (statins): lovastatin, simvastatin		++
+				St. John's wort		++

TABLE 16A (4)

ANTI-INFECTIVE AGENT (A)				OTHER DRUG (B)	EFFECT	SIGNIFICANCE/ CERTAINTY
Del	Efa	Etr	Nev	**Dose change needed:**		
+				Amphetamines	↑ levels of B—**caution**	++
+			+	Antiarrhythmics: amiodarone, lidocaine, others	↓ or ↑ levels of B—**caution**	++
+	+		+	Antifungals: itraconazole, ketoconazole, posaconazole, voriconazole	Potential ↓ levels of B, ↑ levels of A	+
+			+	Antirejection drugs: cyclosporine, rapamycin, sirolimus, tacrolimus	↑ levels of B	++
+			+	Calcium channel blockers	↑ levels of B	++
+			+	Clarithromycin	↑ levels of B metabolite, ↑ levels of A	++
+			+	Cyclosporine	↑ levels of B	++
+				Dexamethasone	↓ levels of A	++
+	+	+	+	Sildenafil, vardenafil, tadalafil	↑ levels of B	++
+				Gastric acid suppression: antacids, H-2 blockers, proton pump inhibitors	↓ levels of A	++
	+		+	Methadone, fentanyl	↓ levels of B	++
	+		+	Oral contraceptives	↑ or ↓ levels of B	++
+	+	+	+	Protease inhibitors—see Table 16B & Table 16C		
+	+	+	+	**Rifabutin, rifampin**	↑ or ↓ levels of rifabutin; ↓ levels of A—**caution**	++
+		+	+	Warfarin	↑ levels of B	++
Pentamidine, IV				Amphotericin B	↑ risk of nephrotoxicity	+
				Foscarnet	↑ risk of hypocalcemia	+
				Pancreatitis-associated drugs, e.g., alcohol, valproic acid	↑ risk of pancreatitis	+

Protease Inhibitors – Anti-HIV Drugs (**Atazan** = ataznavir; **Darun** = Darunavir; **Fosampren** = fosamprenavir; **Indin** = indinavir; **Lopin** = lopinavir; **Nelfin** = nelfinavir; **Saquin** = saquinavir; **Tipran** = tipranavir). For interactions with antiretrovirals see Table 16B & Table 16C. **Only a partial list—check package insert.**

Atazan	Darun	Fosampren	Indin	Lopin	Nelfin	Saquin	Tipran	Also see http://aidsinfo.nih.gov		
								Analgesics		
							+	1. Alfentanil, fentanyl, hydrocodone, tramadol	↑ levels of B	+
	+			+			+	2. Codeine, hydromorphone, morphine, methadone	↓ levels of B	+
+	+	+	+	+	+			**Anti-arrhythmics: amiodarone, lidocaine, mexiletine, flecainide**	↑ levels of B; **do not co-administer**	++
	+		+	+	+	+		**Anticonvulsants: carbamazepine, clonazepam, phenytoin, phenobarbital**	↓ levels of A, ↓levels of B	++
+		+	+				+	Antidepressants, all tricyclic	↑ levels of B	++
+	+						+	Antidepressants, all other	↑ levels of B; **no pimozide**	++
+								Antidepressants: SSRIs	↓ levels of B—avoid	++
+	+	+	+	+	+	+	+	**Benzodiazepines, e.g., diazepam, midazolam, triazolam**	↑ **levels of B—do not use**	++
+	+	+	+	+	+	+	+	Calcium channel blockers (all)	↑ levels of B	++
+	+			+	+	+	+	Clarithro, erythro	↑levels of B if renal impairment	+
			+	+		+	+	Contraceptives, oral	↓ levels of A & B	++
	+	+			+			Corticosteroids: prednisone, dexamethasone	↓ levels of A, ↑ levels of B	+
+	+	+	+	+	+	+	+	Cyclosporine	↑ levels of B, monitor levels	+
							+	Digoxin	↑ levels of B	++
+	+	+	+	+	+	+	+	Ergot derivatives	↑ **levels of B—do not use**	++
		+		+	+			Grapefruit juice (>200ml/day)	↓ indinavir & ↑ saquinavir levels	++
+	+	+	+	+	+	+		H2 receptor antagonists	↓ **levels of A**	++
+	+	+	+	+	+	+	+	HMG-CoA reductase inhibitors (statins): lovastatin, simvastatin	↑ **levels of B—do not use**	++
+								Irinotecan	↑ **levels of B—do not use**	++
+	+	+	+	+	+	+	+	Ketoconazole, itraconazole, ?vori	↑ levels of A,↑ levels of B	+
	+		+				+	Metronidazole	Possible disulfiram reaction, alcohol	+
+	+	+	+	+				**Pimozide**	↑ **levels of B—do not use**	++
+	+		+	+		+		**Proton pump inhibitors**	↓ **levels of A**	++

TABLE 16A (5)

Protease Inhibitors – Anti-HIV Drugs (**Atazan** = ataznavir; **Darun** = Darunavir; **Fosampren** = fosaprenavir; **Indin** = indinavir; **Lopin** = lopinavir; **Nelfin** = nelfinavir).

ANTI-INFECTIVE AGENT (A)	OTHER DRUG (B)	EFFECT	SIGNIFICANCE/ CERTAINTY
Atazan / Darun / Fosampren / Indin / Lopin / Nelfin / Saquin / Tipran	Also see http://aidsinfo.nih.gov		
+ + + + + + + +	Rifampin, rifabutin	↓ levels of A, ↑levels of B **(avoid)**	++ (avoid)
+ + + + + + + +	Sildenafil (Viagra), tadalafil, vardenafil	Varies, some ↑ & some ↓ levels of B	++
+ + + + + + + +	**St. John's wort**	**↓ levels of A—do not use**	++
	Sirolimus, tracrolimus	↑ levels of B	++
+	Tenofovir	↓ levels of B – add ritonavir	++
+ + + +	Theophylline	↓ levels of B	+
+ + + +	Warfarin	↑ levels of B	+
Pyrazinamide	INH, rifampin	May ↑ risk of hepatotoxicity	±
Pyrimethamine	Lorazepam	↑ risk of hepatotoxicity	+
	Sulfonamides, TMP/SMX	↑ risk of marrow suppression	+
	Zidovudine	↑ risk of marrow suppression	+
Quinine	Digoxin	↑ digoxin levels; ↑ toxicity	++
	Mefloquine	↑ arrhythmias	+
	Oral anticoagulants	↑ prothrombin time	++
Quinupristin/ dalfopristin (Synercid)	Anti-HIV drugs: NNRTIs & PIs	↑ levels of B	++
	Antineoplastic: vincristine, docetaxel, paclitaxel	↑ levels of B	++
	Calcium channel blockers	↑ levels of B	++
	Carbamazepine	↑ levels of B	++
	Cyclosporine, tacrolimus	↑ levels of B	++
	Lidocaine	↑ levels of B	++
	Methylprednisolone	↑ levels of B	++
	Midazolam, diazepam	↑ levels of B	++
	Statins	↑ levels of B	++
Raltegravir	Rifampin	↓ levels of A	++
Ribavirin	Didanosine	↑ levels of B → toxicity—**avoid**	++
	Stavudine	↓ levels of B	++
	Zidovudine	↓ levels of B	++
Rifamycins (rifampin, rifabutin) Ref.: ArIM 162:985,2002 **The following is a partial list of drugs with rifampin-induced ↑ metabolism & hence lower than anticipated serum levels: ACE inhibitors, dapsone, diazepam, digoxin, diltiazem, doxycycline, fluconazole, fluvastatin, haloperidol, nifedipine, progestins, triazolam, tricyclics, voriconazole, zidovudine**	Al OH, ketoconazole, PZA	↓ levels of A	+
	Atovaquone	↑ levels of A, ↓ levels of B	+
	β adrenergic blockers (metoprolol, propranolol)	↓ effect of B	+
	Caspofungin	↓ levels of B—increase dose	++
	Clarithromycin	↑ levels of A, ↓ levels of B	++
	Corticosteroids	↑ replacement requirement of B	++
	Cyclosporine	↓ effect of B	++
	Delavirdine	**↑ levels of A, ↓ levels of B—avoid**	++
	Digoxin	↓ levels of B	++
	Disopyramide	↓ levels of B	++
	Fluconazole	↑ levels of A[1]	+
	Amprenavir, indinavir, nelfinavir, ritonavir	↑ levels of A (↓ dose of A), ↓ levels of B	++
	INH	Converts INH to toxic hydrazine	++
	Itraconazole[1], ketoconazole	↓ levels of B, ↑ levels of A[1]	++
	Linezolid	↓ levels of B	++
	Methadone	↓ serum levels (withdrawal)	+
	Nevirapine	**↓ levels of B—avoid**	++
	Oral anticoagulants	Suboptimal anticoagulation	++
	Oral contraceptives	↓ effectiveness; spotting, pregnancy	+
	Phenytoin	↓ levels of B	+
	Protease inhibitors	↑ levels of A, ↓ levels of B— Caution	++
	Quinidine	↓ effect of B	+
	Raltegravir	↓ effect of B	++
	Sulfonylureas	↓ hypoglycemic effect	+
	Tacrolimus	↓ levels of B	++
	Theophylline	↓ levels of B	+
	TMP/SMX	↑ levels of A	+
	Tocainide	↓ effect of B	+
Ritonavir	See Protease inhibitors & Table 16B & Table 16C		
Saquinavir	See Protease inhibitors & Table 16B & Table 16C		

[1] Up to 4wks may be required after RIF discontinued to achieve detectable serum itra levels; ↑ levels associated with uveitis or polymyolysis

TABLE 16A (6)

ANTI-INFECTIVE AGENT (A)	OTHER DRUG (B)	EFFECT	SIGNIFICANCE/ CERTAINTY
Stavudine	Dapsone, INH	May ↑ risk of peripheral neuropathy	±
	Ribavirin	↓ levels of A—**avoid**	++
	Zidovudine	Mutual interference—do not combine	++
Sulfonamides	Cyclosporine	↓ cyclosporine levels	+
	Methotrexate	↑ antifolate activity	+
	Oral anticoagulants	↑ prothrombin time; bleeding	+
	Phenobarbital, rifampin	↓ levels of A	+
	Phenytoin	↑ levels of B; nystagmus, ataxia	+
	Sulfonylureas	↑ hypoglycemic effect	+
Telithromycin (Ketek)	Carbamazepine	↓ levels of A	++
	Digoxin	↑ levels of B—do digoxin levels	++
	Ergot alkaloids	↑ **levels of B—avoid**	++
	Itraconazole; ketoconazole	↑ levels of A; no dose change	+
	Metoprolol	↑ levels of B	++
	Midazolam	↑ levels of B	++
	Oral anticoagulants	↑ prothrombin time;	+
	Phenobarbital, phenytoin	↓ levels of A	++
	Pimozide	↑ **levels of B; QT prolongation—avoid**	++
	Rifampin	↓ **levels of A—avoid**	++
	Simvastatin & other "statins"	↑ levels of B	++
	Sotalol	↓ levels of B	++
	Theophylline	↑ levels of B	++
Tenofovir (Viread)	Atazanavir	↓ levels of B—add ritonavir	++
	Didanosine (ddI)	↑ **levels of B (reduce dose)**	++
Tigecycline	Oral contraceptives	↓ levels of B	++
Trimethoprim	Amantadine, dapsone, digoxin, methotrexate, procainamide, zidovudine	↑ serum levels of B	++
	Potassium-sparing diuretics	↑ serum K$^+$	++
	Thiazide diuretics	↓ serum Na$^+$	+
Trimethoprim/ Sulfamethoxazole	Azathioprine	Reports of leucopenia	+
	Cyclosporine	↓ levels of B, ↑ serum creatinine	+
	Loperamide	↑ levels of B	+
	Methotrexate	Enhanced marrow suppression	++
	Oral contraceptives, pimozide, & 6-mercaptopurine	↓ effect of B	+
	Phenytoin	↑ levels of B	+
	Rifampin	↑ levels of B	+
	Warfarin	↑ activity of B	+
Vancomycin	Aminoglycosides	↑ frequency of nephrotoxicity	++
Zalcitabine (ddC) (HIVID)	Valproic acid, pentamidine (IV), alcohol, lamivudine	↑ pancreatitis risk	+
	Cisplatin, INH, metronid-azole, vincristine, nitro-furantoin, d4T, dapsone	↑ risk of peripheral neuropathy	+
Zidovudine (ZDV)	Atovaquone, fluconazole, methadone	↑ levels of A	+
	Clarithromycin	↓ levels of A	±
	Indomethacin	↑ levels ZDV toxic metabolite	+
	Nelfinavir	↓ levels of A	++
	Probenecid, TMP/SMX	↑ levels of A	+
	Ribavirin	↓ **levels of A—avoid**	++
	Rifampin/rifabutin	↓ levels of A	++
	Stavudine	Interference – do not combine	++
	Valproic Acid	↑ levels of A	++

TABLE 16B: DRUG-DRUG INTERACTIONS BETWEEN PROTEASE INHIBITORS (See footnote1) (Adapted from Guidelines for the Use of Antiretroviral Agents in HIV-Infected Adults & Adolescents; see www.aidsinfo.nih.gov)

NAME (Abbreviation, Trade Name)	Atazanavir (ATV, Reyataz)	Darunavir (DRV, Prezista)	Fosamprenavir (FOS-APV, Lexiva)	Indinavir (IDV, Crixivan)	Lopinavir/Ritonavir (LP/R, Kaletra)	Nelfinavir (NFV, Viracept)	Saquinavir (SQV), (Invirase)	Tipranavir (TPV)
Atazanavir (ATV, Reyataz)		ATV 300 mg once daily with (DRV 600 mg + ritonavir 100 mg bid)		**Do not co-administer;** risk of additive ↑ in indirect bilirubin	RTV 100 mg ↑ ATV AUC¹ 238%		SQV (Invirase) 1600 mg + ATV 300 mg + RTV 100 mg, all q24h	
Darunavir (DRV, Prezista)	ATV 300 mg once daily with (DRV 600 mg + ritonavir 100 mg bid)		No data	Dose unclear	**DO NOT co-administer;** Doses not established	No data	**DO NOT co-administer;** Doses not established	No data
Fosamprenavir (FOS-APV, Lexiva)		No data			↓ serum conc. both drugs; do not co-administer		Insufficient data	Fos APV levels ↓. **Do not co-administer**
Indinavir (IDV, Crixivan)	**Do not co-administer;** risk of additive ↑ in bilirubin	Dose unclear			IDV AUC¹ ↑. IDV dose 600 mg q12h	↑ IDV & NFV levels. Dose: IDV 1200 mg q12h, NFV 1250 mg q12h	SQV levels ↑ 4-7 fold. Dose: Insufficient data	No data
Lopinavir/Ritonavir (LP/R, Kaletra)	RTV 100mg ↑ ATV. AUC¹ 238%	**DO NOT co-administer;** Doses not established	↓ serum conc. both drugs; **do not co-administer**	IDV AUC¹ ↑. IDV dose 600 mg q12h		Dose: LP/R 533/133 mg q12h; NFV 1000 mg q12h	SQV levels ↑. Dose: SQV 1000 mg b.i.d.; LP/R standard	LPV levels ↓. **Do not co-administer**
Nelfinavir (NFV, Viracept)		No data		↑ IDV & NFV levels. Dose: IDV 1200 mg q12h, NFV 1250 mg q12h	LP levels ↓; NFV levels ↑. Dose: LPV/R 533/133 mg q12h; NFV 1000 mg q12h		Dose:SQV 1200 mg b.i.d., NFV 1250 mg b.i.d.	No data
Saquinavir (SQV, Fortovase/Invirase)	SQV (Invirase) 1600 mg + ATV 300 mg + RTV 100 mg, all q24h	**DO NOT co-administer;** Doses not established	SQV (Invirase) 1000 mg q12h + RTV 100-200 mg q12h + FOS-APV 700 mg q12h	SQV levels ↑ 4-7 fold. Dose: Insufficient data	SQV levels ↑. Dose: SQV 1000 mg b.i.d., LP/R-standard	Dose SQV 1200 mg b.i.d., NFV 1250 mg b.i.d.		SQV ↓. **Do not co-administer**
Tipranavir (TPV)		No data	Fos-APV levels ↓. **Do not co-administer**	No data	LPV levels ↓. **Do not co-administer**	No data	SQV ↓. **Do not co-administer**	

1 There is no clear indication to combine protease inhibitors with the exception of "boosting" ritonavir.

TABLE 16C: DRUG-DRUG INTERACTIONS BETWEEN NON-NUCLEOSIDE REVERSE TRANSCRIPTASE INHIBITORS (NNRTIs) & PROTEASE INHIBITORS. (Adapted from Guidelines for the Use of Antiretroviral Agents in HIV-Infected Adults & Adolescents; see www.aidsinfo.nih.gov)

NAME (Abbreviation, Trade Name)	Atazanavir (ATV, Reyataz)	Darunavir (DRV, Prezista)	Fosamprenavir (FOS-APV, Lexiva)	Indinavir (IDV, Crixivan)	Lopinavir/Ritonavir (LP/R, Kaletra)	Nelfinavir (NFV, Viracept)	Saquinavir—softgel (SQV, Invirase)	Tipranavir (TPV)
Delavirdine (DLV, Rescriptor)	No data	No data	**Co-administration not recommended**	IDV levels ↑ 40%. Dose: IDV 600 mg q8h, DLV standard	Expect LP levels to ↑. No dose data	NFV levels ↑ 2X; DLV levels ↓ 50%. Dose: No data	SQV levels ↑ 5X. Dose: SQV 800 mg q8h, DLV standard	No data
Efavirenz (EFZ, Sustiva)	ATV AUC¹ ↓ 74%. Dose: EFZ standard; ATA/RTV 300/100 mg q24h with food	Standard doses of both drugs	FOS-APV levels ↓. Dose: EFZ standard; FOS-APV 1400 mg + RTV 300 mg q24h or 700 mg FOS-APV + 100 mg RTV q12h	Levels: IDV ↓ 31%. Dose: IDV 1000 mg q8h. EFZ standard	Level of LP ↓ 40%. Dose: LP/R 533/133 mg q12h, EFZ standard	Standard doses	Level: SQV ↓ 62%. Dose: SQV softgel 400 mg + RTV 400 mg q12h	No dose change necessary
Etravirine (ETR, Intelence)	↑ ATV & ↑ ETR levels. **Avoid combination.**	No data	↑ levels of FOS-APV. **Avoid combination.**	↓ levels of DV. **Avoid combination.**	↑ levels of ETR, ↓ levels of LP/R. Use caution if combined.	↑ levels of NFV. **Avoid combination.**	↓ ETR levels 33%; SQV/R no change. Standard doses of both drugs.	↓ levels of ETR, ↑ levels of TPV and RTV. **Avoid combination.**
Maraviroc (MVC, Selzentry)	↓ metabolism MVC; use 150 mg po bid							Standard dose
Nevirapine (NVP, Viramune)	No data	Standard doses of both drugs	No data	IDV levels ↓ 28%. Dose: ICV 1000 mg q8h or combine with RTV; NvP standard	LP levels ↓ 53%. Dose: LP/R 533/133 mg q12h; NVP standard	Standard doses	Dose: SQV softgel + RTV 400/400 mg, both q12h	No data

TABLE 17: ANTIMICROBICS IN PREGNANCY

Partial list with emphasis on anti-retrovirals and drugs used for opportunistic infections. For more complete list, see Table 8, The Sanford Guide to Antimicrobial Therapy.

Drug	FDA Pregnancy Categories*	Placental Transfer (%)	Breastfeeding	Adverse Effects: Fetus, Mother
Antibacterial Agents				
Clindamycin	B	6–46	OK	None
Fluoroquinolones	C	80–90	No	Potential arthropathy
Linezolid	C	ND	ND	
Macrolides:				
Azithromycin	B	ND	ND	None
Clarithromycin	C	ND	OK	Fetal toxicity in primates
Erythromycin	B	5–20	OK	None
Metronidazole	B	+	No	None: do not use in 1st trimester
Antifungal Agents:				
Amphotericin B	B	+	OK	None
Caspofungin	C			
Fluconazole, itraconazole	C	ND	ND	NHS
Posaconazole	C	ND	ND	
Voriconazole	D			**Risk of birth defects**
Antiparasitic Agents:				
Nitazoxanide	B	ND	ND	ND
Pentamidine	C	+	No	NHS
Pyrimethamine	C	+	No	None: do not use in 1st trimester
Sulfonamides	C	70–90	No	Potential kernicterus & hem-G6PD
Trimethoprim	C	30–100	OK	None
Antimycobacterial Agents:				
Dapsone	C	+	OK	Hem-G6PD
Ethambutol	ND	30	OK	None
Isoniazid	C	100	OK	None
Pyrazinamide	C	ND	OK	None
Rifabutin	B	ND	ND	–
Rifampin	C	33	OK	Postnatal bleeding in infant
Streptomycin	D	10–40	OK	Ototoxicity (16% deafness)
Thalidomide	X	Presumably	ND	**Major risk birth defects**
Antiviral Agents (Non- HIV Drugs):				
Acyclovir, valacyclovir	B	70	OK ?	None. No data with vala—administer with caution to breast feeding mother
Adefovir	C	ND	No	Not recommended in pregnancy
Cidofovir	C	ND	No	
Entecavir	C	ND	ND	Not recommended in pregnancy
Famcyclovir	B	ND	ND	
Foscarnet	C	ND	ND	
Ganciclovir, valganciclovir	C	No	No	Carcinogenic in animals, NHS
Interferons	C	ND	ND	
Ribavirin	X	ND	No	**Major risk of birth defects**
Antiretroviral Drugs:				
Nucleoside and nucleotide alalogue reverse transcriptase inhibitors (NRTIs):				
Abacavir	C	> 80	No	Teratogen in rats at 35x human exposure
Didanosine	B	50	No	No evidence of teratogenicity
Emtracitabine	B	ND	No	No evidence of teratogenicity
Lamivudine	C	100	No	No evidence of teratogenicity
Stavudine	C	76	No	Tumors in rodents
Tenofovir	B	ND	No	
Zalcitabine	C	30-50	No	Tumors in rodents
Zidovudine	C	85	No	Tumors in rodents
Non-nucleoside reverse transcriptase inhibitors (NNRTIs):				
Delavirdine	C	ND	No	Teratogenic in rats; rodent tumors
Efavirenz	D	ND	No	**High risk of birth defects**
Etravirine	B	ND	No	
Nevirapine	C	100	No	Tumors in rodents
Protease Inhibitors (PIs):				
Amprenavir, fosamprenavir	C	ND	No	Tumors in rodents
Atazanavir	B	ND	No	Tumors in female mice
Darunavir	B	ND	No	Negative
Indinavir	C	ND	No	Tumors in rodents
Lopinavir	C	ND	No	Tumors in rodents
Nelfinavir	B	ND	No	Tumors in rodents
Ritonavir	B	15-100	No	Tumors in rodents
Saquinavir	B	Minimal	No	No evidence of teratogenicity
Tipranavir	C	No	No	No evidence of teratogenicity
Fusion Inhibitors:				
Enfuvirtide	B	ND	No	No evidence of teratogenicity
Chemokine Receptor Antagonist:				
Maraviroc	B	ND	No	
Integrase Inhibitor:				
Raltegravir	C	ND	No	

* **FDA Pregnancy Categories: A**—adequate studies in pregnant women, no risk; **B**—animal studies no risk, but human studies not adequate or animal toxicity but human studies no risk; **C**—animal studies show toxicity, human studies inadequate but benefit of use may exceed risk; **D**—evidence of human risk, but benefits may outweigh; **X**—fetal abnormalities in humans, risk > benefit; **ND** = no data *Abbreviations:* **Hem-G6PD** = hemolysis in individuals with G6PD deficiency; **NHS** = no controlled human studies

TABLE 18: SPECTRUM & TREATMENT OF HIV/AIDS-ASSOCIATED MALIGNANCIES*
(Treatment Review: *Oncologist 10:412, 2005*)

I. **Spectrum of associated malignancies: AIDS-defining neoplasms**
   A. **Kaposi's sarcoma** & other KSHV/HHV8 related neoplasms:
      1. Primary body cavity lymphoma (primary effusion lymphoma)
      2. Multicentric Castleman disease
   B. **HIV-associated lymphoma**
      1. Primary CNS lymphoma (EBV)
      2. Non-Hodgkin's lymphoma (EBV)
      3. Body cavity lymphoma; primary effusion lymphoma (HHV8/EBV)
      4. Plasmablastic lymphoma of the oral cavity (*LnID 8:261, 2008*).
   C. **Cervical carcinoma (human papillomavirus)**
   D. **Other neoplasms with increased incidence in AIDS patients**
      1. Anogenital neoplasia & squamous cell carcinoma of the anus (human papillomavirus)
      2. Basal cell carcinoma of the skin
      3. Hodgkin's disease
      4. Seminoma
      5. Pediatric leiomyosarcoma

II. **Kaposi's sarcoma (KS)—Selected issues:** *CID 37:82, 2003*
   A. **Etiology & pathogenesis**
      1. Human herpesvirus type 8 (HHV8); also called Kaposi's sarcoma-associated herpesvirus (KSHV)
      2. HHV8/KSHV
         a. Viral DNA found in all KS tumors
         b. Infection precedes KS
         c. Seropositivity rate predicts KS rate
         d. Virus latent in most cells; lytic in <5% of cells
         e. Targets spindle cells
   B. **Diagnosis**
      1. Clinical appearance & then biopsy
      2. HHV8/KSHV serology; can now quantitate HHV8 in plasma by PCR
   C. **Treatment** (*Current Topics in Micro & Immun 312:289, 2007*)
      1. **Immune reconstitution** (improvement) with effective antiretroviral therapy of HIV infection leads to:
         a. Reports of clearance of HHV8 from circulating cells; 60–80% response rate
         b. Protease inhibitors have anti-tumor activity in mice & patients: *Nature Med 8:225, 2002*
      2. **Suggest oncology consultation for best local and systemic therapy.**

III. **Primary body cavity lymphoma; primary effusion lymphoma**
   A. Etiology: HHV8/KSHV; some cells also positive for EBV
   B. Diagnosis: Biopsy of tumor masses in pleural space, pericardial space, intraabdominal cavity
   C. Treatment: Suggest oncology consult.
   D. Concomitant ARV RX prolongs survival (*AIDS 17:1787, 2003*).

IV. **Multicentric Castleman disease**
   A. Rare lymphoproliferative disorder
   B. Etiology: HHV8/KSHV
   C. Clinical: Fever, lymphadenopathy, splenomegaly
   D. Treatment: Very effective—Vinblastine or etoposide or rituximab (*AnIM 147:836, 2007*).

V. **HIV-associated lymphoma** (*Curr Opin Oncology 18:449, 2006*)
   A. **General**
      1. Compared to immunocompetent pts, present in advanced stage; median survival only 6 months
      2. HIV-associated non-Hodgkin's lymphomas virtually all of B-cell origin
      3. Viral association
         a. Systemic lymphomas—no viral association
         b. CNS lymphoma—EBV DNA present in 100% but predictive value low (*CID 38:1629, 2004*)
         c. Body-cavity lymphomas—HHV8 genome present in virtually all
      4. Prognosis improving coincident with effective antiretroviral therapy
   B. **Primary CNS lymphoma**
      1. Usually in patients with very low CD4 counts
      2. Detection of EBV DNA by PCR in CSF in >90% pts but predictive value low (*CID 38:1629, 2004*)
      3. Treatment
         a. Whole brain irradiation; prolongs survival 1–3 months; longer survival with concomitant ARV RX (*AIDS 15:2119, 2001*)
         b. Responses to combination of ZDV, ganciclovir, & IL-2 in a few patients (*CID 34:1660, 2002*)
   C. **Non-Hodgkin's lymphoma** (*AIDS Reader 14:605, 2004*)
      1. **Continuous infusion EPOCH** (etoposide, prednisone, vincristine, cyclophosphamide, doxorubicin) leads to 92% probability of remission at 53 months (*Blood 101:4853, 2003*). **No ARV RX** during chemo— controversial.

VI. **Cervical carcinoma:** *JID 188:555, 2003; MMWR 53(RR-15):46, 2004*
   A. Epidemiology: More frequent, more severe in HIV patients.
   B. Etiology: Human papilloma virus.
   C. **Recommendations**
      1. Pap smears x2 in year one & then annually if normal initially; every 3 yrs if CD4 >500/mm^3 (*JAMA 293:1471, 2005*).
      2. More frequent Pap smears if:
         a. Previous abnormal Pap smear
         b. History of papilloma (wart) virus infection
         c. Post-treatment for cervical intraepithelial neoplasia
         d. Symptomatic AIDS or CD4 count <200/mm^3

3. If Pap smear abnormal, refer for colposcopy &/or biopsy.
4. If CD4 count >200 and under age 26, suggest human papilloma virus vaccine.

VII. **Anal neoplasia:** *MMWR 53(RR-15):46, 2004*
   A. Epidemiology
      1. HIV-infected immunodeficient patients at increased risk of human papillomavirus (HPV)-related anal neoplasia.
      2. HPV DNA found in roughly 50% of anal cytology specimens from HIV-infected men.
   B. Recommendations for HIV-infected pts with history of anal intercourse
      1. Anal Pap smear
      2. Routine anoscopy with biopsy as indicated
      3. Wide surgical resection for established neoplasia

TABLE 19: RECOMMENDATIONS FOR ROUTINE IMMUNIZATION OF HIV+ CHILDREN (ASYMPTOMATIC & SYMPTOMATIC)

[Modified from USPHS/IDSA Guidelines (MMWR 49:RR-9, Oct. 6, 2000; MMWR 51:32, 2002; AnIM 137, Nov. 5 [Suppl.]:468, 2002; MMWR 55: Q1, 2007)]

Vaccine	Birth	1 mo.	2 mos.	4 mos.	6 mos.	12 mos.	15 mos.	18 mos.	24 mos.	4–6 yrs.	11–12 yrs.	14–16 yrs.
↓ Recommendations for these vaccines are the same as those for immunocompetent children ↓*												
Hepatitis B[1]	Hep B #1	Hep B #2				Hep B #3					Hep B	
Diphtheria & Tetanus toxoids, Pertussis[2]			DTaP	DTaP	DTaP		DTap			DTap	Tdap	
Hemophilus influenzae type b[3]			Hib	Hib	Hib	Hib					Hib	
Inactivated Polio[4]			IPV	IPV		IPV				IPV	IPV	
Hepatitis A[5]						Hep A series				Hep A series		
Meningo-coccal[10]									MPSV 4	MPSV 4	MCV4	MCV4
Human papilloma virus (HPV)[11]											HPV 3 doses	
↓ Recommendations for these vaccines differ from those for immunocompetent children ↓												
Pneumococcus[6]			PCV	PCV	PCV	PCV			PPV 23	PPV23 (age 5–7yrs)		
Measles, Mumps, Rubella[7]		Do not give to severely immunosuppressed (Category 3) children				MMR				MMR	MMR	
Varicella[8]		Give only to asymptomatic non-immunosuppressed (Category 1) children. Contraindicated in all other HIV-infected children				Var	Var	Var		Var		
Influenza[9]					A dose is recommended every year							

* For detailed recommendations for immunocompetent children see MMWR 57:Q1-4, 2008.

☐ Range of recommended ages for vaccination

▓ Vaccines to be given if previously recommended doses were missed or were given earlier than the recommended minimum age

This schedule indicates the recommended ages for routine administration of licensed childhood vaccines as of Jan. 1, 2006, for children aged birth–18yrs. Additional vaccines might be licensed & recommended during the year. Licensed combination vaccines might be used whenever any components of the combination are indicated & the vaccine's other components are not contraindicated. Providers should consult the manufacturer's package inserts for detailed recommendations.

[1] **Hepatitis B vaccine (HepB).** *AT BIRTH:* **All newborns** should receive monovalent HepB soon after birth & before hospital discharge. **Infants born to mothers who are hepatitis B surface antigen (HBsAg)-positive** should receive HepB & 0.5mL of hepatitis B immune globulin (HBIG) within 12hrs of birth. **Infants born to mothers whose HBsAg status is unknown** should receive HepB within 12hrs of birth. The mother should have blood drawn as soon as possible to determine her HBsAg status; if HBsAg-positive, the infant should receive HBIG as soon as possible (no later than age 1wk). **For infants born to HBsAg-negative mothers,** the birth dose can be delayed in rare circumstances but only if a physician's order to withhold the vaccine & a copy of the mother's original HBsAg-negative laboratory report are documented in the infant's medical record. *FOLLOWING THE BIRTH DOSE:* The HepB series should be completed with either monovalent HepB or a combination vaccine containing HepB. The second dose should be administered at age 1–2mos. The final dose should be administered at age ≥24wks. Administering four doses of HepB is permissible (e.g., when combination vaccines are administered after the birth dose); however, if monovalent HepB is used, a dose at age 4mos is not needed. **Infants born to HBsAg-positive mothers** should be tested for HBsAg & antibody to HBsAg after completion of the HepB series at age 9–18mos (generally at the next well-child visit after completion of the vaccine series).

[2] **Diphtheria & tetanus toxoids & acellular pertussis vaccine (DTaP).** The fourth dose of DTaP may be administered as early as age 12mos, provided 6mos have elapsed since the third dose & the child is unlikely to return at age 15–18mos. The final dose in the series should be administered at age ≥4yrs. **Tetanus toxoid, reduced diphtheria toxoid, & acellular pertussis vaccine (Tdap adolescent preparation)** is recommended at age 11–12yrs for those who have completed the recommended childhood DTP/DTaP vaccination series & have not received a tetanus & diphtheria toxoids (Td) booster dose. Adolescents aged 13–18yrs who missed the age 11–12yr Td/Tdap booster dose should also receive a single dose of Tdap if they have completed the recommended childhood DTP/DTaP vaccination series. **Subsequent Td** boosters are recommended every 10yrs.

TABLE 19 (2)

[3] **Three Hemophilus influenzae type b (Hib) conjugate vaccines** are licensed for infant use. If Hib conjugate vaccine (polyribosylribitol phosphate-meningococcal outer membrane protein [PRP-OMP]) (PedvaxHIB® or ComVax™ [Merck & Company, Inc., Whitehouse Station, NJ]) is administered at ages 2 & 4mos, a dose at age 6mos is not required. Because clinical studies among infants have demonstrated that using certain combination products might induce a lower immune response to the Hib vaccine component, DTaP/Hib combination products should not be used for primary immunization among infants at ages 2, 4, or 6mos, unless approved by the FDA for these ages.

[4] An all-inactivated poliovirus vaccine (IPV) schedule is recommended for routine childhood polio vaccination in the U.S. All children should receive 4 doses of IPV at age 2mos, age 4mos, ages 6–18mos, & ages 4–6yrs. Oral poliovirus vaccine should not be administered to HIV-infected persons or their household contacts.

[5] **Hepatitis A vaccine** (Hep A). HepA is recommended for all children at age 1yr (i.e., 12–23mos). The 2 doses in the series should be administered at least 6mos apart. States, counties, & communities with existing HepA vaccination programs for children aged 2–18yrs are encouraged to maintain these programs. In these areas, new efforts focused on routine vaccination of children aged 1yr should enhance, not replace, ongoing programs directed at a broader population of children. HepA is also recommended for certain high risk groups *(see MMWR 1999;48[No. RR-12])*.

[6] **Heptavalent pneumococcal conjugate vaccine (PCV)** is recommended for all HIV-infected children aged 2–59mos. Children aged ≥2yrs should also receive the **23-valent pneumococcal polysaccharide vaccine (PPV23);** a single revaccination with the 23-valent vaccine should be offered to children after 3–5yrs. Refer to the Advisory Committee on Immunization Practices recommendations *(see CDC. Preventing pneumococcal disease among infants & young children: recommendations of the Advisory Committee on Immunization Practices [ACIP], MMWR 49(RR-9):1–38, 2000)* for dosing intervals for children starting the vaccination schedule after age 2mos.

[7] **Measles, mumps, & rubella (MMR)** should not be administered to severely immunocompromised (Category 3) children. HIV-infected children without severe immunosuppression would routinely receive their 1st dose of MMR as soon as possible after reaching their 1st birthdays. Consideration should be given to administering the 2nd dose of MMR at 1mo (i.e., a minimum of 28 days) after the 1st dose rather than waiting until school entry.

[8] **Varicella-zoster virus vaccine** should be administered only to asymptomatic, non-immunosuppressed children. Eligible children should receive 2 doses of vaccine with a ≥3mo interval between doses. The 1st dose can be administered at age 12mos.

[9] **Inactivated split influenza virus vaccine** should be administered to all HIV-infected children aged ≥6mos each year. For children aged 6mos–<9yrs who are receiving influenza vaccine for the first time, 2 doses administered 1mo apart are recommended. For specific recommendations, *see CDC. Prevention & control of influenza: recommendations of the Advisory Committee on Immunization Practices (ACIP), MMWR 51(RR-4):1–32, 2002.*

[10] **Meningococcal vaccine (MCV4).** Meningococcal conjugate vaccine (MCV4) should be administered to all children at age 11–12yrs as well as to unvaccinated adolescents at high school entry (age 15yrs). Other adolescents who wish to decrease their risk for meningococcal disease may also be vaccinated. All college freshmen living in dormitories should also be vaccinated, preferably with MCV4, although **meningococcal polysaccharide vaccine (MPSV4)** is an acceptable alternative. Vaccination against invasive meningococcal disease is recommended for children & adolescents aged ≥2-10 yrs with terminal complement deficiencies or anatomic or functional asplenia & for certain other high risk groups *(see MMWR 2005;54[No. RR-7])*; use MPSV4 for children aged 2–10yrs & MCV4 for older children, although MPSV4 is an acceptable alternative.

[11] **Human papillomavirus vaccine (HPV).** Minimum age 9 years. Administer the first dose of the HPV vaccine to females at age 11-12 years. Administer second dose 2 months after the first dose and the third dose 6 months after the first dose. Administer HPV vaccine series to females 13-18 years if not previously vaccinated.

For further information, see www.cdc.gov.

TABLE 20: IMMUNIZATION OF HIV+ ADULTS (ASYMPTOMATIC & SYMPTOMATIC)

General Principles/Guidelines:
- In HIV+ individuals, there are activated T-cells (CD25+) & quiescent T-cells (CD25-). Only activated T-cells produce virus & spread infection. In HIV+ adults, significant (2-36 fold) transient (≤6wks) ↑ in plasma viral RNA after pneumococcal, influenzal & tetanus immunization *(NEJM 334:1222, 1996)*. A similar phenomenon occurs with acute infections, i.e., influenza. At present, there are no data suggesting that this is clinically relevant *(AnIM 131:430, 1999; CID 28:548, 1999)*. Concurrently, antibody responses are ↓ in HIV+ individuals. Our recommendations are presented in the following table.
- **Administration of live attenuated vaccines is contraindicated in individuals with advanced HIV infection (AIDS) (MMR is an exception).**
- Immunization (when indicated) with killed whole cell vaccines &/or purified antigens should be done as soon as reasonable after HIV infection diagnosed, before CD4 cells ↓ further *(JID 171:1217, 1995)*.
- Extended primary series &/or more frequent boosters often indicated.
- When specifically indicated, immune globulin (IG) & specific immune globulins can be administered.
- For general reference on licensed vaccine use in immunocompromised hosts, see *Clin Microbiol Rev 11:1, 1998*.

TABLE 20 (2)

RECOMMENDATIONS FOR ROUTINE IMMUNIZATION OF HIV+ ADULTS (United States)
(From Update on Adult Immunization, Centers for Disease Control, MMWR 51:904, 2002; MMWR 54:Q1, 2006; MMWR 55:Q1, 2006)

VACCINE/TOXOID	STAGE OF HIV INFECTION		BOOSTER DOSE	AUTHORS' RECOMMENDATIONS (AIDS Clin Care 8:11, 1996)
	ASYMPTOMATIC HIV+*	SYMPTOMATIC (AIDS)*		
Td (tetanus/ diphtheria)	Yes	Yes	10 yrs	+ (if IDU)
HbCV (Haemophilus influenzae type b conjugate vaccine)	Yes	Yes	None	0
Pneumococcal	Yes	Yes	6yrs	+
Influenza	Yes	Yes	Annual	+
Hepatitis A	Yes	Yes	None	+
HBV (Hepatitis B)	(Yes)**	(Yes)**	None	+
eIPV (polio)	(Yes)**	(Yes)**	(None)	0
MMR (Measles, mumps, rubella)	Yes	(Yes)**	**	NA
Meningococcal	Yes**	Yes**	None	NA
HPV (Human papillomavirus)	Yes	--	3 doses total	NA

Abbreviations: **Td** = tetanus & diphtheria toxoids, adsorbed (for adult use); **MMR** = measles, mumps & rubella vaccine; **HbCV** = Haemophilus influenzae type b conjugate vaccine; **Pneumococcal** = pneumococcal polysaccharide (23 component) vaccine; **HBV** = Hepatitis B vaccine; **eIPV** = enhanced-potency inactivated polio vaccine; **IDU** = injection drug user.

* Asymptomatic-CDC category A1, A2; Symptomatic-CDC A3, B1-3, C1-3
** See Comments; + = benefit > risk, 0 = benefit probably < risk. For further information, see www.cdc.gov.

COMMENTS ON "ROUTINE" VACCINES/TOXOIDS*

VACCINE/TOXOID	COMMENTS
Td	"Injection" drug users at ↑ risk of tetanus
HbCV	Is of unproven benefit & immune responses ↓; although the risk of H. influenzae type b disease is ↑ & adverse reactions are minimal, it is no longer recommended.
Pneumococcal	Risk of bacteremia is ↑ [as high as 9.4/1000/yr (J Inf Dis 162:1012, 1990)]. Revaccination 6yrs after 1st dose is recommended. Benefit appears > risk.
Hepatitis A	In the past several years hep A has ↑ in frequency in homosexual men in the U.S., Canada & Australia (MMWR 45:155, 1992). Outbreaks also reported in injection drug users (IDU) (Am J Pub Health 79:463, 1989). <10% U.S.-born young adults have antibody (Mil Med 157:579, 1992). 2 hep A vaccines, inactivated, are licensed in U.S. FDA-approved indications include: persons engaged in high-risk sexual activity (homosexually active men), IDU (MMWR 47:708, 1998; MMWR 48:RR-12, 1999).
Hepatitis B	If lifestyle or occupation was risk factor for HIV it is also a risk factor for hepatitis B. Series of 3 IM injections in deltoid, using 12-in needle (not into the buttocks), should be given. Test for antibody to HBs Ag 1-6 months after completing series. If anti-HBs is <10 milli-international units, revaccinate with 1 or more doses.
Influenza	Annual immunization with the current vaccine is recommended regardless of age. Benefit appears > risk (AnIM 131:430, 1999). Poor immune response in pts with CD4 count <200. Some recommend use of amantadine, rimantadine or neuraminidase inhibitors instead of immunization in this group (CID 28:548, 1999). Avoid live attenuated vaccine.
eIPV (enhanced-potency inactivated polio vaccine)	In adults ≥18yrs, use only if specifically indicated: travel to developing countries (not Central or South America), prior to (~8wks, time for initial 2 doses) household exposure to individuals given oral polio vaccine.
OPV (oral polio vaccine)	Contraindicated
Specific immunoglobulins: Hepatitis B (HBIG), human rabies (HRIG), tetanus (TIG), vaccinia (VIG), varicella-zoster (VZIG)	Can be used for same indications, same dosage as in non-HIV infected individuals
MMR	Withhold MMR or other measles-containing vaccines from HIV-infected persons with severe immunosuppression
Meningococcal	*Medical indications*: adults with anatomic or functional asplenia or terminal complement component deficiencies. *Other indications*: 1styr college students living in dormitories; microbiologists who are routinely exposed to isolates of *Neisseria meningitides*; military recruits; & persons who travel to or reside in countries in which meningococcal disease is hyperendemic or epidemic (e.g., the "meningitis belt" of sub-Saharan Africa during the dry season [Dec-June]), particularly if contact with local populations will be prolonged. Vaccination required by the government of Saudi Arabia for all travelers to Mecca during the annual Hajj. Meningococcal conjugate vaccine is preferred for adults meeting any of the above indications who are aged ≤55yrs, although meningococcal polysaccharide vaccine MPSV4 is an acceptable alternative. Revaccination after 5yrs might be indicated for adults previously vaccinated with MPSV4 who remain at high risk for infection (e.g., persons residing in areas in which disease is epidemic). See also Table 21B.
Varicella zoster	Contraindicated in immunocompromised HIV+ patients: live virus vaccine.
Vaccinia (smallpox)	Contraindicated: live virus vaccine
Rotavirus	Contraindicated: live virus vaccine

• For further details, see *Wilson, et al., AnIM 114:582, 1991; Topics in HIV Medicine 14:154, 2007; MMWR 57:Q1, 2008.*

TABLE 21A: MEASURES TO BE TAKEN BY PHYSICIANS IN PREPARING HIV+ PATIENTS & INDIVIDUALS LIKELY TO HAVE "RISKY" BEHAVIOR FOR OVERSEAS TRAVEL*[1]

The likelihood of developing an illness during a 3-wk vacation in a tropical area is about 50% *(J Travel Med 6:71, 1999)*.

Since illnesses are likely to be more serious &/or become chronic in the HIV+ patient, there is advice to be given & measures to be taken to minimize risks. These include:

- If the traveler is likely to engage in risky behavior during travel, ascertain the HIV antibody status before travel, especially if travel is planned to a developing country.

- If the traveler is known to be HIV+, take account of legal restrictions on travel for persons with HIV infection[2] (e.g., ability to transport ARV medications into the country). Assess the immune status (CD4 cell count) in infected persons.

- Review planned itinerary & activities in light of the patient's immune status & review the added risks for travel, especially to developing or tropical countries. In some instances, it may be prudent to recommend a change in itinerary or activities because of serious risks that cannot be eliminated or reduced.

- Recommend the following measures to reduce exposure to pathogens:
  Assiduously avoid food & beverages that may be contaminated, especially raw or undercooked shellfish, fish, meat, or eggs; raw, unpeeled fruits & vegetables; tap water & ice; as well as unpasteurized milk & milk products (cheese). Insist on eating only well-cooked foods & on drinking only very hot or bottled beverages.
  Reduce contact with vectors, for example, by using insect repellent & avoiding outdoor exposure at dusk or other times & places of increased insect activity.
  Frequent handwashing, ideally with alcohol based hand cleanser gels.

- Urge the patient to obtain prompt evaluation of symptoms of illness & early treatment of infection. Where possible, identify a physician knowledgeable about HIV infection at the destination prior to departure[3]. Arrange for continuation of medical management during travel (for example, prophylaxis for Pneumocystis carinii pneumonia).

- Use vaccine & prophylactic therapy as indicated by the planned itinerary & activities. Avoid live vaccines in pts with profound immunodeficiency not on ARV therapy. Prescribe antimicrobial agents (with or without antimotility drugs) & counsel the patient on their use for early treatment of diarrheal disease.[4]

---

* *Reproduced with permission from Wilson ME, von Reyn CF, Fineberg HV: Infections in HIV-infected travelers: risks & prevention (Table 2). AnIM 114:582, 1991. USPHS/IDSA Guidelines CID 21(Suppl. 1):520, 1999*

---

[1] The most up-to-date source is: Health Information for the International Traveler, 1995. HHS Publication (CDC) No. 93-8280. Available from U.S. Government Printing Office, Washington, DC 20402. See also www.travmed.com; www.fitfortravel.scot.nhs.uk.

[2] Duckett M., Orkin AJ: AIDS-related migration & travel policies & restrictions: a global survey. *AIDS 3:(Suppl 1) S231-252, 1989.*

[3] For a list of English-speaking doctors abroad & health information: International Association for Medical Assistance to Travelers (IAMAT), 417 Center St., Lewiston, NY 14092.

[4] For suggestions regarding a medical kit & advice (for all travelers): Sanford JP: Self-help for the traveler who becomes ill. *Inf Dis Clin NA 6:405, 1992.*

TABLE 21B: IMMUNIZATION OF HIV+ ADULTS TRAVELING TO DEVELOPING COUNTRIES*

VACCINE/TOXOID	STAGE OF HIV INFECTION		COMMENTS
	ASYMPTOMATIC HIV+*	SYMPTOMATIC (AIDS)*	
"Routine" for All Developing Countries			
eIPV	Yes	Yes	*See Table 19 & Table 20.* OPV contraindicated
Hepatitis A	Yes	Yes	*See Table 20 (2).*
Typhoid Vi polysaccharide vaccine (Connaught)	Yes	Yes	Boosters recommended q2yrs. Live attenuated (eg, Ty21a) oral typhoid vaccine contraindicated
Immune globulin (IG)	Yes	Yes	For 2–3mos travel, 0.02ml/kg IM single dose
"Special" Depending on Itinerary: Country & Activity			
Cholera (inactivated vaccine)	See Comments	See Comments	Vaccine does not prevent transmission, efficacy ~50%, risk to U.S. travelers very low. WHO does not recommend, but some countries require (check with Health Dept.). If required, have vaccination completed, signed, dated & validated to avoid risk of revaccination & quarantine.
Rabies (pre-exposure) (inactivated vaccine)	Yes, if indicated (Animal handlers, travelers spending 1mo or more in country where rabies is a constant threat)	Yes, if indicated	Course: Three 1ml of HDCV or RVA IM on days 0, 7, 28. Test serum for antibodies 2wks after 3rd dose.
Meningococcal (polysaccharide vaccine)(Menomune) or polysaccharide-protein conjugate (Menactra)	Yes, if traveling to area where meningococcal disease is epidemic or endemic (sub Sahara Africa)		Note recent CDC advisory: 5 cases of Guillain-Barre syndrome reported after Menactra vaccination. Causal relationship NOT clear (www.phppo.cdc.gov)
Yellow Fever (live attenuated)	Yes (±); offer choice if potential exposure unavoidable	No (contra-indicated)	
Japanese Encephalitis	Yes, if indicated: travel to Asia, in monsoon (summer) months, staying in rural areas		Requires 3 injections: day 0, 7, & 30. An abbreviated schedule at days 0, 7, 14 can be used but less effective *(MMWR 42:RR-1, 1993).*
Plague (inactivated)	Yes, if indicated: to areas of endemic plague, esp. if staying in rural areas, not in tourist hotels		
BCG (Bacillus Calmette-Guerin) vaccine	No	No	Is live attenuated vaccine

* All travelers should have current routine immunizations, *Table 20.*
** Asymptomatic-CDC category A1, A2; Symptomatic-CDC A3, B1-3, C1-3 *(Table 4A).*
For further information, see www.travmed.com; www.fitfortravel.scot.nhs.uk.

TABLE 22: BIOLOGICS IN TREATMENT OF HEMATOCYTOPENIAS*

DRUG NAME, GENERIC (TRADE) COST	COMMENTS ON USE, ADVERSE EFFECTS
Erythropoietin (Epogen, Procrit) 4000 units **Darbepoetin** (Aranesp, Nesp) = long-acting erythropoietin. 0.025 mg	Not FDA approved for Rx of anemia in HIV. FDA advisory warning: ↑ risk of death, thromboembolic, and cardiovascular events. Monitor red blood cell levels (hemoglobin) and adjust dose to maintain the lowest hemoglobin level needed to avoid the need for blood transfusions (Hgb >12 assoc. with increased events) *(see Lancet 369:381, 2007 and JAMA 299:914, 2008).* Antibody to erythropoietin can lead to red cell aplasia *(AJG 100:1415, 2005).* **Erythropoietin Dose:** 100units/kg IV or subQ 3x/wk for 8wks. If no response, can increase dose 50–100units/kg increments to a max. dose of 300units/kg 3x/wk. 40,000–60,000units subQ once weekly may equal efficacy of 3x/wk. rx. **Dose of darbepoetin:** 0.45 mcg/kg IV or subQ **q wk**.
Granulocyte-CSF or G-CSF, Filgrastim (Neupogen), 300mcg Pegfilgrastim (Neulasta), 6 mg $3 **Granulocyte-monocyte-CSF or GM-CSF,** Sargramostim (Leukine), 250mcg	**G-CSF:** Standard dose 5mcg/kg/day subQ; lower doses may work in HIV pts, i.e., 1mcg/kg/day subQ until ANC >1000 cells/dl, then 1–2x/wk. No effect on HIV replication. Pegylated G-CSF—pegfilgrastim: 6 mg subQ once per chemotherapy cycle. **GM-CSF:** Dose 5mcg/kg/day subQ → ↑ PMNs. Trend toward ↑ CD4 and slightly lower VL. Adverse effects: fever, myalgia, fatigue, malaise, headache, bone pain.
Intravenous immune serum globulin (IVIG) (Gamimune N, Gammar, & others). General dosage: (1) Adults: 200–400 mg/kg q21 days; (2) Children: 400 mg/kg/ month	Example uses: (1) Parvovirus **B-19 infection**. Effective. Dose: 400 mg/kg/day x10 days. (2) **Immune thrombocytopenia**. Use IVIG only if pt bleeding &/or immediate invasive procedure. Rapid effects but transient. Dose: 1–2 gm/kg over 2–5 days. Anti-Rh immune globulin *(see below)* more cost effective and may be more clinically effective. (3) **Autoimmune neutropenia**. 1–2mo. benefit in pts who failed G-CSF. Dose: 20–25gm/day x 4–6 days. *(See Transfusion 46:741, 2006 for review of uses.)*
Rho (D) Immune Globulin (Anti-Rh immunoglobulin), intravenous (human) (WinRho). 1500 intl units (equals 300 mcg)	Treatment for **HIV-induced ITP** in non-splenectomized Rh+ pts. Coats Rh+ RBC with antibody; competes with antibody-coated platelets for binding sites on splenic macrophages. Some RBC hemolysis. Effective AIDS pts. Dose: 25–50 mcg/kg/day x7 days, then q3wks. One small study of 9 patients found that rho immune globulin produced higher platelet counts and a longer duration of effect than IVIG *(Am J Hematol 82:335, 2007).*

* **NOTE**: Majority of hematologic problems resolve, or substantively improve, with control of HIV replication. In general, treat HIV first before using drugs outlined above.

TABLE 23: AIDS INFORMATION & REFERRAL SERVICES

- AIDS/HIV Clinical Trials conducted by National Institutes of Health & FDA-approved efficacy trials: 1-800-874-2572

- For a wide variety of AIDS/HIV information, resources, publications, call the National AIDS Clearinghouse: 1-800-458-5231

- To find out about AIDS resources in your area, call the National AIDS Hotline: 1-800-342-2437

- The AIDS/HIV Treatment Directory is published by the American Federation for AIDS Research (AmFAR) & is updated semi-annually; 733 Third Ave., 12th Floor, New York, NY 10017-3204. Telephone: 1-800-392-6327

- The HIV/AIDS Treatment Information Service (Public Health Coordinating Group): 1-800-HIV-0440

- Travel information for patients: www.travmed.com & www.fitfortravel.scot.nhs.uk

- The National Clinicians' Post-Exposure Prophylaxis Hotline, for the latest information on post-exposure protocols and preventative therapy: http://www.ucsf.edu/hivcntr/Hotlines/PEPline.html

- The Francis J. Curry National Tuberculosis Center, for information on educational programs and phone consultation (415-502-4700 or 877-390-NOTB(6682)) on prevention and management of tuberculosis: http://www.nationaltbcenter.edu/.

Helpful Websites for Information / Questions About HIV/AIDS:
CDC National Information Prevention Network: www.cdcnpin.org
amFAR (American Foundation for AIDS Research): www.amfar.org
The HIV/AIDS Treatment Information Service (ATIS): www.hivatis.org
IAS-USA (International AIDS Society-USA) www.iasusa.org
NATAP (National AIDS Treatment Advocacy Project) www.natap.org
San Francisco General Hospital: http://hivinsite.ucsf.edu
Stanford HIV Drug Resistance Database: http://hivdb.stanford.edu
University of Liverpool HIV Drug Interactions Assessment: www.hiv-druginteractions.org
Johns Hopkins AIDS Service: www.hopkins-aids.edu
WHO Treatment Guidelines: www.who.org

TABLE 24: LIST OF GENERIC & COMMON TRADE NAMES

GENERIC NAME: TRADE NAMES

Abacavir: Ziagen
Abacavir + 3TC: Epzicom
Abacavir + 3TC + ZDV: Trizivir
Acyclovir: Zovirax
Adefovir: Hepsera
Amikacin: Amikin
Amphotericin B: Fungizone
Ampho B cholesteryl complex: Amphotec
Ampho B lipid complex: Abelcet
Ampho B liposomal: AmBisome
Atazanavir: Reyataz
Atovaquone: Mepron
Azithromycin: Zithromax
Capreomycin: Capastat
Caspofungin: Cancidas
Cidofovir: Vistide
Ciprofloxacin: Cipro
Clarithromycin: Biaxin, Biaxin XL
Clindamycin: Cleocin
Clofazimine: Lamprene
Cycloserine: Seromycin
Darunavir: Prezista
Daunorubicin-liposome: DaunoXome
Delavirdine: Rescriptor
Didanosine (ddI): Videx
Dronabinol: Marinol
Efavirenz: Sustiva
Emtricitabine:
Emtracitabine + Efav + Teno: Atripla
Emtriva
Enfuvirtide: Fuzeon

GENERIC NAME: TRADE NAMES

Erythropoietin: Epogen, Procrit
Ethambutol: Myambutol
Ethionamide: Trecator
Etravirine: Intelence
Famciclovir: Famvir
Filgrastim (G-CSF): Neupogen
Fluconazole: Diflucan
Flucytosine: Ancobon
Fomivirsen: Vitravene
Fosamprenavir: Lexiva
Foscarnet: Foscavir
Ganciclovir: Cytovene
Human growth hormone (rHGH): Serostim
Imipenem: Primaxin
Indinavir: Crixivan
Interferon alfa: Roferon-A, Intron A
Iodoquinol: Yodoxin
Isoniazid: INH, Laniazid, Tubizid
Itraconazole: Sporanox
Ketoconazole: Nizoral
Lamivudine (3TC): Epivir, Epivir-HBV
Linezolid: Zyvox
Maraviroc: Selzentry
Megestrol: Megace
Nelfinavir: Viracept
Nevirapine: Viramune
Norfloxacin: Noroxin
Ofloxacin: Floxin
Palivizumab: Synagis
Paromomycin: Humatin
PAS: Paser
Pegylated interferon alfa-2a: Pegasys

GENERIC NAME: TRADE NAMES

Pegylated interferon alfa-2b: PEG Intron
Pentamidine: Pentam 300
Pentamidine aerosol: NebuPent
Posaconazole: Noxafil
Primaquine: Primachine
Pyrazinamide: Pyrazinamide
Pyrimethamine: Daraprim
Quinupristin/dalfopristin: Synercid
Raltegravir: Isentress
Ribavirin: Virazole, Rebetol
Rifabutin: Mycobutin
Rifampin: Rifadin, Rimactane
Saquinavir: Invirase (hard cap) Fortovase (softgel)
Sargramostim (GM-CSF): Leukine, Prokine
Stavudine (d4T): Zerit
Tenofovir: Viread
Tenofovir + Emtricitabine: Truvada
Thiacetazone: Tibione
Tipranavir: Aptivus
Trimethoprim: Proloprim, Trimpex
Trimethoprim/Sulfamethoxazole: Bactrim, Septra
Trimetrexate: Neutrexin
Valacyclovir: Valtrex
Valganciclovir: Valcyte
Vidarabine: Vira-A
Voriconazole: Vfend
Zidovudine (ZDV): Retrovir

TRADE NAME: GENERIC NAME

Abelcet: Ampho B lipid emulsion
AmBisome: Ampho B liposomal
Amikin: Amikacin
Amphotec: Ampho B cholesteryl complex
Ancobon: Flucytosine
Aptivus: Tipranavir
Atripla: Emtricitabine + Efav + Teno
Bactrim: TMP/SMX
Biaxin, Biaxin XL: Clarithromycin
Cancidas: Caspofungin
Capastat: Capreomycin
Cleocin: Clindamycin
Cipro: Ciprofloxacin
Combivir: Zidovudine + lamivudine
Crixivan: Indinavir
Cytovene: Ganciclovir
Daraprim: Pyrimethamine
DaunoXome: Daunorubicin-liposome
Diflucan: Fluconazole
Doxil: Doxorubicin- liposome
Emtriva: Emtricitabine
Epivir, Epivir-HBV: Lamivudine
Epogen: Erythropoietin
Epzicom: Abacavir + 3TC
Famvir: Famciclovir
Floxin: Ofloxacin
Fortovase: Saquinavir softgel
Foscavir: Foscarnet
Fungizone: Amphotericin B
Fuzeon: Enfuvirtide
Hepsera: Adefovir
Humatin: Paromomycin

TRADE NAME: GENERIC NAME

Intelence: Etravirine
Intron A: Interferon alfa
Invirase: Saquinavir hard cap
Isentress: Raltegravir
Kaletra: Lopinavir + ritonavir
Lamprene: Clofazimine
Leukine: Sargramostim (GM-CSF)
Lexiva: Fosamprenavir
Marinol: Dronabinol
Megace: Megestrol
Mepron: Atovaquone
Myambutol: Ethambutol
Mycobutin: Rifabutin
NebuPent: Pentamidine aerosol
Neupogen: Filgrastim (CSF)
Neutrexin: Trimetrexate
Noroxin: Norfloxacin
Noxafil : Posaconazole
Paser: PAS
PEG Intron: Pegylated interferon alfa-2b
Pegasys: Pegylated interferon alfa-2a
Pentam 300: Pentamidine
Prezista: Darunavir
Primachine: Primaquine
Primaxin: Imipenem + cilastatin
Procrit: Erythropoietin
Prokine: Sargramostim (GM-CSF)
Proloprim: Trimethoprim
Rebetol: Ribavirin + interferon alfa-2b
Rescriptor: Delavirdine
Retrovir: Zidovudine
Reyataz: Atazanavir
Rifadin: Rifampin

TRADE NAME: GENERIC NAME

Rimactane: Rifampin
Roferon-A: Interferon alfa
Selzentry: Maraviroc
Septra: TMP/SMX
Seromycin: Cycloserine
Serostim: Human growth hormone [HGH(m)]
Sporanox: Itraconazole
Sustiva: Efavirenz
Synagis: Palivizumab
Synercid: Quinupristin/ dalfopristin
Tibione: Thiacetazone
Trecator: Ethionamide
Trimpex: Trimethoprim
Trizivir: Abacavir + zidovudine + lamivudine
Truvada: Tenofovir + emtricitabine
Valcyte: Valganciclovir
Valtrex: Valacyclovir
Vfend: Voriconazole
Videx: Didanosine (ddI)
Viracept: Nelfinavir
Viramune: Nevirapine
Virazole: Ribavirin
Viread: Tenofovir
Vistide: Cidofovir
Vitravene: Fomivirsen
Yodoxin: Iodoquinol
Zerit: Stavudine (d4T)
Ziagen: Abacavir
Zithromax: Azithromycin
Zovirax: Acyclovir
Zyvox: Linezolid

INDEX TO MAJOR ENTRIES

Abacavir 9, 14, 15, 16, 18, 19, 24, 25, 27, 28, 29, 38, 41, 44, 47, 48, 60, 61, 172, 181, 190, 199
Abacavir/Lamivudine 24
Acanthamoeba 116
Acute infectious diarrhea 93, 94, 95, 96
Acute loss of vision 85
Acute retroviral (HIV) syndrome (symptomatic primary HIV infection) 74
Acute retroviral syndrome 81, 89, 92, 115
Acyclovir 44, 67, 92, 100, 149, 152, 156, 157, 158, 168, 172, 178, 190, 199
Adefovir 44, 149, 152, 168, 172, 178, 190, 199
Adenovirus 94, 96, 106, 149
Adrenal 83, 84
AIDS cholangiopathy 59
AIDS dementia complex 75, 76, 79, 105
Albendazole 146, 148, 165, 171
Amantadine 149, 187
Amikacin 127, 128, 142, 163, 174, 175, 199
Amphotericin B, ampho B 44, 60, 100, 136, 137, 138, 139, 141, 142, 143, 144, 159, 160, 171, 176, 181, 182, 183, 185, 190, 199
  lipid ampho B preps 159, 176, 182
Analgesics 185
Anemia 38, 42, 100, 120
Anidulafungin 137, 138, 160, 171, 181
Aphthous ulcers 158
Arthritis 97, 112
Ascites 113
Aspergillosis 78, 110, 136
Aspergillus flavus 135
Aspergillus fumigatus 115, 135
Aspergillus terreus 135
Atazanavir 14, 17, 24, 25, 26, 28, 31, 33, 39, 44, 46, 47, 57, 63, 172, 181, 182, 185, 186, 187, 188, 189, 190, 199
Atazanavir + ritonavir 24, 57
Atovaquone 44, 54, 67, 68, 72, 146, 147, 165, 171, 177, 182, 186, 187, 199
Atripla 25, 30, 178, 199
Azithromycin 44, 66, 122, 127, 128, 130, 133, 134, 147, 165, 181, 184, 190, 199

Babesiosis 146
Bacillary angiomatosis 20, 116, 122
Bacterial meningitis 80
Bacterial vaginosis 4, 99, 147
Bartonella 7, 78, 86, 88, 101, 115, 116, 122
BCG 7, 116, 123, 197
BK virus, post-renal transplant 149
Black molds 143
Blastocystis hominis 145
Blastomyces dermatitidis 135
Blastomycosis 109, 137
Bowel perforation 93
Bronchitis 103

Calymmatobacterium granulomatis 97, 122
Campylobacter 94, 97, 98, 122
Campylobacter jejuni 94, 122
Candida 4, 58, 59, 73, 135, 137, 138, 148, 162
  albicans 99, 135, 137, 148
  glabrata 135, 137, 148, 160
  krusei 135, 137, 160, 162
  lusitaniae 135
Candidemia, candidiasis 20, 89, 91, 116, 137, 138, 148
Candidiasis 20, 89, 91, 116, 137, 138, 148
Capreomycin 163, 182, 199
Carcinoma 90

Cardiomyopathy 59
Caspofungin 60, 136, 137, 138, 147, 160, 171, 181, 182, 186, 190, 199
CD4 cell count 28, 56, 121, 125, 141, 196
CD4/CD8 antigen 13
Cervical carcinoma 191
Cervical dysplasia 20
Cervicitis 5, 97
Chancroid 97
Chlamydia 97, 106, 122, 130, 131
Cidofovir 44, 67, 149, 151, 156, 157, 167, 178, 190, 199
Ciprofloxacin 122, 123, 124, 127, 128, 129, 131, 145, 146, 164, 175, 181, 183, 199
Clarithromycin 44, 57, 66, 68, 73, 122, 127, 128, 129, 130, 147, 164, 175, 184, 185, 186, 187, 190, 199
Clindamycin 44, 130, 133, 146, 147, 165, 181, 183, 190, 199
Clofazimine 66, 87, 127, 129, 130, 164, 199
Clostridium difficile 94, 122
Coccidioides immitis 109, 121, 135
Coccidioidomycosis 20, 109, 138
Combivir 26, 27, 30, 61, 199
Community-acquired pneumonia 104, 105
Condyloma acuminatum 157
Congestive heart failure 59
Contraception 50
Crusted (Norwegian) scabies 118
Cryptococcal meningitis 21, 60, 80
Cryptococcemia 140
Cryptococcosis 20, 59, 86, 90, 108, 116, 139, 140
Cryptococcus 108, 120, 131, 135
Cryptococcus neoformans 108, 120, 131, 135
Cryptosporidia 95
Cryptosporidiosis 20, 120
Cryptosporidium 118, 145, 166
Cunnilingus 4
Cycloserine 124, 163, 183, 199
Cyclospora 95, 145
Cytomegalovirus (CMV) 7, 20, 58, 67, 73, 74, 75, 77, 78, 81, 82, 83, 84, 85, 86, 87, 88, 90, 91, 92, 93, 95, 97, 98, 99, 102, 110, 111, 113, 115, 117, 120, 121, 149, 150, 151, 156, 167, 168, 179
  CMV pneumonia 150

Dalfopristin 199
Dapsone 44, 52, 54, 66, 72, 73, 130, 146, 147, 165, 171, 177, 183, 187, 190
Darunavir 14, 17, 33, 39, 44, 55, 63, 172, 181, 185, 186, 188, 189, 190, 199
Delavirdine 14, 16, 31, 39, 44, 62, 172, 181, 183, 184, 186, 189, 190, 199
Delirium 161
Dematiaceous fungi 143
Dematiaceous molds 135
Depression 76
Diarrhea 34, 38, 39, 40, 44, 58, 93, 96, 97, 120, 165
Didanosine (ddI) 14, 15, 18, 24, 26, 29, 38, 41, 42, 44, 47, 61, 172, 178, 182, 183, 186, 187, 190, 199
Didanosine + (emtricitabine or lamivudine) 24
Dirithromycin 181, 184
Disulfiram 184
Doxorubicin 199
Doxycycline 122, 123, 132, 133, 134, 181
Drug Resistance Testing 9, 14
Drug-drug interactions 37, 160, 161, 162
Dysphagia 58, 91, 93

Echinocandin 135, 137
Efavirenz 14, 16, 24, 25, 26, 28, 32, 33, 37, 39, 41, 43, 44, 46, 47, 48, 50, 51, 61, 62, 71, 85, 136, 172, 181, 182, 183, 184, 185, 189, 190, 199
Ehrlichiosis 106
Emtricitabine 14, 15, 24, 25, 28, 30, 38, 61, 62, 172, 178, 199
Encephalitis 77, 78, 150, 197
Encephalitozoon hellum 85, 146
Endocarditis 122
Enfuvirtide 14, 36, 40, 55, 57, 65, 172, 181, 190, 199
Entamoeba histolytica 95, 97, 145
Entecavir 149, 152, 153, 168, 172, 178, 190
Enteroadherent E. coli 94
Eosinophilia 100
Eosinophilic folliculitis 115, 118, 120
Epzicom 25, 30, 60, 61, 199
Erythromycin 122, 123, 131, 133, 134, 175, 184, 190
Ethambutol 44, 66, 123, 124, 125, 126, 127, 128, 129, 162, 171, 177, 183, 190, 199
Ethionamide 124, 130, 163, 177, 199
Etravirine 14, 16, 32, 39, 55, 62, 172, 181, 183, 184, 189, 190, 199

Famciclovir 149, 156, 157, 168, 172, 178, 199
Fever of Unknown Origin (FUO) 88, 122
Filgrastim (G-CSF) 42, 167, 197, 199
Fluconazole 44, 60, 80, 91, 137, 138, 139, 140, 143, 148, 160, 162, 169, 170, 171, 177, 182, 186, 190, 199
Flucytosine 44, 135, 140, 160, 171, 177, 199
Fluoroquinolones 122, 125, 126, 128, 129, 130, 131, 164, 183, 190
Focal brain dysfunction 77, 78, 79
Fosamprenavir 14, 17, 24, 25, 26, 34, 39, 44, 46, 57, 63, 151, 172, 181, 182, 185, 186, 188, 189, 199
Fosamprenavir + ritonavir 24
Foscarnet 44, 67, 83, 149, 150, 151, 156, 157, 167, 172, 179, 183, 185, 190, 199
Fungal meningitis 80
Fusariosis 141
Fusarium sp. 135, 162

Ganciclovir 44, 67, 83, 97, 100, 149, 150, 151, 167, 172, 179, 183, 190, 199
Gastritis 92
Gatifloxacin 164, 183
Gemifloxacin 133, 164, 175, 183
Genital ulcers 4, 97, 98
Genotype resistance testing 9, 15
Gentamicin 174, 175, 183
Giardia 95, 146, 166
Giardia lamblia 146, 166
Giemsa stain 96, 107
Gingivitis 158
Gonads 85
Gonorrhea 130
Granulocytopenia 167
Granuloma inguinale 97, 122
Griseofulvin 161
Guillain-Barre syndrome 38, 81, 197

Haemophilus influenzae pneumonia 103, 105, 115, 195
Hairy leukoplakia 90, 152
Headache 31, 33, 38, 74, 78, 81, 152
Heart failure 111
Hep B Co-infection 37, 101
Hepatitis 7, 23, 37, 39, 40, 69, 101, 102, 120, 149, 152, 153, 154, 156, 168, 169, 193, 194, 195, 197
Hepatitis A 101, 102, 152, 193, 194, 195, 197
Hepatitis B 7, 23, 30, 31, 37, 38, 39, 42, 69, 71, 101, 102, 113, 120, 149, 152, 153, 169, 193, 195
Hepatitis C 7, 42, 69, 71, 87, 101, 102, 113, 117, 120, 149, 154, 156
Hepatitis D 101, 102
Hepatitis E 102
Hepatitis G 102
Herpes infections 106, 156, 191
Herpes simplex 4, 7, 20, 67, 77, 78, 86, 91, 92, 97, 117, 120, 149, 156
Herpes zoster 21, 86, 87, 120, 157
Heterosexual transmission 50
Histoplasma capsulatum 109, 118, 121, 135
Histoplasmosis 20, 73, 90, 97, 109, 110, 111, 116, 141
HIV aseptic meningitis 80
HIV Testing 6
HIV-1 antibody tests 10
HIV-2 9, 10, 11, 13, 104
HIV-associated cottonwool spots (CWS) 58, 87
HIV-associated gingivitis & periodontitis 90
HIV-associated IgA nephropathy 114
HIV-associated nephropathy 23, 114
Human herpesvirus 8 89, 108, 156
Human papillomavirus (HPV) 50, 90, 97, 116, 157, 192, 193, 194, 195
Hyperkalemia 83
Hyperuricemia 164
Hypocalcemia 83
Hypoglycemia 85
Hyponatremia 83

Idiopathic (aphthous) esophageal ulceration (IEU) 92
Imidazoles 161
Imipenem 128, 131, 142, 165, 183, 199
Imiquimod 157, 170
Immune reconstitution inflammatory syndrome (IRIS) 80, 81, 88, 101, 102, 104, 111, 113, 114, 119, 140, 157
Immunization 7, 10, 13, 57, 106, 194, 195
Impetigo 59
Indinavir 7, 14, 17, 18, 34, 40, 42, 44, 46, 63, 84, 126, 130, 172, 179, 181, 183, 185, 186, 188, 189, 190, 199
Inflammatory demyelinating polyneuropathy (IDP) 81
Influenza 7, 102, 106, 149, 195
Influenza A 149
Interferon alfa 157, 169, 170, 199
Interferons 170, 190
Iodoquinol 145, 165, 199
Isentress 36, 40, 66, 199
Isoniazid (INH) 44, 66, 68, 72, 82, 101, 104, 123, 124, 125, 126, 128, 129, 162, 163, 171, 177, 182, 183, 184, 186, 187, 190, 199
Isospora belli 93, 95, 96, 146
Itraconazole 44, 60, 73, 115, 136, 138, 139, 140, 141, 142, 143, 144, 161, 171, 177, 181, 184, 186, 187, 199
Ivermectin 115, 118, 148, 165, 171

Kaletra 25, 26, 34, 40, 46, 64, 181, 188, 189, 199
Kaposi's sarcoma 20, 58, 84, 89, 91, 92, 97, 108, 110, 111, 116, 117, 118
Karnofsky Scale 21
Ketoconazole 44, 100, 142, 161, 185, 199

Lactic acidosis 41, 50, 83, 168
Lamivudine (3TC) 15, 16, 25, 26, 27, 29, 30, 37, 38, 42, 44, 45, 47, 48, 51, 55, 56, 57, 61, 71, 82, 84, 93, 102, 113, 149, 153, 169, 172, 179, 184, 190, 199
Lamivudine/Stavudine 47, 48
Lamivudine/Zidovudine 47, 48
Lamivudine/Zidovudine/ Nevirapine 48
Legionella 105
Leiomyosarcoma 59
Leishmania 117

Leishmaniasis 90, 93
Levofloxacin 122, 124, 133, 164, 175, 183
Linezolid 44, 125, 131, 142, 176, 181, 184, 186, 190, 199
Lipid-based ampho B 144, 159
Lipodystrophy 83, 102
Lipomatosis 102
Listeriosis 122
Lobomycosis 142
Lopinavir 14, 17, 18, 24, 25, 26, 27, 34, 40, 44, 46, 57, 64, 65, 80, 81, 90, 126, 172, 181, 184, 185, 186, 188, 189, 190, 199
Lopinavir/ritonavir 24, 27, 44, 57, 64, 65, 181, 188, 189
Lymphogranuloma venereum (LGV) 97, 98, 123
Lymphoid interstitial pneumonia (LIP) 59, 108
Lymphoma 20, 83, 90, 92, 108, 111

M. avium 20, 88, 105, 110, 111, 116, 162
Malaria 88
Maraviroc 14, 15, 17, 36, 40, 42, 44, 55, 57, 65, 172, 179, 181, 184, 189, 190, 199
Measles 106, 193, 194, 195
Mefloquine 171, 186
Meningitis 79, 80, 81, 108, 120, 133, 139, 140, 141
Meningovascular syphilis 81, 98
Menstrual dysfunction 50
Metronidazole 115, 122, 145, 146, 147, 148, 166, 176, 184, 185, 190
Micafungin 136, 137, 138, 160, 171, 181, 184
Miconazole 161
Microsporidia 96
Microsporidiosis 146
Minocycline 130, 181
Molluscum contagiosum 80, 85, 86, 116, 120, 157
Mononeuritis multiplex (MM) 81, 82, 150
Movement disorders 81, 82
Moxifloxacin 125, 164, 181, 183
MRSA 59, 112, 132, 133
MSSA 132, 133
Mucormycosis 145
Mutations 14, 16, 17, 107, 146
Mycobacterium avium 57, 66, 68, 73, 86, 88, 96, 111, 115, 117, 118, 120, 127
Mycobacterium avium- intracellulare complex
    (MAC or MAI) 66, 73, 75, 83, 84, 88, 91, 93, 98, 103, 110, 111, 113, 115, 117, 118, 119, 121, 127, 128,129, 164
Mycobacterium celatum 128
Mycobacterium chelonae, ssp. abscessus, chelonae 128
Mycobacterium fortuitum 128
Mycobacterium genavense 109, 128
Mycobacterium gordonae 128
Mycobacterium haemophilum 128
Mycobacterium kansasii 109, 129
Mycobacterium leprae 116, 129
Mycobacterium marinum 129
Mycobacterium scrofulaceum 129
Mycobacterium simiae 129
Mycobacterium tuberculosis 68, 72, 80, 97, 110, 111, 118, 123
Mycobacterium ulcerans (Buruli ulcer) 129
Mycobacterium xenopi 129
Myelopathy 81
Myopathy 82, 113

Nafcillin 181
Neisseria gonorrhoeae 97, 130
Nelfinavir 14, 17, 27, 34, 40, 44, 46, 56, 57, 64, 126, 181, 184, 185, 186, 187, 188, 189, 190, 199
Nephropathy 59
Netilmicin 175
Neuropathy 44, 74, 81, 167

Neutropenia 42, 100, 137, 146, 167
Nevirapine 14, 16, 24, 27, 32, 39, 41, 42, 44, 47, 48, 62, 101, 173, 181, 184, 185, 186, 189, 190, 199
Nitazoxanide 95, 145, 146, 166, 171, 190
Nocardiosis 108, 142
Norwegian scabies 100, 148
NRTIs 14, 16, 29, 31, 32, 37, 38, 39, 41, 42, 43, 46, 55, 60, 61, 65, 83, 113, 190
Numbness/burning 82
Nystatin 138, 148, 161

Occupational exposure 69
Odynophagia 92
Ofloxacin 122, 124, 127, 130, 164, 183, 199
Oral lesions 89, 91, 117
Oseltamivir 149, 172, 173
Osteonecrosis 43, 112

p24 antigen 5, 9, 11, 12, 52, 53, 74, 93
Pancreatitis 29, 31, 38, 40, 42, 44, 84, 93, 113, 185
Pap smear 7, 50, 157, 191, 192
Papulosquamous lesions 117, 118
Paracoccidioidomycosis 109, 142
Paromomycin 166, 199
Parvovirus B-19 157, 197
Parvovirus B-19 infection 197
PCP pneumonia 106, 107
Pediatric AIDS 52, 59
Pegylated interferon 199
Peliosis hepatis 101, 122
Pelvic inflammatory disease (PID) 50, 98, 105, 130
Penciclovir 168
Penicilliosis 142
Penicillium marneffei 88, 90, 109, 116, 142
Pentamidine 44, 67, 85, 100, 147, 166, 177, 183, 185, 190, 199
Pericarditis 99
Pets 7, 85
Phaeohyphomycosis 143
Phthirus pubis 148
Pituitary 84
Plasma HIV RNA Testing 9, 11
Pleural effusion 104, 108, 110, 111
Pneumococcal pneumonia 104, 105
Pneumococcal vaccine 7
Pneumocystis carinii pneumonia (PCP) 10, 20, 52, 54, 59, 66, 83, 85, 88, 91, 99, 104, 105, 106, 107, 108, 109, 110, 111, 116, 121, 146, 147, 165,166, 196
Pneumocystis jiroveci (carinii) 88, 93, 103, 110, 116
Pneumonia 20, 103, 105, 106, 107, 108, 133
    adult 7, 54, 55, 60, 61, 62, 63, 64, 65, 66, 67, 159, 165, 173, 195
Pneumothorax 107, 111
Podofilox 157, 170
Podophyllin 157
Polyenes 135
Polymyositis 113
Porphyria cutanea tarda 117
Posaconazole 135, 136, 138, 139, 141, 143, 145, 161, 171, 182, 190, 199
Prednisone 92, 147
Primaquine 44, 166, 199
Primary CNS lymphoma 76, 78, 191
Proctitis 97, 98
Progressive multifocal leukoencephalopathy (PML) 20, 58, 75, 76, 77, 79, 121, 157
Prostatitis 131
Protease inhibitors (PI) 14, 15, 17, 23, 25, 28, 31, 32, 34, 35, 37, 38, 39, 40, 42, 43, 51, 55, 57, 64, 65, 82, 85, 113, 126, 181, 182, 184, 185, 186, 191
Protein S 59
Proteinuria 114

Pseudomonas aeruginosa 96, 105, 115
Psoriasis 112, 118, 158
Pulmonary tuberculosis 21, 103, 104, 105, 121
Pyomyositis 111
Pyrazinamide (PZA) 66, 72, 123, 124, 125, 126, 128, 129, 162, 163, 171, 177, 186, 190, 199
Pyrimethamine 44, 100, 146, 147, 166, 171, 177, 181, 183, 186, 190, 199

QTc prolongation 33, 39, 45
Quinupristin/dalfopristin 186, 199

Raltegravir 14, 17, 36, 40, 55, 66, 173, 181, 186, 190, 199
Recurrent aphthous ulcers (RAU) 91, 158
Recurrent bacteremia 115
Retinitis 120, 151, 152
Rheumatoid arthritis 112
Rhodococcus 86, 88, 110, 115, 131
Ribavirin 44, 100, 106, 149, 155, 169, 172, 181, 183, 186, 187, 190, 199
Rifabutin 44, 57, 66, 72, 73, 87, 100, 123, 124, 125, 126, 127, 128, 129, 130, 164, 178, 181, 182, 183, 185, 190, 199
Rifamate 163
Rifampin 44, 66, 68, 72, 100, 122, 123, 124, 125, 126, 127, 128, 129, 130, 131, 132, 133, 162, 163, 164, 171, 178, 182, 183, 184, 186, 187, 190, 199
Rifater 163
Rifaximin 181
Rimantadine 172
Ritonavir 14, 17, 25, 26, 33, 35, 40, 42, 44, 46, 57, 63, 65, 126, 173, 179, 181, 186, 188, 189, 190

Salivary gland enlargement 91
Salmonella 20, 94, 115, 131
Saquinavir 14, 17, 24, 28, 35, 40, 46, 57, 65, 126, 173, 181, 186, 188, 189, 190, 199
Sarcoidosis 121
Sargramostim (GM-CSF) 167, 197, 199
Scabies 98, 115, 165
Scedosporium 135, 143, 161
Scedosporium apiospermum (Pseudoallescheria boydii) 135
Scedosporium prolificans 135, 143
Seborrheic dermatitis 117, 158
Secondary syphilis 90, 98
Seizures 79
Sepsis 59, 103, 114, 115
Septata intestinalis 96
Septic arthritis 112
Shigella 94, 97
Shigellosis 131
Sinusitis 115
Skin 26, 30, 39, 41, 59, 80, 115, 116, 117, 118, 120, 142, 143, 158, 163, 164, 165, 166
Splenomegaly 118
Sporotrichosis 116, 143, 144
Staphylococcus aureus 105, 132, 133
Stavudine (d4T) 14, 15, 16, 28, 31, 38, 41, 43, 44, 47, 51, 61, 84, 173, 179, 186, 187, 190, 199
Stevens-Johnson syndrome 34, 39, 40, 41, 49, 62, 115, 117, 166
Stomach 92, 93, 94, 95, 96
Stomatitis 138
Streptococcus pneumoniae 80, 104, 133
Streptomycin 66, 163, 171, 174, 177, 190
Strongyloidiasis 165
Sulfadiazine 44, 147, 166, 176
Sulfamethoxazole 176, 187, 199
Syphilis 87, 97, 98, 116, 134

Telbivudine 169, 172
Tenofovir 4, 14, 15, 16, 18, 24, 25, 28, 29, 30, 31, 33, 37, 38, 42, 44, 47, 51, 55, 56, 57, 62, 71, 113, 153, 169, 173, 179, 183, 186, 187, 190, 199
Tenofovir + Emtracitabine 37, 199
Terbinafine 143, 161
Testes 85
Testosterone 85
Tetracycline 134, 175, 182
Thalidomide 91, 92, 96, 130, 158, 190
Thrombocytopenia 57, 89, 100, 161
Thyroid 84, 183
Tigecycline 181, 187
Tinidazole 146, 148, 171
Tipranavir 14, 17, 35, 40, 44, 55, 65, 173, 181, 185, 186, 188, 189, 190, 199
Tobramycin 174, 175
Toxic neuropathy 82
Toxoplasma gondii 73, 84, 110, 147
Toxoplasmic encephalitis 76, 78
Transmission of HIV 50
Trichomonas vaginalis 148
Trichomoniasis 99, 148
Trifluridine 168
Trimethoprim 72, 83, 166, 176, 183, 187, 190, 199
Trimethoprim (TMP)/Sulfamethoxazole (SMX) 21, 41, 52, 54, 66, 67, 68, 72, 73, 78, 83, 92, 94, 95, 100, 101, 105, 107, 113, 115, 117, 122, 128, 129, 131, 132, 133, 142, 145, 146, 147, 165, 166, 176, 186, 187, 199
Trimetrexate 44, 199
Trizivir 27, 29, 60, 61, 199
Truvada 25, 30, 61, 62, 153, 168, 199
Tuberculosis 7, 59, 77, 97, 104, 111, 113, 198
Tuberculous meningitis 80
Typhlitis 96

Urethritis 97
Uveitis 87, 164

Vacuolar myelopathy 82
Vaginitis 147, 148
Valacyclovir 149, 156, 157, 168, 172, 180, 199
Valganciclovir 44, 67, 73, 100, 149, 150, 151, 167, 172, 180, 183, 199
Vancomycin 122, 131, 132, 133, 176, 182, 187
Varicella (chickenpox) 158
Varicella zoster virus (VZV) 68, 75, 77, 78, 82, 85, 86, 87, 102, 157, 158
Vinblastine 191
Voriconazole 44, 60, 135, 136, 137, 138, 139, 140, 141, 143, 162, 171, 177, 181, 182, 190, 199
Vulvovaginitis 138

Warts 90, 170
Wasting syndrome 20, 58
Weakness 82
Western blot 7, 9, 10, 12, 20, 53

Xerostomia 91
Xerotic eczema 117

Zalcitabine (ddC) 14, 15, 44, 56, 79, 82, 84, 91, 101, 113, 123, 180, 184, 187, 190
Zanamivir 149
Zidovudine (ZDV, AZT) 6, 14, 15, 16, 24, 25, 26, 27, 28, 29, 30, 31, 38, 42, 44, 47, 48, 50, 51, 55, 56, 57, 58, 61, 71, 79, 82, 93, 94, 99, 100, 101, 102, 113, 118, 127, 173, 180, 182, 183, 184, 186, 187, 190, 191, 199
Zidovudine/ Lamivudine 24
Zygomycetes 135

DATE DUE			

DEMCO